CARDIORESPIRATORY DISORDERS DURING SLEEP

Second Revised Edition

Edited by

Richard J. Martin, M.D.

CARDIORESPIRATORY DISORDERS DURING SLEEP

Second Revised Edition

Edited by

Richard J. Martin, M.D.

Director, Sleep Disorders Program
Staff Physician, Department of Medicine
National Jewish Center for Immunology and
Respiratory Medicine
Associate Professor of Medicine
University of Colorado Health Sciences Center
Denver, Colorado

FUTURA

**Futura Publishing
Company, Inc.**
Mount Kisco, NY
1990

Library of Congress Cataloging-in-Publication Data
Cardiorespiratory disorders during sleep / edited by Richard J. Martin. — 2nd ed.
p. cm.
Rev. ed. of: Cardiorespiratory disorders during sleep / Richard J. Martin. 1984.
Includes bibliographical references.
ISBN 0-87993-380-1
1. Sleep apnea syndromes. 2. Sleep disorders. 3. Sleep. 4. Respiration 5. Respiratory organs—Diseases. 6. Cardiovascular system—Diseases. I. Martin, Richard J. (Richard Jay), 1946– II. Martin, Richard J. (Richard Jay), 1946– Cardiorespiratory disorders during sleep.
[DNLM: 1. Respiration Disorders—complications. 2. Sleep Disorders—complications. WF 140 C2676]
RC737.5.C37 1990
DNLM/DLC
for Library of Congress 89-23723
CIP

Published by:
Futura Publishing Company, Inc.
2 Bedford Ridge Road, P.O. Box 330
Mount Kisco, New York 10549

LC #: 89-23723
ISBN #: 0-87993-380-1

Printed in the United States of America.

To all who have dedicated themselves
for the better understanding and advancement
of cardiorespiratory function during sleep.

Contributors

Robert D. Ballard, M.D,
Director, Adult Special Care Unit
National Jewish Center for Immunology
and Respiratory Medicine
Assistant Professor of Medicine
University of Colorado Health Sciences Center
Denver, Colorado

Eugene C. Fletcher, M.D.
Director, Pulmonary Physiology and Sleep Research Laboratory
Houston V.A. Medical Center
Associate Professor of Medicine
Baylor College of Medicine
Houston, Texas

Kevin S. Hara, M.D.
Pulmonary Fellow
Division of Thoracic Diseases
Mayo Clinic
Rochester, Minnesota

Richard J. Martin, M.D.
Director, Sleep Disorders Program
Staff Physician, Department of Medicine
National Jewish Center for Immunology
and Respiratory Medicine
Associate Professor of Medicine
University of Colorado Health Sciences Center
Denver, Colorado

Gary C. Prechter, M.D.
Pulmonary Fellow
Division of Thoracic Diseases
Mayo Clinic
Rochester, Minnesota

Mark H. Sanders, M.D.
Director, Pulmonary Sleep Evaluation Laboratory
Presbyterian University Hospital
Associate Professor of Medicine
University of Pittsburgh
School of Medicine
Pittsburgh, Pennsylvania

John W. Shepard, Jr., M.D.
Medical Director, Sleep Disorders Center
Mayo Clinic
Associate Professor of Medicine
Mayo Medical School
Rochester, Minnesota

David P. White, M.D.
Chief, Respiratory Care
Denver V.A. Medical Center
Associate Professor of Medicine
University of Colorado Health Sciences Center
Denver, Colorado

Foreword

Blessings on him that first invented sleep!
–Cervantes, Don Quixote, II

As Richard Martin says in his Chapter 1, History and Comments, mankind has probably had many questions about sleep since the origin of the species.

Poets have used the theme "sleep" for various purposes. Who doesn't remember:

Hush a bye baby on the tree top,
When the wind blows the cradle will rock;
When the bough breaks the cradle will fall,
And down will come baby, cradle, and all.

Sleep has often been likened to death, e.g.,

How wonderful is death,
Death and his brother sleep.

–Shelly, Queen Mab.

Indeed it has been sudden and unexpected death, such as sudden infant death syndrome and deaths in adults as a result of sleep apnea and associated fatal arrhythmias, which has been a major stimulus in sleep research aimed at understanding pathological consequences of sleep in search of preventive therapy.

Martin's second edition on the phenomenon of sleep in relation to cardiorespiratory disease, now considerably expanded from the first edition, is an excellent work. Historical perspectives, advances in technology, classifications of disease, new clinical science resulting in understandings of sleep phenomena in relation to disease, and the systematic physiologically oriented treatment for sleep disorders breathing are all discussed in an eminently readable manner in this edition.

Having been interested in one limited aspect of pathological sleep responses, i.e., the hematopoietic response to postural and nocturnal hypoxemia (*Am J Med* 1968; 48:880), I continue to marvel at the technological advances that have made sleep studies a reality not only in formal sleep laboratories but also on a limited basis in the home. Certainly the recording pulse oximeter has been one of these advances. Many other technological advances resulting in integrative assessment of sleep in relation to cardiorespiratory diseases have also marked the past nearly quarter of a century.

Those who read and study the second edition will be enlightened and thrilled over our improved understanding of sleep and its implications in both health and disease, as I was.

Thomas L. Petty, M.D.
Director
Academic and Research Affairs
Presbyterian/St. Lukes Center
for Health Sciences Education
Denver, Colorado

Preface

It has been six years since the first edition of this book was published. Over this period of time, significant advances in our understanding of the pathophysiology and treatment of cardiopulmonary problems during sleep have occurred. However, as stated in the Preface of the first edition, "many areas of nocturnal changes in cardiopulmonary disease still need to be further investigated." What additionally holds true is the statement of over 30 years ago by Eugene Robin that "the sleeping patient is still a patient. His disease not only goes on while he sleeps, but indeed may progress in an entirely different fashion from its progression during the waking state."

This second edition of *Cardiorespiratory Disorders During Sleep* has been expanded significantly. Examples of this can be seen by the division of the sleep apnea syndrome from one to three chapters. A new chapter on Cardiopulmonary Disorders in the Elderly has been added and other information has been updated. Finally as the wealth of information expands, no longer can one individual write an entire textbook. Thus, there are now eight contributing authors.

The book is still directed to clinicians and investigators interested in cardiopulmonary problems associated with sleep. Each chapter stands on its own in developing the discussed topic. Where appropriate, similar information may be found in different chapters. This text is intended to be an up-to-date evaluation of specific cardiopulmonary problems and abnormalities in regard to physiology, pathology, clinical course, and therapy.

Richard J. Martin, M.D.
Denver, Colorado

Acknowledgments

Publications of this nature need the support of many individuals. I wish to thank in particular two of these people. Deep appreciation goes to Patricia Kelly for her research and technical assistance and to Judy Tisdale for secretarial support.

Contents

1

History and Comments

Richard J. Martin, M.D.

History of Sleep Studies

The history of evaluating sleep physiology and, in particular, respiratory disorders during sleep is still in its relative infancy compared to other medical specialties. Approximately 40 years ago, sleep was still thought to be a simple, homogeneous state of little clinical importance. A change in this concept came about when Loomis et al.[1] described distinct electroencephalographic stages during sleep. It took almost another two decades before the next major advance in sleep studies occurred. Aserinsky and Kleitman showed that bursts of rapid eye movement (REM) sleep occurred at repetitive intervals.[2] Subsequently, this stage of sleep was associated with dreaming.[3] Indeed, most physiologic processes are different during REM sleep compared to non-REM sleep.

Until the advent of the electroencephalogram, by which sleep staging could be clearly defined, sleep was a perplexing process to the investigator. Was it a totally benign, quiescent time of the day for the body to recover from the waking stresses and strains, or was there an active process going on during sleep that expressed itself in dreaming? With the relatively recent development of the electroencephalogram, it has become evident that sleep functions in both capacities.

The questions that mankind has about sleep probably occurred with the first of the human species. Thus, it is not surprising that

Martin RJ: Cardiorespiratory Disorders During Sleep, 2nd Edition. Futura Publishing Company, Inc., Mount Kisco, NY, © 1990.

biases and misguided reasoning hindered the early development of scientific research into the area of sleep. Sleep research can be divided into two phases. The first phase began in approximately the 1860s and continued until the development of the electroencephalograph (1935), when the second phase was instituted and is still undergoing an explosive expansion up to the present time. The first period of development produced many theories, which mostly hindered the understanding of sleep. The postelectroencephalographic period, which is of rather short duration, has produced a wealth of information to aid our understanding of the physiologic aspect of sleep.

The pre-electroencephalographic sleep researchers measured many variables that are still used today to describe sleep. These included measurements of threshold arousals to sound, heart rate, pupil size, body temperature, respiration, metabolic rate, electromyogram, galvanic skin response, and body movement. Of interest, particular attention was focused on position change during sleep.

In 1860, Kohlschuter[4] started experiments on threshold response during sleep. That same year, Fechner[5] attempted to delineate the strength of sound necessary to awaken a person from sleep, which was thought to be indicative of the depth of sleep. Investigators today are still trying to determine the arousal phenomenon or lack of it in certain disease states such as sleep apnea or nocturnal ventilatory failure in asthma. The device that has helped present-day researchers look at this complex issue that exhibits variable patterns and reveal it as a meaningful and important facet is the electroencephalogram. Whereas great intrasubject variability was thought to be present, this type of response can now be directly related to sleep staging (Fig. 1a,b).

One can appreciate the difficulties that the pre-electroencephalogram researchers had by looking at a very common sleep index: sleep duration. Even if the investigators controlled for variables such as laboratory adaptation, previous nights' sleep, and daytime activities, how could these variables be accurately measured if there was no way to objectively determine when the subject fell asleep? Basically, a subject with closed eyes may be awake or asleep. It was not until the 1960s that a description of sleep time was fully investigated.[6]

Other earlier investigators had similar problems trying to explain observations that appeared inconsistent even in the same individual. As early as the late 1800s, it was thought that certain physiologic functions tend to change during sleep. These included blood pressure, respiration, and heart rate.[7] However, these "inconsistent" changes were thought to be due to artifactual laboratory influences until the electroencephalograph helped to delineate sleep (Table 1).

Interestingly, brain wave activity was reported in 1875 by Caton[8] using rabbits and monkeys. Seventeen years later, work was done with humans.[9] Both of these endeavors and the work of Hans Berger[10] (who used scalp electrodes to record electroencephalographic activity in 1924 from humans) were essentially ignored.

The use of the electroencephalogram in sleep research began in 1935 when Loomis et al.[1] described the electrical brain wave activity during sleep. Their staging system was thought to be related to different levels of sleep; the levels were lettered A through E. Then, in 1953[2] and 1955,[3] Aserinsky and Kleitman reported on the division of sleep between REM and non-REM sleep and related the REM sleep to dreaming. When normal subjects were awakened during REM phases, 20 of 27 respondents described dreaming. During non-REM sleep, 19 of 23 denied dreaming. These studies have been repeated many times with slightly different results but with each investigation showing that dreaming is linked to REM sleep.

With the new emphasis on two totally different types of sleep, researchers' interest into the confusing nocturnal physiologic patterns was rekindled. Essentially all types of physiologic patterns have been investigated during sleep. During REM sleep, autonomic ner-

Table 1
Alterations in Cardiorespiratory Patterns

	Respiratory rate	*Heart rate*	*Blood pressure*
Stages 1–2 (light sleep)	Can be irregular	Decrease	Slight decrease
Stages 3–4 (deep sleep, slow wave sleep)	Regular	As above or further decrease	Falls further
Rapid eye movement sleep	Fluctuates	Fluctuates	Fluctuates

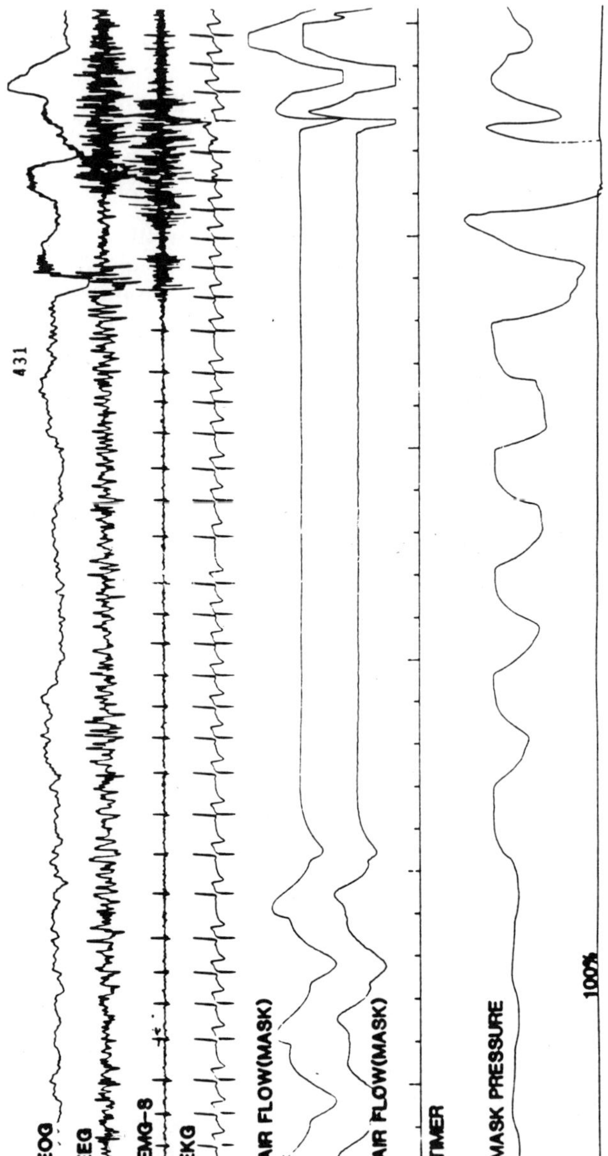
431
EOG
EEG
EMG-S
EKG
AIR FLOW(MASK)
AIR FLOW(MASK)
TIMER
MASK PRESSURE
100%
50%
SaO₂
A

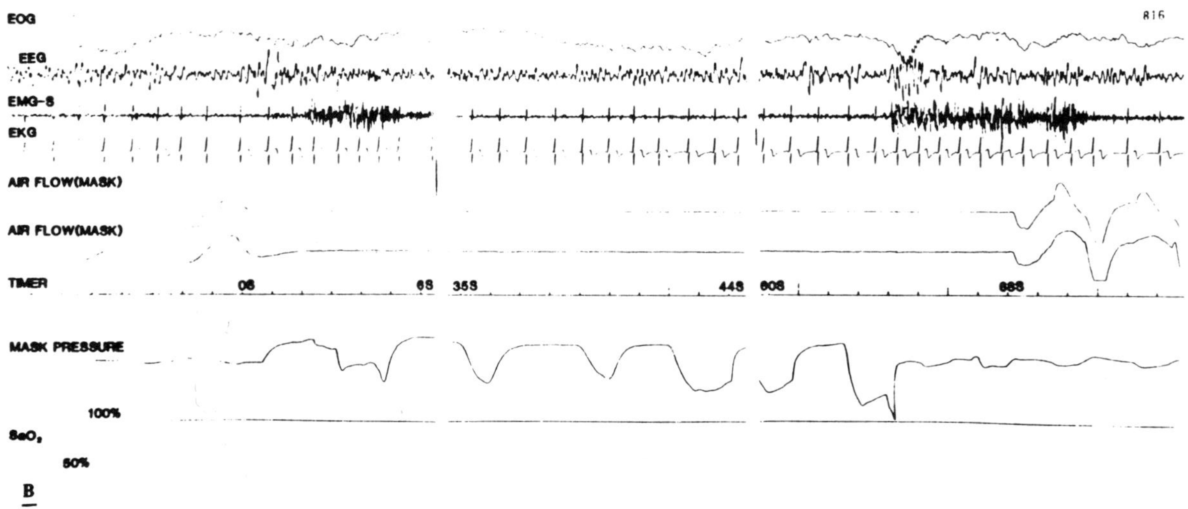

Figure 1 a,b: These figures demonstrate the intrasubject variability that is present due to sleep stages. Figure 1a is an external occlusion of the airway, in a patient with severe nocturnal asthma, during stage 2 with arousal in 13 seconds. The occlusion is placed outside the mask and thus the two flow signals read zero. The pressure inside the mask represents effort to breathe. During REM sleep (Fig. 1b) the external occlusion was released at 68 seconds when the patient awoke. EOG = electroocculogram; EEG = electroencephalogram; EMG-S = submental electromyogram; EKG = electrocardiogram; SaO_2 = oxygen saturation; S = seconds.

vous system activity is increased and irregular with respect to respiratory and cardiac rate as well as systolic blood pressure.[11] Autonomic activity during REM sleep has been shown to affect penile erection.[12,13] An increase in oxygen consumption was seen during REM sleep,[14] as well as increases in cerebral blood flow,[15] an elevation of brain temperature,[16] a fall in body temperature,[17] and changes in the circulating hydroxycorticoids.[18] An important physiologic variable that decreases during sleep and in particular during REM sleep is muscle activity.[19,20] As discussed in following chapters, this decrement in tone is an important step in the initiation of upper airway obstruction. Thus, the major breakthrough in the study of all aspects of sleep occurred with the advent of the electroencephalogram in the laboratory.

Sleep Staging

Briefly, sleep staging[21] (Figs. 2 to 7) can be divided into non-REM movement (stages 1–4) and REM sleep. The staging is as follows:

> *Stage W (wakefulness)*—The electroencephalogram shows alpha activity (8–12 cycles per second) and/or low voltage, with mixed frequency activity.

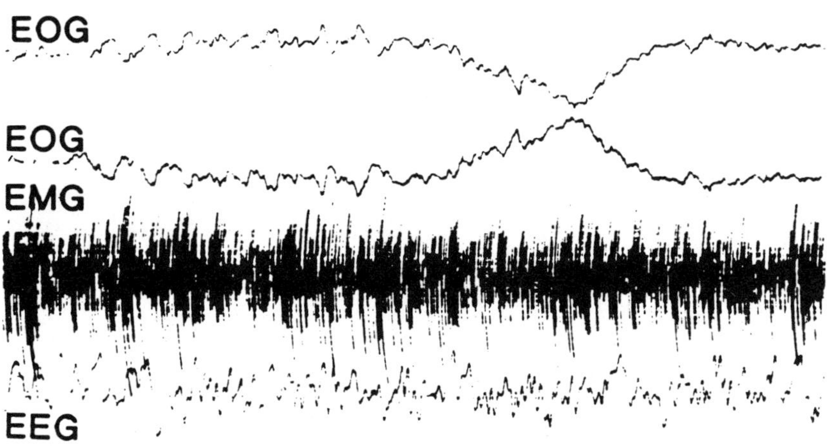

Figure 2. Wakefulness. Alpha wave activity, low voltage, mixed frequency EMG activity.

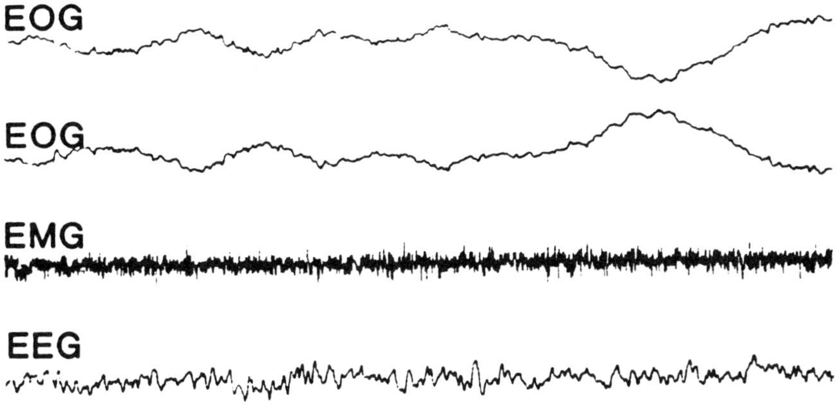

Figure 3. Stage 1. Low voltage, mixed frequency, less than 50% alpha wave.

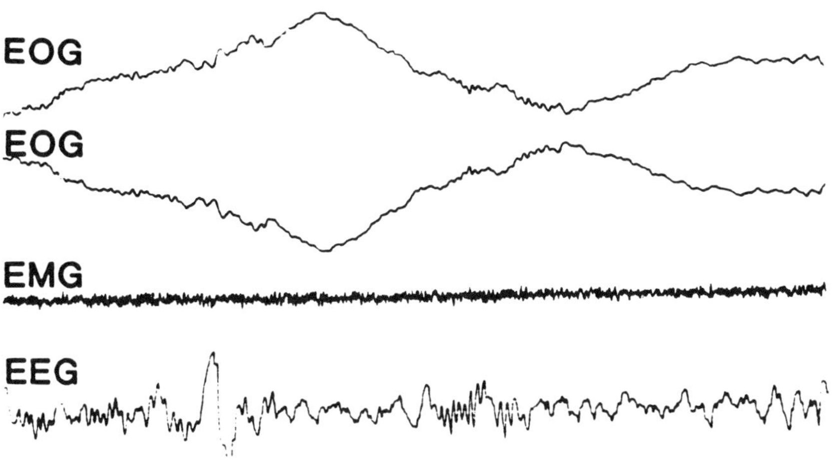

Figure 4. Stage 2. K complexes and sleep spindles.

Stage 1—Low voltage, mixed frequency with majority of activity in the 2–7 cycles per second range, less than 50% alpha per epoch (page).
Stage 2—Presence of sleep spindles (12–14 cycles per second) and/or K complexes (well-defined positive–negative wave).

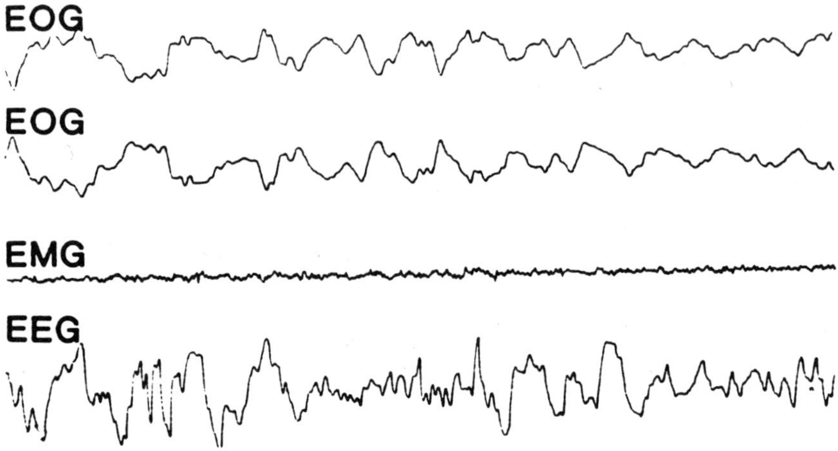

Figure 5. Stage 3. Slow, large delta waves, 20–50%.

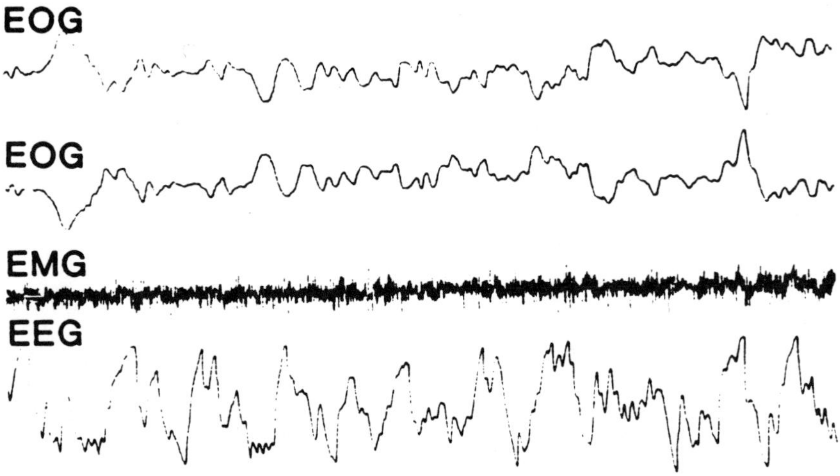

Figure 6. Stage 4. Delta activity greater than 50%.

Stage 3—Delta wave activity (slow, large waves of two cycles per second) that is present on 20%–50% of a given epoch.
Stage 4—Delta wave activity is greater than 50% of the epoch.
Rapid eye movement—EEG shows low voltage, mixed frequency with episodic rapid eye movements. Phasic REM with eye movements. Tonic REM without eye movements.

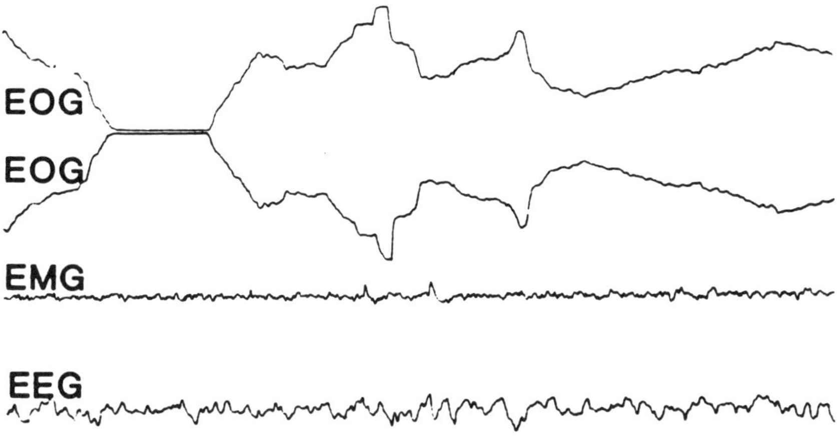

Figure 7. Rapid eye movement. Low voltage, mixed frequency.

The REM stage occurs approximately every 90 minutes during sleep and with each successive occurrence is longer in duration.

History of Respiratory Sleep Studies

Although much was known about obesity and respiratory problems during wakefulness, such as hypercapnia, it was not until the mid-1960s that Gastaut et al.[22] added a new dimension to the evaluation. This was the study of respiratory parameters during sleep, from which a description of sleep apnea emerged. Since that time many descriptive studies have been done to delineate the cardiorespiratory effects of sleep apnea. More recently, respiratory patterns and oximetry during sleep were reported in a group of normal subjects.[23] Presently, the pathophysiologic aspects are being investigated to unravel this intriguing problem as well as many other cardiopulmonary problems during sleep. These studies will be discussed in chapters to follow.

There is an ever-increasing wealth of information on respiratory sleep disorders. The scant data that were available to the practicing clinician only a few short years ago is now becoming a formidable array of information to help understand and treat these problems. Included in this picture is the close link of pulmonary to cardiac function during sleep. This book will focus on the respiratory–cardiac sleep physiology in normals and individuals with the sleep apnea syndrome, lower airway obstructive disease, and the effects of "nonpulmonary" disease on the pulmonary system.

The Problem of Literary and Vogue Terms in Respiratory Sleep Studies

There are three terms frequently used to classify certain respiratory abnormalities during sleep. They are the Pickwickian syndrome, obesity–hypoventilation syndrome and Ondine's curse. The terms are catchy and in the past called the attention of the medical field to these respiratory disorders. Now, however, we need to be very particular in classifying any sleep-related respiratory disorder in order to better understand the mechanisms involved and thus the appropriate treatment.

The term Pickwickian syndrome was adapted from Charles Dickens' *The Posthumous Papers of the Pickwick Club* and was initially coined for the medical literature by William Osler[24] in 1918 and brought to prominence by Burwell et al.[25] The latter described the syndrome to include obesity, hypersomnolence, periodic breathing with hypoventilation, and cor pulmonale. At least three editorials have coaxed the medical profession to abandon this term. Comroe[26] pointed out that the term was incorrect in content because Joe the Fat Boy was not a member of the Pickwick Club and scientifically incorrect because Joe was not described as having apnea, irregular breathing, or cyanosis. Phillipson,[27] in a humorous yet penetrating editorial, felt that in order to keep the "ties" between medicine and the literary arts, the sleep apnea syndrome should be called the Fee-Fi-Fo-Fum syndrome after the giant in *Jack and the Beanstalk* who frequently uttered that phrase. The giant would, perhaps, be scientifically more correct than Joe the Fat Boy. Martin[28] stated that the four types of respiratory disorders during sleep (primary alveolar hypoventilation, central apnea, upper airway obstruction, and mixed apnea) can present with the exact same symptoms and physical complex, yet the treatment is different. Thus, to better understand the evolution of these physiologic processes and to lead to the proper noninvasive treatment regimens, we need to classify each entity appropriately. Perhaps in the future there may even be subclassification of each entity.

Much the same can be said for the "obesity–hypoventilation"

term. There are many nonobese patients with sleep apnea and hypersomnolence as well as obese people who do not "hypoventilate."

Ondine's curse is another term used in medicine that suffers both from literary and clinical errors.[26] Ondines were mermaids. If they fell in love with a human, an undesirable ending would occur if the romance ended. However, in the many variations of the story, the Ondines never placed a curse on their lovers. Indeed, they always tried to help their male mortals. The one reference usually quoted for Ondine's curse is the story by Jean Giraudoux.[28] In this story the curse is said to have involved the loss of all automatic sensory and motor functions. This loss included respiratory and nonrespiratory muscle activity. Unless the male lover (Hans) forces his body to see, hear, move, etc., existence would cease. Thus, "it's an exhausting stewardship." By no stretch of the imagination is Ondine's curse solely related to "forgetting to breathe" and thus it is a clinically confusing term that does not aid the medical profession in understanding this process. Classifications (Table 2) used in this text will

Table 2

Classifications of Sleep-Related Respiratory Disorders

Sleep Apnea Syndrome

- *Upper airway obstruction*—Cessation of airflow of at least 10 seconds with continued respiratory attempts.
- *Partial upper airway obstruction (obstructive hypopnea)*—Decrease in airflow while respiratory efforts are maintained.
- *Central apnea*—Cessation of airflow of at least 10 seconds with no respiratory attempts.
- *Mixed apnea*—Cessation of airflow of at least 10 seconds with no respiratory attempts followed by attempts at respiration in the same apneic episode. The pattern may be reversed with initial attempts followed by no effort. This latter pattern is rare.

Hypoventilation—Decreased minute ventilation (decreased tidal volume and/or frequency) to produce hypercapnia. This process can produce the exact signs and symptoms as attributed to the previously described apneas.

Hypopneas—Decrease in the tidal volume which produces oxygen desaturation. Hypercapnia may or may not be present and if present does not account for the degree of hypoxemia that develops. This pattern is commonly seen in chronic obstructive pulmonary disease patients.

Ventilation-to-Perfusion Mismatching—This process is inferred when oxygen desaturation occurs in the absence of the previously defined patterns. It is usually seen in asthmatic patients with a nocturnal exacerbation.

attempt to be specific in describing the physiologic aspect so that the reader can separate the entities and treatments.

References

1. Loomis AL, Harvey EN, Hobart G. Potential rhythms of the cerebral cortex during sleep.*Science* 1935; 81:597–598.
2. Aserinsky E, Kleitman N. Regularly occurring periods of eye motility and concomitant phenomena during sleep. *Science* 1953; 118:273–274.
3. Aserinsky E, Kleitman N. Two types of ocular motility occurring in sleep. *J Appl Physiol* 1955; 8:1–10.
4. Kohlschuter E. *Z Ration Med 3 Reihe* 1863; 17:209.
5. Fechner G. Elemente der Psychophysik. Leipzig, Breitkopf & Hartel, 1860.
6. Webb WB, Agnew HW Jr. Measurement and characteristics of nocturnal sleep. *In* LE Abto, BF Riess (eds). Progress in Clinical Psychology, Dreams and Dreaming. New York, Grune & Stratton, 1968; pp 2–27.
7. Howell WH. A contribution to the physiology of sleep, based upon plethysmographic experiments. *J Exp Med* 1897; 2:313–345.
8. Caton R. The electric currents of the brain. *Br Med J* 1875; 2:278.
9. Ladd GT. Contribution to the psychology of visual dreams. *Mind* 1892; 1:299–304.
10. Berger H. Uber das Elektroenkephalogramm des Menschen. *Arch Psychiatr Nervenkr* 1929; 87:527–570.
11. Snyder F, Hobson JA, Morrison DF, et al. Changes in respiration, heart rate, and systolic blood pressure in human sleep. *J Appl Physiol* 1964; 19:417–422.
12. Fisher C, Gross J, Zach J. Cycle of penile erection synchronous with dreaming (REM) sleep. Preliminary report. *Arch Gen Psychiatry* 1965; 12: 29–45.
13. Kahn E, Fisher C. Some correlates of rapid-eye movement sleep in the normal aged male. *J Nerv Ment Dis* 1969; 148: 495–505.
14. Brebbia DR, Altshuler KZ. Oxygen consumption rate and electroencephalographic stage of sleep. *Science* 1965; 150:1621–1623.
15. Kanzow E, Krause D, Kuhael H. Die Vasomotorik der Hirnrinde in den Phasen desynchronisierter EEG-Aktivitat in naturlichen Schlaf der Katze. *Pfluegers Arch* 1962; 274:593–607.
16. Baker MA, Hayward JN. Autonomic basis for the rise in brain temperature during paradoxical sleep. *Science* 1967; 157:1586–1588.
17. Verdone P. Temporal reference of manifest dream content. *Percept Motor Skills* 1965; 20:1253–1256.
18. Weitzman ED, Schaumburg H, Fishbein W. Plasma 17-hydroxycorticosteroid levels during sleep in man. *J Clin Endocrinol Metab* 1966; 26:121–127.
19. Berger RJ. Tonus of extrinsic laryngeal muscles during sleep and dreaming. *Science* 1961; 134:840.
20. Jacobson A, Kales A, Lehmann D, et al. Muscle tonus in human subjects during sleep and dreaming. *Exp Neurol* 1964; 10:418–424.

21. Rechtschaffen A, Kales A. A Manual of Standardized Terminology, Techniques and Scoring System for Sleep Stages of Human Subjects. U.S. Department of Health, Education and Welfare, Public Health Service, National Institutes of Health, National Institute of Neurology Disease and Stroke, Neurological Information Network, Bethesda, Maryland, 1968, pp 1–12.
22. Gastaut H, Tassinari CA, Duron B. Polygraphic study of the episodic diurnal and nocturnal (hypnic and respiratory) manifestations of the Pickwick syndrome. *Brain Res* 1966; 2:167–186.
23. Block AJ, Boysen PT, Wynne JW, et al. Sleep apnea hypopnea and oxygen desaturation in normal subjects. *N Engl J Med* 1979; 300:513–517.
24. Osler W. The Principles and Practice of Medicine, 8th ed. New York, Appleton, 1918.
25. Burwell CS, Robin ED, Whaley RD, et al. Extreme obesity associated with alveolar hypoventilation; a Pickwickian syndrome. *Am J Med* 1956; 21: 811–818.
26. Comroe JH Jr. Frankenstein, Pickwick and Ondine. *Am Rev Respir Dis* 1975; 111:689–692.
27. Phillipson EA. Pickwickian, obesity-hypoventilation or Fee-Fi-Fo-Fum syndrome? *Am Rev Respir Dis* 1980; 121:781–782.
28. Martin RJ. The problems of sleep-related respiratory disorders. *J Am Med Assoc* 1981; 245:1250–1251.
29. Giraudoux J. Ondine. 1939 (French); English adaptation by Maurice Valency, New York, Random House, 1954.

2

Physiologic Cardiopulmonary Monitoring and Assessment during Sleep

Richard J. Martin, M.D.

Over the last 10–15 years, there has been an explosion of clinical reports and scientific investigation into the area of respiratory problems during sleep. The obvious conclusion is that the more the medical profession looks for this problem, the more common it becomes. Unfortunately, the vast majority of patients are never questioned about sleep-related symptoms or signs. The patient who is being treated for congestive heart failure is asked if he gets short of breath at night. A positive response immediately elicits an association to paroxysmal noctural dyspnea and cardiac dysfunction. Rarely is any question asked relative to possible sleep apnea as the primary cause of the "dyspnea" and heart failure. It is important to realize that sleep-related respiratory disorders affect many organ systems (Table 1).

Cerebral function can be greatly altered in several types of pulmonary-related abnormalities, such as the sleep apnea syndrome,[1] chronic obstructive pulmonary disease,[2,3] and asthma.[4] The changes that have been observed relate to alertness, thought process, personality changes, problem solving, short- and long-term memory and motor skills. Since there is no known anatomic brain abnormality, the changes in cerebral function are most likely related to changes in

Martin RJ: Cardiorespiratory Disorders During Sleep, 2nd Edition. Futura Publishing Company, Inc., Mount Kisco, NY, © 1990.

Table 1
Organ Systems Affected by Nocturnal Respiratory Disorders

I.	Brain
	A. Thought process
	B. Personality changes
	C. Problem solving
	D. Memory
II.	Cardiac
	A. Arrhythmias
	B. Heart failure
	1. Left sided
	2. Cor pulmonale
	C. Nocturnal angina
III.	Pulmonary
	A. Mechanics
	B. Airflow—lower airways
	C. Pulmonary hypertension
	D. Apnea
IV.	Hemopoietic
	A. Erythrocytosis
V.	Gastrointestinal
	A. Reflux
VI.	Sexual
	A. Impotence
VII.	Neuromuscular
	A. Weakness
	B. Fatigue
	C. Nocturnal seizures

pulmonary function producing cerebral hypoxia. The altered respiratory system, as will be seen in specific chapters related to each disease, is worse during sleep. The common denominator is significant hypoxemia.[5–7] As the disorder is treated or the hypoxia improves, marked improvement can be seen in the cerebral functioning of the patient. In fact, oxygen therapy was administered to a group of elderly normal subjects who professed to have problems with memory, and their neuropsychologic functioning was improved after four weeks on oxygen.[8] Treated patients with sleep apnea are no longer lethargic or forgetful and are able to return to gainful employment.[9] These patients have been diagnosed as being "paranoid" or "schizophrenic" and rapidly revert to a normal personality once the apnea/hypoxia is corrected. Similarly, in patients with asthma or chronic obstructive pulmonary disease, cerebral functioning is improved as the hypoxia is improved.[10–12]

The cardiopulmonary changes during sleep will be more fully documented in other chapters under the specific disease entities. However, certain aspects need to be stressed here. Deaths in the general population and in patients with diseases such as asthma or chronic obstructive pulmonary disease occur most frequently during the night.[13–15] Cardiac arrhythmias and nocturnal angina are common events that occur during sleep in patients with coronary heart disease.[16–18] Also, not surprisingly, electrocardiographic changes are more common during sleep in chronic obstructive pulmonary disease.[19] These high incidences of mortality and morbidity can be explained by nocturnal hypoxia and resultant cardiac damage.

Alterations in the hemopoietic system are associated with changes in the respiratory system during sleep. As hypoxemia develops secondary to apneas, hypopneas, or other alterations producing changes in ventilation-to-perfusion, erythropoietin is stimulated and erythrocytosis develops. On several occasions we have seen patients given many tests to determine the cause of erythrocytosis before a sleep history is taken or nocturnal abnormalities considered.

Although respiratory disorders do not play a known role in relation to the gastrointestinal system, nocturnal reflux and aspiration may alter respiratory function.[20,21] Where reflux exists and careful histories are taken, all types of pulmonary disorders are noted to be worsened during sleep. As an example, asthmatics commonly complain of reflux symptoms (due to decreased tone of the lower gastroesophageal sphincter by theophylline and steroid preparations or hiatal hernias) and, as a result, experience nocturnal worsening of their wheezing or cough. If antireflux regimens are followed, improvement in the asthmatic symptoms is also noted.

Sexual impotence in chronic obstructive pulmonary disease may even be related to the day–night hypoxemia. Fletcher and Martin[22] showed in a study of patients with chronic obstructive pulmonary disease that the group without nocturnal penile tumescence (organic impotence) tended to have lower arterial oxygen tensions. One patient was placed on low-flow home oxygen for 20 weeks and began to have erections and intercourse.

As with any disease process, normality must be understood before shades of abnormality are defined. For example, we are in our relative infancy in understanding precisely the hows, whys, and whats of normality with regard to the heart–lung system during sleep. Much of the information about the normal state was derived from animal studies, which are of great value but may not be precisely applicable to the human condition. The following information represents the normal human population unless otherwise noted.

Normal Respiratory Pattern and Oxygen Saturation

Three studies that investigated the normal respiratory pattern during sleep have helped to establish normality (Table 2). Webb[23] studied a group of normal male subjects aged 19–63 years. He found periodic breathing with apnea that was associated with increasing age in a "surprising number of subjects." Nine of 11 men older than 45 years had one or more episodes of periodic breathing with apneas lasting 20–233 minutes per night. These episodes were not seen during slow-wave sleep (stages 3–4), but they were observed during light sleep (stages 1–2) and rapid eye movement (REM) sleep. Bulow[24] reported, from a study of 53 healthy men and women, that periodic breathing was present to some extent in all but eight subjects. Apneas were not mentioned. Four men and two women, age range from 20 to 60 years, had marked periodic breathing. Slow-wave sleep breathing was regular and breathing during REM sleep was described as being irregular. This irregular breathing during REM has been noted by many investigators. REM breathing is associated with frequent changes in the depth of a tidal breath and respiratory rate.

Table 2
Normal Sleep Respiratory Patterns

I. Sleep onset
   A. Carbon dioxide set point shift may cause periodic respiration
   B. Arousals
II. Non-REM sleep
   A. Stages 1 and 2 (light sleep)
      1. Irregular to regular respiration
      2. Hypopneas
      3. Apneas
   B. Stages 3 and 4 (deep sleep, slow-wave sleep)
      1. Regular respiration
      2. Rare apneas
III. REM sleep
   A. Respiratory frequency and tidal volume may be regular or irregular
   B. If apneas occur, they are more common during REM than non-REM sleep

A more recent study[25] that consisted of 30 asymptomatic men and 19 asymptomatic women showed similar findings to the aforementioned publications and determined the incidence of oxygen desaturation. Twenty males accounted for 264 episodes of nocturnal desaturation (fall in saturation via ear oximetry by at least 4%) or abnormal breathing. The abnormal breathing was divided into hypopneas (decreased flows at mouth and nose, decreased chest movement and desaturation) and apneas (total cessation of flow). There were 105 hypopneic episodes lasting 6–74 seconds (mean 26 seconds) and 51 apneic episodes of 10–54 seconds (mean 20 seconds). There were 251 episodes of desaturation, of which 43% were not associated with hypopneas or apneas, i.e., a normal breathing pattern persisted. The episodes of desaturation and hypopneas were significantly associated with increased age and weight. Apneas were correlated to weight, but not age. Of the 19 females, none had oxygen desaturation and only three had a total of nine apneic episodes of short duration (mean 14 seconds, range 10–24 seconds). However, this does not exclude the possibility that young adult females can have as frequent irregular breathing episodes as males. This has been evident on occasion in our laboratory.

Once again, the stage of sleep was found to be important with respect to the hypopneic, apneic, and oxygen-desaturation episodes discussed above. The respiratory abnormalities and oxygen desaturations were more common as a percent of the time spent in REM sleep. Also, as previously noted, abnormalities were frequent in light sleep but not in slow-wave sleep.

Basically, during light sleep there tends to be periodic-type breathing and at times short apneic episodes. This type of ventilatory change is probably related to a state change from wakefulness to sleep. As a person becomes drowsy and goes into stage 1 or 2 sleep, the arterial carbon dioxide tension set point for ventilation shifts. That is, as the normal ventilatory response during wakefulness starts to diminish at sleep onset, the alveolar ventilation decreases, and there is a slight rise in the arterial carbon dioxide tension with a decrease in the arterial oxygen tension. At this point an arousal, but not necessarily an awakening, can occur that will then increase the ventilatory drive and decrease the carbon dioxide. The arousal is then blunted and slightly deeper sleep ensues. This cycle can be repeated, causing the periodic-type breathing that is seen in the lighter stages of sleep. Perhaps this is a more common phenomenon in older subjects because it takes them longer to establish sleep and to stabilize breathing.

During slow-wave sleep, breathing is typically regular with rare apneas. During REM sleep, ventilatory responses to chemical stimuli are markedly decreased (see below). The decreased responsiveness to chemical and other stimuli during REM sleep probably causes the irregular, though not the periodic, pattern of breathing as well as the more frequent and longer apneas.

Why do normal females have less periodic/irregular breathing and apneas than males? Additionally, a male predominance is seen during the abnormal state of the sleep apnea syndrome.[5] The most striking difference would be hormonal in nature. Does progesterone and/or estrogen help to block this phenomenon or does testosterone promote these respiratory sleep abnormalities? Block et al.[26] showed that postmenopausal females develop a marked increase in sleep-related respiratory abnormalities. In addition, the sleep apnea syndrome is usually more prevalent in postmenopausal females than in premenopausal females. However, no exact cause and effect has been demonstrated and if postmenopausal females are given progestational hormone therapy, there is no decrease in the hypopneas-apneas-desaturations.[26]

We have evaluated a patient on supplemental testosterone who also had severe sleep apnea associated with upper airway obstruction. Ten years prior to this diagnosis the patient had a pituitary tumor surgically removed. The pituitary gland was totally evacuated and this left the patient panhypopituitary and on supplemental hormonal therapy. Approximately seven years after the surgery, hypersomnolence started and progressed over a three-year period with a weight increase of 20 kg. He was euthyroid on supplemental medication. At that time a polysomnographic evaluation showed 348 apneas of which 333 were upper airway obstructions, 14 were mixed apneas (upper airway obstruction and a central component during each episode) and one was a central apnea. The mean duration of the apneas was 19.6 seconds. The sleep time during this study was 4.63 hours. Forty-one percent of the sleep time was spent in an apneic pattern. Although the ear oximeter loses some accuracy below 60%, oxygen saturations were commonly recorded between 10% and 30%. The most frequent range of apnea-related oxygen desaturation was in the 50%–60% range. The patient was then taken off of his testosterone for a period of eight weeks. The serum testosterone level was essentially zero at this time, and his daytime symptoms of hypersomnolence, depression, memory loss and headaches were not improved in spite of a 25-kg weight loss mainly due to fluid loss. A repeat polysomnographic study of 3.48 hours showed similar results. There were 241 upper airway obstructive episodes, three mixed apneas, and two central apneas. The mean duration of the apneas was 18 seconds and 35% of the sleep time was spent apneic. The oxygen desaturation was in the same range as the initial study. Thus, although it appears that there is some hormonal control over nocturnal respiration, the exact relationship is not clear.

There is a slight but significant rise in arterial carbon dioxide (or alveolar carbon dioxide) during sleep in the normal population.[27–30] This increase in carbon dioxide may be due to either of two mechanisms: an increase in CO_2 production or a decrease in alveolar ventilation. Sleep is usually accompanied by a decrease rather than an increase in carbon dioxide production.[28] Thus, the mild hypercapnia of sleep is secondary to a primary alveolar hypoventilation. This is true if the alveolar ventilation is not impaired by increased mechanical impedance to breathing even in the face of augmented respiratory drives.[31] The possibility of increased airway resistance or decreased pulmonary compliance during sleep in normal man was considered (though only in three subjects) by Robin et al.[28] There was an absence of mechanical changes in pulmonary mechanics, which supports the concept of decreased ventilatory drives and alveolar hypoventilation. Associated with the hypoventilation is a small but significant decrease in arterial pH of 0.03–0.05 units.[28–30] Hudgel et al.[32] also showed that lung compliance and resistance did not change in normal man, but resistance in the upper airway was increased during sleep (see below).

The discussion, to this point, on sleep-induced alveolar hypoventilation has been related to non-REM sleep. During REM sleep, the measurement of alveolar ventilation is difficult because of the non-steady state of ventilation. That is, tidal volume and rate vary considerably within a REM period. Thus, different conclusions have been reached by various investigators from hypoventilation to no change to hyperventilation during this sleep stage.

Chemical Control of Breathing

The exact relationship of the chemical control of breathing, i.e., hypercapnic and hypoxic ventilatory responses, during sleep, to these irregular respiratory changes, is unknown. Controversy exists about the exact control of breathing responses themselves.

In the awake state, breathing is controlled by two systems that are physically separate but function as an integrated process.[33,34] The systems are the behavioral (voluntary) control system and the metabolic (chemical) control system. The behavioral system arises in the cortical and forebrain areas. It is mainly involved with processes that use the respiratory system for nonventilatory purposes, e.g., phonation. However, this system can override the metabolic system. The metabolic system is involved with acid–base and oxygen control. The location of this control system is in the brain stem (pons and medulla) and the carotid bodies. The study of ventilatory control during sleep has mainly focused on the chemical control of breathing because it is assumed that the behavioral system is not active. The assumption may be incorrect, however.

The early reports[28,35–37] of ventilatory responses during sleep to hypercapnia concluded that there was blunting of chemosensitivity during sleep. However, these studies suffered from a lack of sleep staging (probably all were non-REM studies) and failure to provide supplemental oxygen during the testing. Without the addition of oxygen to the testing system, a distinction cannot be made between a hypercapnic response and a hypercapnic–hypoxic interaction. Subsequent investigations[38,39] using a steady-state hypercapnic response with supplemental oxygen in non-REM sleep showed little decrease in the slope of the ventilatory response to hypercapnia. There was, rather, more of a parallel shift of the slope so that a higher carbon dioxide was needed to elicit the same ventilatory response. Using this steady-state technique, many subjects aroused from sleep and were excluded from the study. In an extensive study, Bulow[24] found, while using a rebreathing technique, that the mean slope of change in ventilation to the change in the alveolar carbon dioxide response line decreased progressively from 1.25 L/min/mm Hg during wakefulness to 0.5 L/min/mm Hg in slow-wave sleep. He reported only one carbon dioxide response test in one subject during REM sleep that was similar to stage 1.

Phillipson et al.,[40] using a dog model, studied the effect of hypercapnia in all sleep stages. During REM sleep, the hypercapnic ventilatory response was markedly decreased in comparison to the non-REM stages. In addition, the length of the carbon dioxide rebreathing was longer and the alveolar carbon dioxide level reached was higher during REM sleep due to a lack of arousal. The highly irregular REM breathing pattern persisted. This suggests that the progressive hypercapnia had little influence on the ventilatory control system during REM sleep, and apparently there is a change in the central respiratory control aspect to breathing during this sleep stage. Anatomically, the structure of the pontine reticular formation that is involved in REM sleep[41] is closely situated to the pontine pneumotaxic center,[42] which could lead to a change in the initiating process. Another possibility that explains the irregularities of respiration is fluctuating supraspinal inhibitory and excitatory stimuli, which act on the phrenic neurons of the cervical cord rather than acting centrally. It is known that other spinal motoneurons are influenced by these inhibitory–excitatory impulses occurring during REM sleep.[43]

In 12 adult human subjects (six male, six female; no difference between male and female response), the awake ventilatory response to progressive hypercapnia was 1.60 L/min/mm Hg ± 0.19 SE.[43] This response was measured at 0.69 ± 0.08 during stage 2, at 0.81 ± 0.10 during slow-wave sleep, and at 0.45 ± 0.10 during REM. All sleep stages were significantly different from the awake state, and the response during REM was different from the non-REM stages. The relationship of the hypercapnia to the irregular REM breathing patterns was not investigated. As evidenced in this study, there is marked blunting of the ventilatory response to hypercapnia during sleep.

The ventilatory response during sleep to hypoxia has not been studied as much as the hypercapnic response. Until recently, the most complete study was in dogs.[45] There was no difference in the ventilatory response from awake to all stages of sleep, although the waking response from REM sleep developed at a lower arterial oxygen saturation as compared to non-REM sleep (70.5 ± 3.4% vs. 87.5 ± 2.6%, respectively). These investigators felt that the maintenance of an intact hypoxic ventilatory response may be of importance in maintaining adequate ventilation during this stage of sleep. However, Douglas et al.[46] showed that the hypoxic drive in adult human male subjects falls progressively and significantly from the awake state (1.07 L/min/% sat ± 0.19 SE) to stage 2 (0.64 ± 0.1) to slow-wave sleep (0.62 ± 0.09) to REM sleep (0.33 ± 0.04). The different findings in the two studies appear to be species-related and obviously changes conclusions about ventilatory responses during REM and non-REM sleep in humans. It appears that a sex difference is present to some degree in human hypoxic response during sleep.[47] The isocapnic hypoxic ventilatory response in premenopausal women was found to be similar during the awake state and non-REM sleep. During REM sleep, the response fell to 70% of the waking value ($P < 0.05$). This hypoxic response tended to be greater in the luteal than in the follicular phase of the menstrual cycle, both awake and asleep. Of interest, these women demonstrated significantly less awake hypoxic responses than males even when corrected for body surface area. During sleep, both men and women exhibited similar responses, but there was a large decrement from waking values in the men, while in the women there was little change. Thus, it appears that for both hypoxic (particularly in males) and hypercapnic ventilatory responses, there is a progressive decrease from the awake state to light sleep to slow-wave sleep to REM sleep. This may be the reason that apneas and desaturation are more pronounced in REM, but it does not explain why slow-wave sleep has very regular respiratory patterns. Other factors, such as arousal (see below), must be taken into consideration.

The possibility that low awake ventilatory drives lead to further respiratory sleep disorders is an interesting hypothesis. Martin et al.[48] studied a family with low awake ventilatory drives to determine if this factor leads to serious sleep-related respiratory problems. The contact patient was a 16-year-old male with primary alveolar hypoventilation. The rest of the family included both parents, three brothers, and a sister. None of the family members had significant respiratory problems during sleep except for the contact patient. Initially he weighed 200% of ideal body weight and had frequent and severe bouts of desaturation secondary to a breathing pattern that was so irregular that an adequate description could not be given. In addition, he had 32 upper airway obstructive episodes per night. After weight loss to 133% of ideal body weight, his awake blood gases returned to almost normal and all of the respiratory sleep disorders improved greatly. In this family, where low awake ventilatory drives predominated, there was no correlation with sleep-related respiratory disorders in the absence of obesity.

We have evaluated a 26-year-old patient who had carotid body resections for asthma and was having difficulty determining when her asthma was worsening because of decreased awareness of dyspnea. Her awake ventilatory response to hypoxia and mouth occlusion pressure (a reflection of neural output) were flat. It was assumed that her respiratory pattern and oxygen saturation would be significantly compromised during sleep. She was studied during sleep at a time when her asthma was well controlled. Both her respiratory pattern and oxygen saturation were maintained throughout the night. The only respiratory rhythm disturbance was one central apnea of 30 seconds during REM sleep with a 2% fall in saturation. This nocturnal polysomnographic study was well within normal limits. This patient was at her ideal body weight and without other stresses to her respiratory system at the time of the study, which, again, suggests that under these conditions other factors may play an important role in the maintenance of respiration during sleep.

Arousal

It appears that weight, age and, to some extent, sex play an important part in the regulation of breathing and oxygen saturation during sleep. However, for normal or disease states, not all sleep-related disorders are associated with obesity, age, or sex. Furthermore, not all elderly, overweight males have breathing disorders. Perhaps arousal or a lack of it plays an important part in the scheme (Table 3). For example, both hypoxia and hypercapnia stimulate the reticular activating system and produce arousal.[49,50] But, with abnor-

Table 3
Arousal Responses

Changes in arousal/perception pattern in normals			
Hyperventilation	Awake →	Breathing rhythm maintained	
	Sleep, anesthesia →	Apnea	
Laryngeal stimulation	Awake →	Cough	
	Sleep →	Apnea	
Hypoxia or Hypercapnia	Non-REM →	RAS →	Arousal
	REM →	RAS →	Arousal
Patients with sleep-related respiratory problems			
Hypoxia or Hypercapnia	Non-REM —//→	RAS —//→	Arousal
	REM —///→	RAS —///→	Arousal

REM = rapid eye movement sleep; RAS = reticular activating system; // or /// = delay of response which may occur at either point.

malities of respiration and apneas that lead to significant hypoxia and hypercapnia, the question of why there is failure to arouse needs to be answered. Fink[51] demonstrated in the awake state that after a period of significant hyperventilation, subjects did not lose the normal rhythmicity of breathing. However, during sleep or anesthesia, this rhythmicity posthyperventilation is lost. Sullivan et al.[52] found that in dogs laryngeal stimulation could produce apnea during sleep without any demonstration of the cough reflex. It is interesting that during wakefulness, coughing was always present, but apneas could not be induced. These two studies demonstrate that the awake state is a potent stimulus to breathing. Thus, with arousal or wakening, an appropriate overall response to respiratory stimuli can occur.

It is important that either a change in the sleep stage or total wakening occur if a respiratory problem is to be overcome. If an event such as an upper airway obstruction occurs, it would not be feasible just to exert more respiratory effort to overcome the obstruction as this would actually potentiate the problem. With arousal or awakening, the obstructing factors could be alleviated. The arousal response should be regarded as a separate reflex and not simply an action that is similar to the ventilatory response. In other words, patients with abnormal ventilatory drives may awaken appropriately if abnormal nocturnal events occur. Alternatively, it was shown, in dogs, that hypoxia causes a similar ventilatory response whether awake, during REM or non-REM sleep, but there is a sharp difference in the ability of hypoxia to produce arousal between those sleep stages.[45] In non-REM sleep, hypoxia led rapidly to arousal at a mean saturation of 87.5 $\pm$ 2.6% (SE), whereas it took severe hypoxia to produce arousal during REM sleep, 70.5 $\pm$ 3.4%. Perhaps this is the reason why sleep apnea patients have longer apneas with more severe desaturation during REM sleep. To strengthen the theory that ventilatory control and arousal are not linked, it has been shown that the hypercapnic ventilatory response is progressively diminished during sleep, but the arousal response is sustained.[40]

Asthma is another process in which arousal from sleep plays a very important role. Some asthmatic patients have severe nocturnal bronchospasm from which they only awaken by the time severe distress has developed and then quickly progress to cardiopulmonary arrest. In one study,[53] two adolescent males with nocturnal arrests were studied for arousal response during a stable period in their disease and compared to three healthy males plus the identical twin of one of the patients who had asthma without the nocturnal arrests.

The subjects wore a tight-fitting face mask to which a pneumotachograph and an occlusion device were attached. The external airway was occluded at end-expiration and released when alpha waves, indicating wakefulness, appeared on the electroencephalogram. Although there was individual variability of response in each of the patients and control subjects, the two patients had lengthened arousal time of greater than 20 seconds in various sleep stages, while none of the subjects had arousal times of more than 9 seconds. Thus it appears that these patients have suppressed arousal responses that then can lead to further worsening of their asthma before they finally awaken. In general, the exact relationship of arousal or the lack of it to disordered breathing and nocturnal oxygen desaturation needs to be developed to better understand these problems.

Snoring

The relationship between snoring and heart–lung abnormalities is an interesting one (Fig. 1). Snoring should first be defined. It is an acoustic process caused by the vibration of the soft palate and the faucial pillars. Both anatomical factors and sleep-related physiologic events play a role in the development of snoring. The anatomic process is related to the thickness of the faucial tissue, the size of the adenoids and tonsils, any mandibular malformation, and mucosal edema. The physiologic factors relate to the hypotonia of the oral pharyngeal muscles that develops during sleep. The physical conditions whereby air passes through a narrow orifice causing the soft palate to vibrate are created by the relative positions of the tongue and soft palate.[54] The snore is an almost exclusively inspiratory noise that arises during sleep onset and intensifies progressively with the deepening of non-REM sleep. During rapid eye movement it becomes discontinuous and less intense but persists during bursts of eye movement.[55] The prevalence of habitual snoring is greater in males than females. From 10–30 years of age, the habitual snorers in both groups comprise less than 15% of the population. From 30–60 years old, there is a progressive increase in the incidence of snoring. At approximately 60 years, the male population has an incidence of about 60% and female 40%, after which the incidence of snoring levels off.[56]

Lugaresi et al.[27,55,56] have shown changes in the cardiocirculatory system and arterial gas tensions in subjects who are heavy snorers but

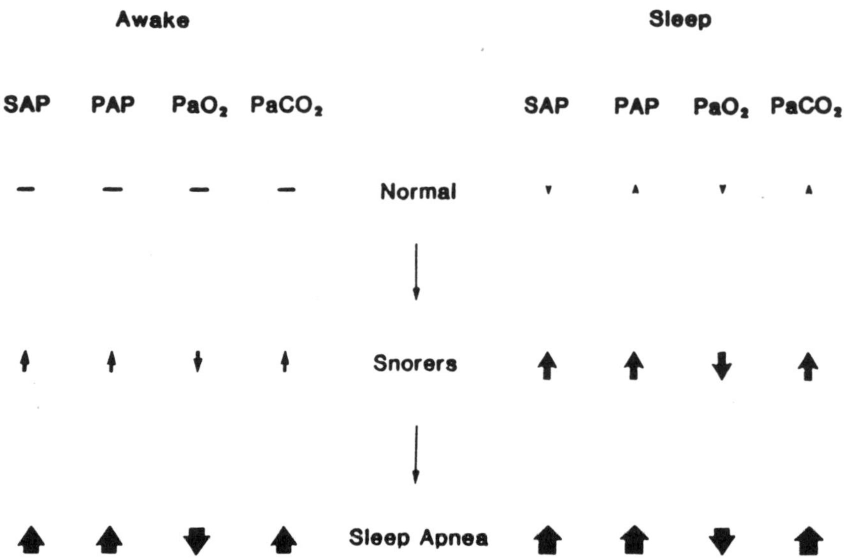

Figure 1: This shows the continuum from normals to habitual snorers to the sleep apnea patients. There is a progressive worsening of hemodynamic and gas exchanged variables. SAP = systemic arterial pressure; PAP = pulmonary artery pressure; PaO_2 = partial pressure of arterial oxygen; $PaCO_2$ = partial pressure of arterial carbon dioxide; size of arrow = degree of involvement.

otherwise normal. These subjects have a higher incidence of systemic hypertension than nonsnorers even when obesity is taken into account. In addition, the pulmonary artery pressures are also higher than in nonsnorers both during wakefulness and sleep. The arterial oxygen and carbon dioxide tensions are similar during the awake state in the two groups, but the oxygen level is decreased and carbon dioxide level increased in the snorers more than in the nonsnorers during sleep.

Heavy snoring is a relatively common finding, particularly with increasing age. Heavy snoring is associated with sleep apnea syndrome, but this problem is not as common with respect to the total population. Habitual snoring may represent a middle ground between nonsnorers and sleep apnea. This is exemplified in the heart–lung findings of the heavy snorers who fall between the nonsnorers and the sleep apnea group.

Hemodynamics

Only a few studies have been done that delineate the specific changes between the awake and sleep states in regard to cardiac function, pulmonary artery pressures, and system blood pressure in normal nonsnoring individuals. The arterial blood pressure tends to fall progressively from the awake state to stage 4 by 5%–23%, depending on the study.[27,57] During REM sleep, the blood pressure returns to the awake baseline value but can fluctuate greatly.[27,57,58] The exact cause of the fall in pressure during non-REM sleep and the increase during REM sleep is not known but is probably related to the changes in sympathetic nervous system activity and vasomotor tone.[59] The pulmonary artery pressure rises slightly but significantly during sleep,[26] although the physiologic range is never exceeded. The mean awake value in 10 subjects was 18/8 mm Hg, while during sleep it rose to 23/12 mm Hg.

The cardiac output also appears to fall progressively from the awake state to REM sleep.[57,60] One study attributed this fall to a decreased heart rate[57] and another study to decreased stroke volume.[60] Of interest, the cardiac output appears to decrease further as the sleep time increases.[60] That is, in any sleep stage, cardiac output is lower during each successive sleep cycle throughout the night. The lowest cardiac output was during the last REM period before arousal, which was 26% below the waking value. This could be of great importance in developing an understanding of why both normal individuals and patients with cardiac and/or pulmonary disease have the highest mortality during the early morning hours.[61] During this portion of the night, periodic breathing with oxygen desaturation is the greatest. With the addition of decreased cardiac output, myocardial oxygen supply can be greatly compromised, leading to arrhythmias and possible death.

Pulmonary Mechanics

The last aspect of pulmonary function during sleep is pulmonary mechanics. This, again, has not been well documented. Robin et al.[28] found a small decrease in pulmonary resistance during sleep. Sleep staging techniques were not applied, therefore the exact stages cannot be stated, but in all probability this decrease occurred during non-REM sleep. The pulmonary compliance appeared unchanged. In contrast, Hudgel et al.[32] found that although dynamic compliance did not change from the awake state to sleep, airflow resistance increased significantly. This latter study used a tight-fitting face mask with a pneumotachograph, an esophageal balloon, and mask pressure to determine resistance and compliance. An inductance vest was used to determine any changes in end-expiratory lung volumes. Airflow resistance increased from an awake value of 3.93 ± 0.56 cm H_2O/L/sec to 7.96 ± 0.95 in stage 2 sleep and to 8.66 ± 1.43 in REM sleep (P = 0.02). These investigators placed a catheter in the retroepiglottic space, thus dividing the airway into upper and lower zones. By doing this, the location of the increase in resistance could be determined. The resistance was found to be increased almost entirely below the retroepiglottic space. The additional information found in this study was that lung volume only minimally changed during the various stages of sleep.

From the above discussion of the current knowledge concerning the cardiopulmonary physiologic sleep processes that normal subjects undergo, one can see that we are at a new frontier in medicine. Although a great deal has been learned about the normal functioning of the cardiopulmonary system during sleep, there is a tremendous amount of knowledge yet to be gained. As in any field, as normality is fully understood, the abnormal states can be better delineated, treated, and prevented.

Monitoring of Respiratory Problems during Sleep

Monitoring devices have evolved over the last 15 years to the extent that important clinical information can be obtained with little discomfort to the patient. For the vast majority of situations, the following relatively simple full-night polysomnographic studies can answer the basic questions about cardiorespiratory function during sleep. However, in some situations more extensive monitoring is required to obtain sufficient information in order to treat the patient. In conjunction with the monitoring devices, a sleep laboratory requires a room where the sound, light, temperature, and, if possible, humidity can be controlled for the patient's comfort. This ability to control the environmental conditions will then enable the clinicians and investigators to obtain the needed information during sleep.

Full-Night Respiratory Polysomnographic Evaluation

There are four basic variables (Table 4) that should be measured during a complete study. These include: sleep staging, cardiac rate and rhythm, oxygen levels (saturation or oxygen tension), and respiratory patterns. A fifth variable may be the electromyogram (EMG) of the leg to determine if myoclonus is present, but this needs further investigation before mandating it to be included in a complete study.

Table 4
Respiratory Polysomnographic Evaluation

I. Sleep staging
   A. Electroencephalogram
      1. One or two leads are needed
      2. Interference usually from fluorescent light source
   B. Electromyogram
   C. Electrooculogram
II. Cardiac monitoring
   A. Rate and rhythm
   B. Single chest lead
      1. Multiple leads indicated if more involved rhythm or ST-segment T-wave changes
III. Oxygen saturation or tension
   A. Ear oximetry
   B. Transcutaneous monitoring
   C. Indwelling arterial line
IV. Respiratory patterns
   A. Air movement
      1. Qualitative
         a. Thermistors
         b. Carbon dioxide sensors
      2. Quantitative
         a. Pneumotachograph
   B. Effort
      1. Qualitative
         a. Strain gauge
         b. Pneumobelt
      2. Quantitative
         a. Esophageal balloon

Sleep Staging

Since the sleep electroencephalogram is important, the patient's room should be relatively free of ambient electromagnetic radiation.

Although some investigators feel that the sleep room should be totally shielded to block all interference, this is not usually necessary. Probably the most frequent source of electroencephalographic interference is fluorescent lamps. This type of lighting can easily be avoided with the use of incandescent fixtures for lighting where needed. If interference is a major problem, then methods for shielding a room have been well described.[62]

Essentially any electroencephalographic machine of recent manufacture is acceptable for the acquisition of the electroencephalograph and other endosomatic potentials necessary for sleep staging (EMG and electrooculogram, EOG). These potentials are characterized by amplitudes of 5 μV or more. It is important that these recorders have a paper supply compartment that is adequate for continuous runs of 6–8 hours. This requires that the paper drive mechanism be capable of a heavy-duty performance without attention for continuous operation over the expected time intervals. Some portable electroencephalographic recorders will not be able to perform an all-night study.

The question frequently arises about the unfamiliarity of the sleep laboratory for the patient and its effect on the first night of sleep. In normal subjects there appears to be some effect in the time it takes to fall asleep, the amount of REM sleep, and the amount of stage 4 sleep.[63,64] Even though there is suppression of these two sleep stages, it is not severe enough to cause a rebound effect the following night. Although some laboratories consider the first night as an adjustment night and use succeeding nights for documentation of patterns, there is no study that shows cardiorespiratory patterns to be significantly altered unless there is a very minimal number of apneas. Therefore, only one night is needed as long as all sleep stages are obtained.

The variables obtained from sleep staging are numerous and useful even when the main emphasis is on cardiopulmonary effects. For a complete description, refer to the book by Williams et al.[65]

1. *Time in Bed.* The time from when the subject is settled in bed with the electrodes on and the light turned off until the study is terminated.
2. *Sleep Period Time.* Time in bed less the time it took the subject to fall asleep after the lights were out and less the time he lay in bed after awakening in the morning.
3. *Total Sleep Time.* Sleep period time less any time the subject spent awake during the night after initial sleep onset.
4. *Percentage of Each Stage.* This is generally computed as the

percentage of sleep period time since it is then possible to compute the percentage of time awake during the night as well as the percentage of each of the sleep stages.

5. *Sleep Onset Latency.* The time from lights out until the appearance of the first sleep stage.
6. *Number of Stage Shifts.* This variable is measured because there are indications that the number of times sleep changes from one stage to another is a measure of subjective sleep "disturbance."
7. *Number of Awakenings, Amount of Awake Time.* These are measures of the amount of sleep disturbance present.
8. *Latency of Each Stage.* This is defined as the length of time from sleep onset to the appearance of each stage. But since sleep must start with one of the stages (usually stage 1), the latency of the first stage to appear is computed from the beginning of time in bed and is equal to sleep latency.
9. *Sleep Efficiency Index.* This measure is derived by dividing the total sleep time by time in bed.

Computer printouts of this information are easy to obtain and useful. An example is seen in Figure 2.

Electrode placement and interpretation of wave forms are well described in a pamphlet by Rechtschaffen and Kales.[66] To ensure a good signal throughout the night without waking the patient, two or three different leads should be placed at the start of the study. Even if only one EEG is recorded, the other leads can be turned on if the initial lead has come loose or if a poor signal develops.

Since the advent of electroencephalographic, electromyographic, and electrooculographic monitoring in addition to documentation of the respiratory patterns and the use of a well-taken history, a classification of sleep and arousal disorders has been established.[67] Table 5 outlines this classification.

Cardiac Monitoring

Cardiac rate and rhythm are usually obtained from one chest lead. Important information regarding the presence or absence of potentially lethal arrhythmias is documented in this manner. If more precise information on cardiac activity is desired, multiple leads can be placed. Since the paper speed for a polysomnographic evaluation

Data is saved in file RASSO DAT

Patient name:

Study title: APNEA DOCUMENTATION SLEEP STAGING
Date of test: 06-23-83
The program is using 2 pages per minute.
Comments:
POST WEIGHT LOSS

First page of the recording	: 23
Last page of the recording	: 885
Page of AWAKE onset	: 28
Page of REM onset	: 321
Page of STAGE 1 onset	: 26
Page of STAGE 2 onset	: 39
Page of STAGE 3 onset	: 46
Page of STAGE 4 onset	234
Page of undefined epochs	: 0
Page of LAST sleep epoch	875
Total number of AWAKE epochs	: 111
Total number of REM epochs	: 95
Total number of STAGE 1 epochs	: 207
Total number of STAGE 2 epochs	: 424
Total number of STAGE 3 epochs	: 24
Total number of STAGE 4 epochs	2
Total number of UNDEFINED epochs	: 0
Number of pages EQUALS number of epochs	
Total time awake	: 55.50
Total sleep time	: 376.00
Total time in bed	: 431.50
Sleep efficiency	: 87.14%
(total sleep time/time in bed)	
Sleep latency	: 1.50
Arise latency	: 5.00
Sleep period time	: 425.00
(time in bed-sleep and arise latencies)	

STAGE	LATENCY FROM LIGHTS OUT	TOTAL MINUTES	PERCENT OF SLEEP PERIOD TIME	PERCENT OF TOTAL SLEEP TIME
AWAKE *	1.00	49.00	11.53	———
REM *	147.50	47.50	11.18	12.63
STAGE 1	1.50	103.50	24.35	27.53
STAGE 2	8.00	212.00	49.88	56.38
STAGE 3	11.50	12.00	2.82	3.19
STAGE 4	105.50	1.00	0.24	0.27
undefined	0.00	0.00	0.00	0.00

* Latency from sleep onset

Figure 2: A computer printout of data obtained from a polysomnographic evaluation.

Table 5
Classification of Sleep and Arousal Disorders

I. Insomnias: disorders of initiating and maintaining sleep (DIMS)
  A. Psychophysiological
    1. Transient and situational
    2. Persistent
  B. Associated with psychiatric disorders
    1. Affective disorders
    2. Personality disorders
    3. Other functional psychoses
  C. Associated with use of drugs and alcohol
    1. Tolerance to or withdrawal from CNS depressants
    2. Sustained use of CNS stimulants
    3. Sustained use of or withdrawal from other drugs
    4. Chronic alcoholism
  D. Associated with sleep-induced respiratory impairment
    1. Sleep apnea DIMS syndrome
    2. Alveolar hypoventilation DIMS syndrome
  E. Associated with sleep-related (nocturnal) myoclonus and "restless legs"
    1. Sleep-related (nocturnal) myoclonus DIMS syndrome
    2. "Restless legs" DIMS syndrome
  F. Associated with other medical, toxic, and environmental conditions
  G. Childhood-onset DIMS
  H. Associated with other DIMS conditions
    1. Repeated REM sleep interruptions
    2. Atypical polysomnographic features
II. Hypersomnias: Disorders of excessive somnolence (DOES)
  A. Psychophysiological
    1. Transient and situational
    2. Persistent
  B. Associated with psychiatric disorders
    1. Affective disorders
    2. Other functional disorders
  C. Associated with use of drugs and alcohol
    1. Tolerance to or withdrawal from CNS stimulants
    2. Sustained use of CNS depressants
  D. Associated with sleep-induced respiratory impairment
    1. Sleep apnea DOES syndrome
    2. Alveolar hypoventilation DOES syndrome
  E. Associated with sleep-related (nocturnal) myoclonus and "restless legs"
    1. Sleep-related (nocturnal) myoclonus DOES syndrome
    2. "Restless legs" DOES syndrome
  F. Narcolepsy
  G. Idiopathic CNS hypersomnolence
  H. Associated with other medical, toxic, and environmental conditions
  I. Associated with other DOES conditions
    1. Intermittent DOES (periodic) syndromes
      a. Kleine-Levin syndrome
      b. Menstrual-associated syndrome

continued

Table 5 (*continued*)
Classification of Sleep and Arousal Disorders

2. Insufficient sleep
3. Sleep drunkenness

J. No DOES abnormality
1. Longer sleeper
2. Subjective DOES complaint without objective findings

III. Disorders of the sleep–awake schedule

A. Transient
1. Rapid time-zone change (jet lag) syndrome
2. Work-shift change in conventional sleep–awake schedule

B. Persistent
1. Frequently changing sleep–awake schedule
2. Delayed sleep phase syndrome
3. Advanced sleep phase syndrome
4. Non-24-hour sleep–awake syndrome
5. Irregular sleep–awake pattern

IV. Dysfunctions associated with sleep, sleep stages, or partial arousal (parasomnias)

A. Sleepwalking (somnambulism)

B. Sleep terror (pavor nocturnus, incubus)

C. Sleep-related enuresis

D. Other dysfunctions
1. Dream anxiety attacks (nightmares)
2. Sleep-related epileptic seizures
3. Sleep-related bruxism
4. Sleep-related head banging (jactatio capitis nocturna)
5. Familial sleep paralysis
6. Impaired sleep-related penile tumescence
7. Sleep-related painful erections
8. Sleep-related cluster headaches and chronic paroxysmal hemicrania
9. Sleep-related abnormal swallowing syndrome
10. Sleep-related asthma
11. Sleep-related cardiovascular symptoms
12. Sleep-related gastroesophageal reflux
13. Sleep-related hemolysis (paroxysmal nocturnal hemoglobinuria)
14. Asymptomatic polysomnographic finding
15. Not otherwise specified

is slower than for a routine cardiogram, specific types of rhythm disturbances may not always be definable.

Oxygen–Carbon Dioxide

Oxygen saturation can be measured by an oximeter, while tension can be determined by an arterial blood sample from an indwelling line or by transcutaneous surface measurements. Although carbon dioxide has not been a standard measurement in the past, with the advent of transcutaneous measurements, it may be measured more frequently in the future if the response time can be enhanced.

The oximeter is a reliable means of obtaining oxygen saturation by colorimetric analysis via light wavelengths of blood flow through the ear (Fig. 3) or finger. However, there are several drawbacks to using the oximeter. The first is discomfort. Over a 5- to 7-hour study period, discomfort is a common complaint. It also restricts the patient's mobility in that there is difficulty sleeping on the side (if ear probe used) where the oximeter is placed. Second, the oximeter is not accurate in very dark-skinned or in deeply jaundiced patients.[68] Third, below a saturation of approximately 60%, accuracy is not as well maintained,[69,70] but adequate trends are still preserved. Fourth, there is a delay of 10–30 seconds from the initiating event until a maximal change is seen by the oximeter. This delay is not a significant problem, however.

An indwelling arterial line will certainly give precise information about oxygen, carbon dioxide, and acid–base (pH) status, but the

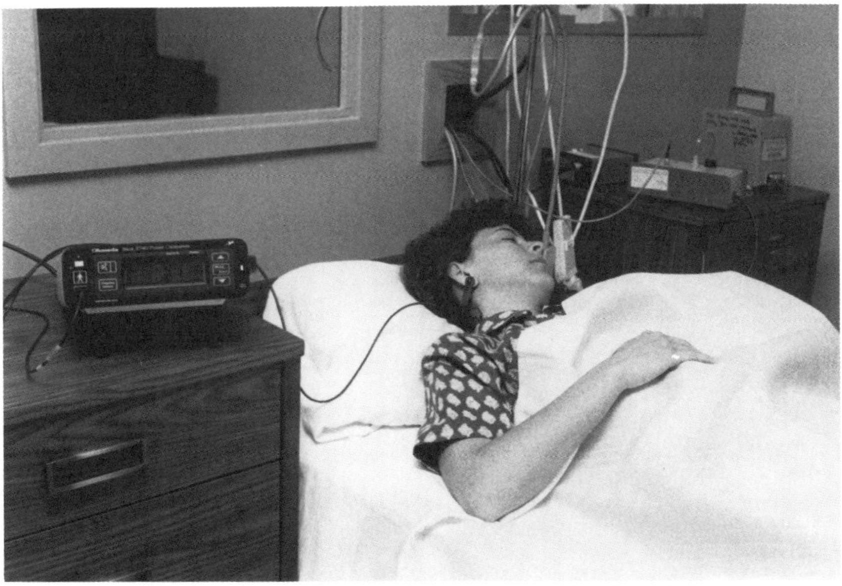

Figure 3: Ear oximetry measures oxygen saturation.

drawbacks are numerous. At present, there is no clinically available means of continuously measuring blood samples throughout the night. Thus, only intermittent values can be obtained and severe hypoxemia or hypercapnia may be missed by chance alone. There is some risk of arterial thrombosis and infection associated with an arterial line. The incidence of these complications increases the longer the catheter is in place. Over a 5- to 7-hour study, however, the risk is minimal. Another problem may occur when the line is flushed with heparin solution after a sample is taken. The heparin can give a painful, burning sensation in the hand, which could awaken the patient. This problem can be somewhat overcome by a slow infusion to clear the line.

The transcutaneous oxygen and carbon dioxide monitoring system is a relatively new means of measuring continuous gas tension by a noninvasive mechanism (Fig. 4). Both oxygen and carbon dioxide diffuse through the skin and can be measured at that point. The electrode leads of this system are heated to 44–45°C. This will increase perfusion in that area and shift the oxyhemoglobin dissociation curve to the right, which helps the unloading of oxygen from hemo-

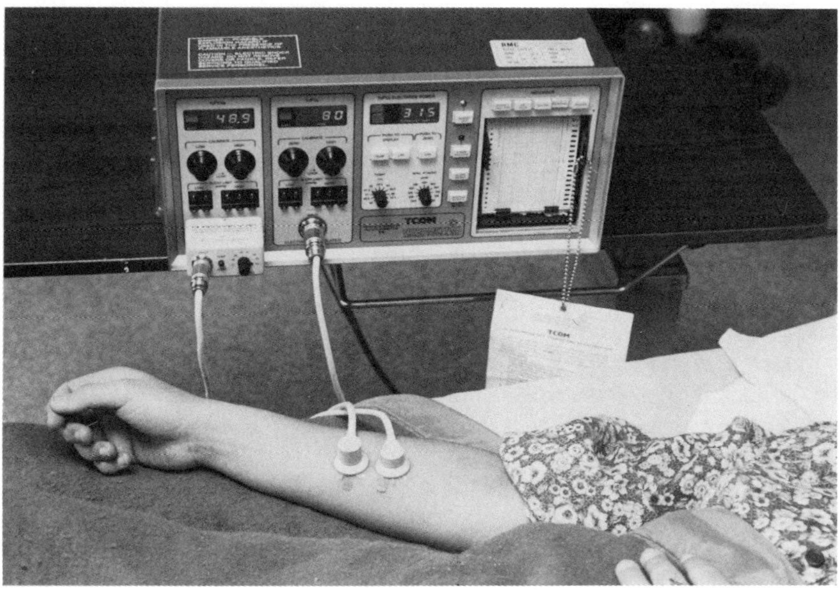

Figure 4: Transcutaneous carbon dioxide and oxygen monitoring.

globin. The oxygen sensor works on a Clark-type polarographic electrode with an oxygen-permeable membrane. The oxygen molecules diffuse through the membrane and create an electrochemical reaction. The current is converted into a value proportional to the oxygen tension at the electrode membrane. The carbon dioxide sensor utilizes a pH electrode based on the Stow-Severinghaus principle. As the carbon dioxide molecules pass through the permeable membrane, there is a reaction with a specific electrolyte solution. This reaction alters the pH of the solution, which changes the voltage across the pH and reference electrodes. The voltage change is converted into a value corresponding to the carbon dioxide tension at the skin surface.

Since the transcutaneous sensor is measuring tissue levels of oxygen and carbon dioxide, the levels are not exactly the same as in an arterial sample. The transcutaneous oxygen level will be within a value of 10% lower than the corresponding arterial oxygen tension.[71–73] The carbon dioxide level will be approximately 1.1–1.5 times the arterial value.[74–76]

The transcutaneous system was used only in infants initially but is now being used more frequently in adults. For sleep studies, it has many advantages over the other systems described. The patient's movement is not hindered, and there is no discomfort compared to the ear oximeter.

The drawbacks of the transcutaneous system are few. The main safety problem is the possibility of a mild skin burn if the heated electrode heads are left in place too long. Changing the position approximately every 4 hours will prevent skin surface damage and the patient is left at times with only an area of erythema that fades during the next day. Another problem that rarely occurs is a leak around the sensor head at the skin surface. With room air between the skin and electrode, the transcutaneous oxygen levels will read falsely high and the carbon dioxide will be falsely low. The oxygen tension in the room air is higher and the carbon dioxide tension lower than at tissue levels. This will then change the transcutaneous readings. Another factor to be considered is that of cardiac output. Changes in cardiac output change the transcutaneous oxygen and carbon dioxide values.[72,73,75] As cardiac output falls by approximately 40%, the skin perfusion will fall and therefore relatively less oxygen is available for consumption at the skin sensor. The false elevation in carbon dioxide occurs because of vasoconstriction of the skin capillaries and a "trapping" of CO_2; thus, the transcutaneous value rises. The reverse occurs with an increase in cardiac output. Unless a patient has significant heart disease, these large alterations in cardiac output do not usually occur during sleep. A final point to be considered is the time delay from an actual event to the initial change in transcutaneous values. This can range from 10 to 25 seconds, with maximal changes occurring in several minutes, resulting in the necessity of back extrapolation.

Respiratory Effort and Flow

Great emphasis should be placed on the accurate determination of sleeping respiratory patterns because treatment varies with the type of abnormality found. The two basic variables necessary for pattern interpretation are air movement and chest wall or abdominal movement. This will allow for the determination of apneas and type of apnea, hypopneas, and hyperpneas.

Air movement at the mouth and/or nose can be qualitatively or quantitatively measured using several different systems. Qualitative measurement is done by thermistors or carbon dioxide sensors. Quantitative flow is measured with a pneumotachograph.

Thermistors (Fig. 5) are heat sensors that detect changes in heat

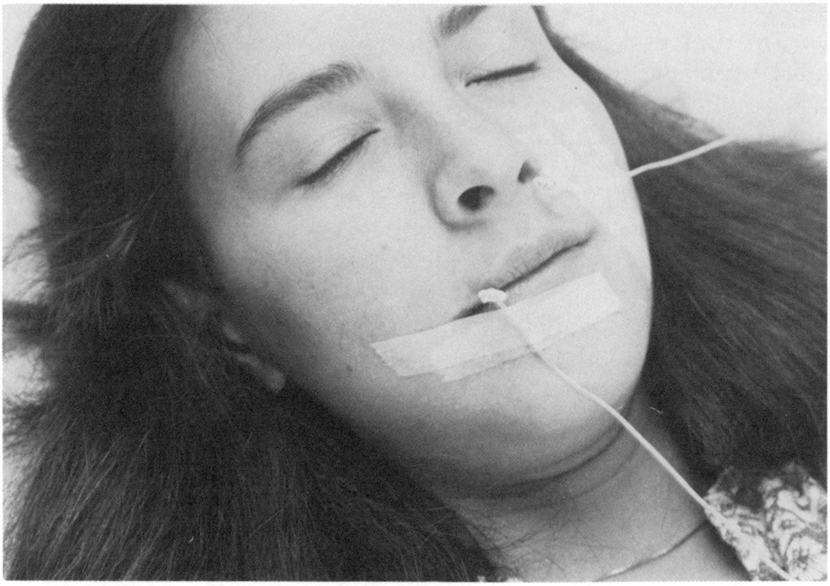

Figure 5: Thermistors qualitatively measure air movement.

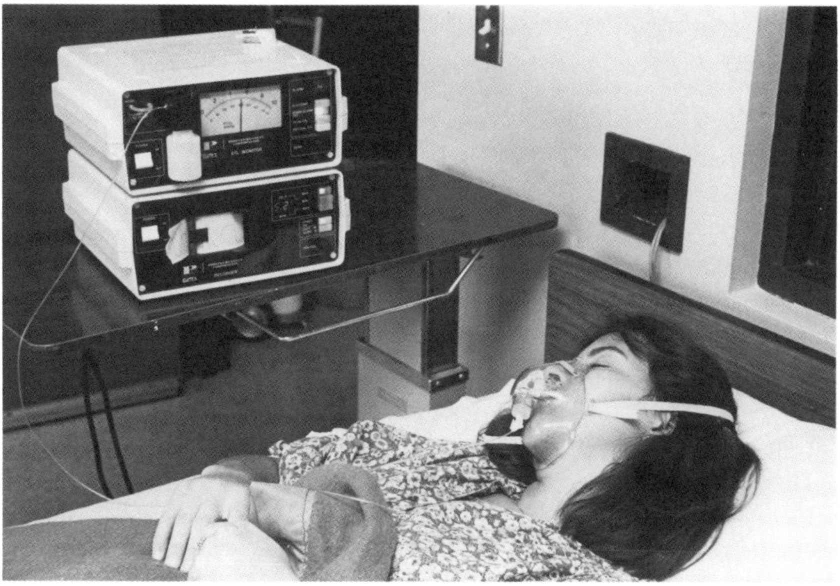

Figure 6: A capnograph measures expired carbon dioxide as an indicator of airflow.

between inspiration (cooler room air) and expiration (warmer body air). The thermistor must be clipped onto the lip and naris so as to detect either mouth or nose breathing. Another way to use the thermistor is to place it in a comfortable, loose-fitting mask, e.g., oxygen mask, and when done this way, only one thermistor is needed. This method will also eliminate the need for an additional channel on the recorder. The major difficulty in this system involves upper airway obstructions. Not uncommonly, the obstruction is not complete, i.e., there is an expiratory leak of air and the thermistor system will show an unusual air movement pattern.

A capnograph (Fig. 6) detects the expiration of carbon dioxide as a measurement of air movement. The set-up must be able to detect both nasal and oral flow so as not to give a falsely apneic pattern. Again, the easiest way to accomplish this is with a comfortable, loose-fitting mask with the sensor inside. The advantage to this system is that if hypoventilation occurs, the end-tidal carbon dioxide will be higher if an alveolar plateau is reached.

Quantitative measurement of flow can be determined by a pneumotachograph placed at the end of a tight-fitting face mask (Fig. 7).

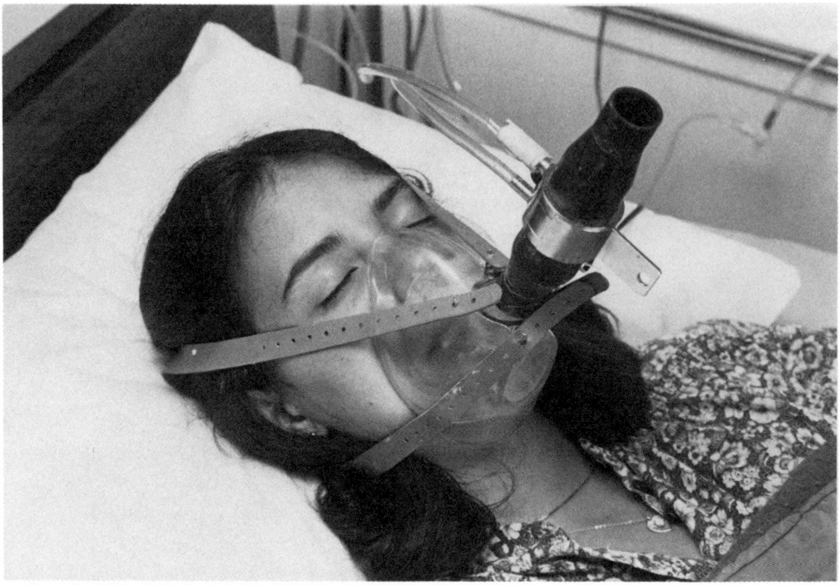

Figure 7: A pneumotachograph quantitatively measures airflow. This can then be integrated to volume.

The advantage of this system is that flow can be integrated to an accurate measurement of volume. Thus the extent of hypo- or hyperventilation can be determined. Clinically, this is seldom necessary and is used more frequently on a research basis. However, when a questionable pattern of upper airway obstruction or partial obstruction (obstructive hypopnea) occurs (see Chapter 4), the pneumotachograph helps to delineate the true process. The major drawback is a tight-fitting face mask with the additional weight of the pneumotachograph on a port opening.

Respiratory effort can be measured either qualitatively or quantitatively. The qualitative measure is achieved with a thoracic or abdominal strain gauge or pneumobelt. The quantitative measure is made with an inductance vest (Respitrace vest), magnetometers, or esophageal pressures.

The strain gauge (Fig. 8) works on the principle that a change in length, i.e., stretching the instrument, is proportional to a change in resistance, which in turn is proportional to a voltage change resulting in the signal. When stretched, the pneumobelt produces changes in

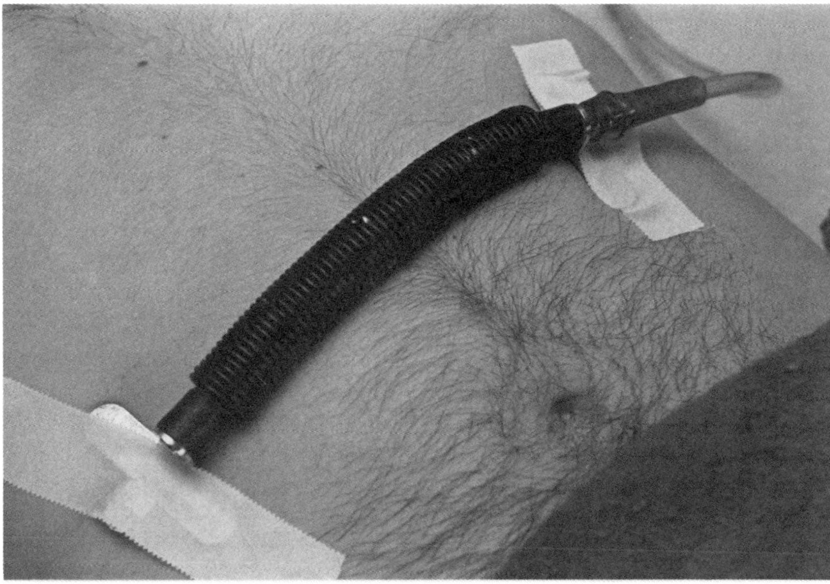

Figure 8: A strain gauge qualitatively measures respiratory effort.

pressure which then causes a voltage change. These instruments are placed over the area of maximum displacement of the chest wall or abdomen. The placement is usually halfway between the xyphoid and umbilicus. Although the exact amount of effort cannot be quantitated, increasing or decreasing efforts can be seen. In very obese people, small efforts may be missed because of a lack of enough stretch on the system. Furthermore, as a patient changes position during sleep, the same effort that produced a good signal before may produce very little signal. In certain situations, if one is not careful to take into account these possibilities when interpreting a signal from a strain gauge or pneumobelt, an upper airway obstruction apnea may be mistaken for a central apnea. Many centers use both a thoracic and an abdominal strain gauge.

The inductance vest (Fig. 9) can be used to measure the volume of air moved by the chest and abdomen. Considering both volumes, the tidal volume of a given breath can then be calculated.[77] Therefore, if larger or smaller efforts are made, this will be reflected in the volume of that breath. If there is a central apnea, then no volume will be

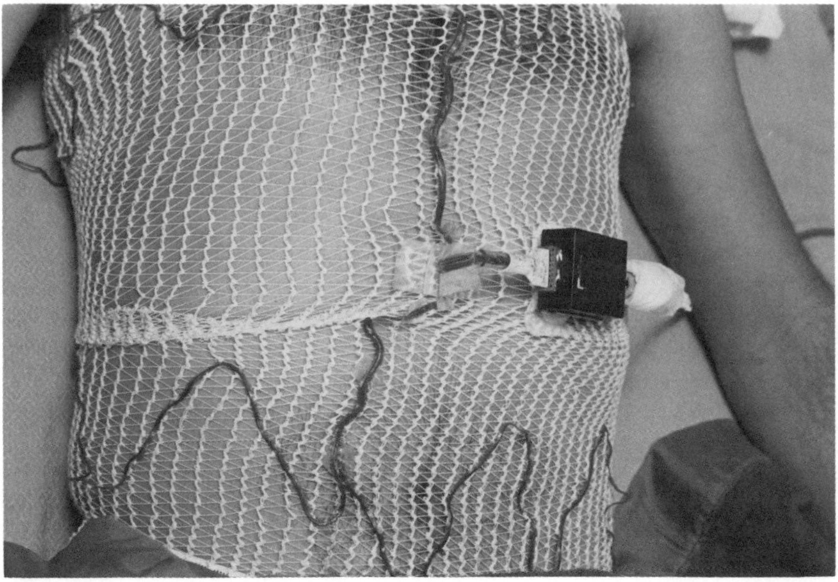

Figure 9: An inductance vest can quantitatively measure volume and divide this into chest wall and abdominal components.

moved. If there is a total upper airway occlusion, then paradoxic breathing can be seen between the chest wall and abdominal movements. The drawback to this system is the expense and the length of accurate calibration time needed for various positions. The time involved for calibration is 45 minutes to an hour. The cost of the system is approximately $5000.

Magnetometers measure the anteroposterior and lateral diameters of the chest wall and abdomen. The signal is linearly related to and capable of calibration in terms of linear displacement or volume change. This system has been used accurately in sleep apneas.[78] Again, the major drawbacks are cost and calibration time. The cost of this system is approximately $3000.

An inexpensive means of accurately measuring respiratory effort with little calibration time is with an esophageal balloon. This measurement reflects pleural pressure and thus effort. With proper explanation and topical anesthesia, there is only minimal discomfort to the patient. Occasionally a patient will not tolerate this procedure and an alternate means of respiratory effort is necessary.

Recording Systems

The recording system used for polysomnographic studies is usually a Grass (Grass Instruments, Quincy, MA), Nihon Kohden (Irvine, CA), Beckman (Beckman Instruments, Schiller Park, IL), or Gould (Gould Inc., Dayton, OH) recorder. Obviously, any recording system can be used that processes alternating current signals for the electroencephalogram and electromyogram and direct current signals for the saturation, gas tensions, pressure, volume, and flow signals. Figure 10a,b shows two recordings with different variables.

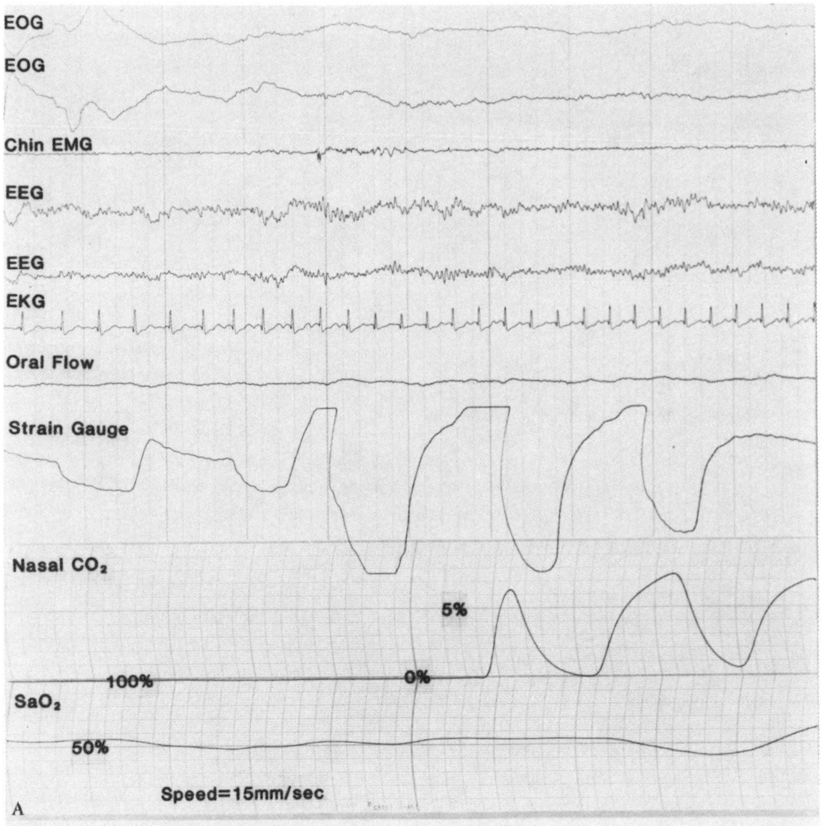

Figure 10a: This is an example of a typical polysomnographic evaluation.

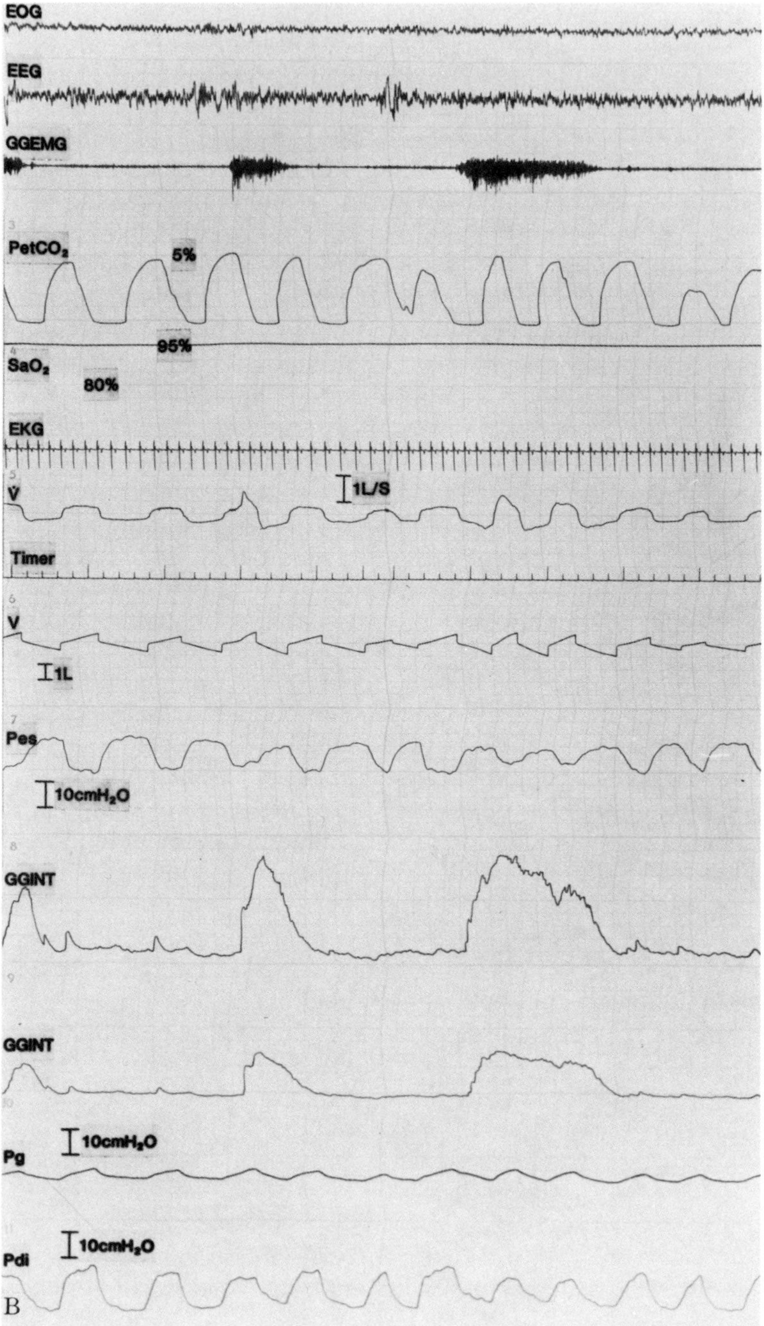

Figure 10b: More involved measurement during sleep can be made as compared to Figure 10a.

Screening Studies

A screening study can be defined in a number of ways. Here it will be defined as any study that is not a full-night polysomnographic evaluation for respiratory disorders. Thus, included in screening evaluations are individual studies of oxygen saturations, transcutaneous gas tension, arterial gas tension, direct observations, short-term nap studies, or home monitoring.

When should a short-duration nap study take the place of a more expensive all-night study to determine if respiratory abnormalities exist? First, the patient population must be defined. If patients with diseases such as chronic obstructive pulmonary disease, most of the severe cardiopulmonary dysfunction occurs during REM sleep. This stage of sleep does not usually occur during a short nap period. On the other hand, in patients with a strong history and physical examination and laboratory data supportive of sleep apnea or primary alveolar hypoventilation (see Chapter 4), a diagnosis can be made with a daytime nap study.

The second consideration for the nap-type study is the extent of information desired about the patient. That is, how representative is the nap study versus an entire night study? As stated previously, during a daytime nap, REM sleep is not usually obtained. Apneas and hypoventilation during REM are usually of longer duration, increased frequency, and are associated with greater oxygen desaturation. Overall, the type of apneas (upper airway obstruction, mixed, or central) changes very little from a nap study to a full-night study. Martin et al.[79] showed that four of five sleep apnea patients maintained essentially the same type of apneas when comparing a one-half-hour nap study with a full-night evaluation. However, the fifth patient went from 10% upper airway obstruction, 40% mixed apneas, and 50% central apneas during the half-hour nap to 51% upper airway obstruction, 43% mixed apneas, and 6% central apneas for the entire night.

Treatment is not solely based on the severity of sleep abnormalities. Daytime symptoms are of equal importance, and thus a full-night polysomnographic study may not always be needed.

Home monitoring systems are starting to be evaluated. They would reduce the cost of the testing, but may eliminate certain variables that could be of importance. That is, with a compact portable unit only certain parameters can be studied. Some units have only three channels, while others have up to eight channels. Investigation is needed to determine the usefulness of such monitoring systems.

Would direct observation of the sleeping patient be an appropriate screening test for sleep apnea? In the more severe cases of upper airway obstruction, one can see chest wall movement in an attempt to breathe. This is not true for all of the cases though. Many times, physicians or family members state that no effort is made, indicating a central apnea. Only when these patients are formally studied does the upper airway obstructive pattern become clear. Therefore, prolonged direct observation helps the physician determine if a respiratory disorder is present, but it does not delineate the type.

Not uncommonly, the question arises as to whether changes in oxygen and/or carbon dioxide tension occur during sleep. In this case, all that is necessary is a means of measuring the desired variables. This includes an oximeter for oxygen desaturation, an indwelling arterial catheter, or a transcutaneous oxygen–carbon dioxide monitor. These monitoring devices have been discussed above under "Full-Night Respiratory Polysomnographic Evaluation."

References

1. Guilleminault C, van den Hoed J, Mitler MM. Clinical overview of the sleep apnea syndromes. *In* C Guilleminault, WC Dement (eds). Sleep Apnea Syndromes. New York, Alan R. Liss, 1978, pp 1–12.
2. Dudley DL, Glasner EM, Jorgenson BN, et al. Psychosocial concomitants to rehabilitation in chronic obstructive pulmonary disease. *Chest* 1980; 77:413–420.
3. Grant I, Heaton RK, McSweeney AJ, et al. Brain dysfunction in COPD. *Chest* 1980; 77(S):308–309.
4. Schraa JC, Dirks JF, Jones NF, et al. Bender-Gestalt performance and recall in an asthmatic sample. *J Asthma* 1981; 18:7–9.
5. Guilleminault C, Tilkian A, Dement WC. The sleep apnea syndromes. *Annu Rev Med* 1976; 27:464–484.
6. Flick MR, Block AJ. Continuous in-vivo monitoring of arterial oxygenation in chronic obstructive lung disease. *Ann Intern Med* 1977; 86:725–730.
7. Montplaisir J, Walsh J, Malo JL. Nocturnal asthma: Features of attacks, sleep and breathing patterns. *Am Rev Respir Dis* 1982; 125:18–22.
8. Krop HD, Block AJ, Cohen E, et al. Neuropsychologic effects of continuous oxygen therapy in the aged. *Chest* 1977; 72:737–743.
9. Martin RJ, Sanders MH, Gray BA, et al. Acute and long-term ventilatory effects of hyperoxia in the adult sleep apnea syndrome. *Am Rev Respir Dis* 1982; 125:175–180.
10. Block AJ, Castle JR, Keitt AS. Chronic oxygen therapy. Treatment of chronic obstructive pulmonary disease at sea level. *Chest* 1974; 65:279–288.

11. Krop HD, Block AJ, Cohen E. Neuropsychologic effects of continuous oxygen therapy in chronic obstructive pulmonary disease. *Chest* 1973; 65:317–322.
12. Eckert CR. Personal communication.
13. Smolensky M, Halberg F, Sargent F II. Chronobiology of the life sequence. *In* S Itoh, K Ogata, H Yoshimura (eds). Advances in Climatic Physiology. New York, Springer-Verlag, 1972, pp 281–318.
14. Cochrane GM, Clark TJH. A survey of asthma mortality in patients between ages 35 and 64 in the Greater London Hospitals in 1971. *Thorax* 1975; 30:300–305.
15. Hetzel MR, Clark TJH, Branthwaite MA. Asthma: Analysis of sudden death and ventilatory arrests in hospital. *Br Med* 1977; 1:808–811.
16. Rosenblatt G, Hartmann E, Zwilling GR. Cardiac irritability during sleep and dreaming. *J Psychosom Res* 1973; 17:129–134.
17. Lown B, Tykocinski M, Garfein A, et al. Sleep and ventricular premature beats. *Circulation* 1973; 48:691–701.
18. Nowlin JB, Troyer WG Jr, Collins WS, et al. The association of nocturnal angina pectoris with dreaming. *Ann Intern Med* 1965; 63:1040–1045.
19. Tirlupur VG, Mir MA. Nocturnal hypoxemic and associated electrocardiographic changes in patients with chronic obstructive airways disease. *N Engl J Med* 1982; 306:125–130.
20. Mays EE. Intrinsic asthma in adults: Associated with gastroesophageal reflux. *J Am Med Assoc* 1976; 236:2626–2628.
21. Goodall RJR, Euris JE, Looper DN, et al. Relationship between asthma and gastro-oesophageal reflux. *Thorax* 1981; 36:116–121.
22. Fletcher EC, Martin RJ. Sexual dysfunction and erectile impotence in chronic obstructive pulmonary disease. *Chest* 1982; 81:413–421.
23. Webb P. Periodic breathing during sleep. *J Appl Physiol* 1974; 37:899–903.
24. Bulow K. Respiration and wakefulness in man. *Acta Physiol Scand Suppl* 1963; 209:1–110.
25. Block AJ, Boysen PG, Wynne JW, et al. Sleep apnea, hypopnea and oxygen desaturation in normal subjects. *N Engl J Med* 1979; 300:513–517.
26. Block AJ, Wynne JW, Boysen PG, et al. Menopause, medroxyprogesterone and breathing during sleep. *Am J Med* 1981; 70:506–510.
27. Lugaresi E, Coccagna G, Cirignotta F, et al. Breathing during sleep in man in normal and pathological conditions. *Adv Exp Med Biol* 1978; 99: 33–45.
28. Robin ED, Whaley RD, Crump CH, et al. Alveolar gas tensions, pulmonary ventilation and blood pH during physiologic sleep in normal subjects. *J Clin Invest* 1958; 37:981–989.
29. Birchfield RI, Sicker HO, Heyman A. Alterations in blood gases during natural sleep and narcolepsy. *Neurology* 1958; 8:107–112.
30. Birchfield RI, Sicker HO, Heyman A. Alterations in respiratory function during nocturnal sleep. *J Lab Clin Med* 1959; 54:216–222.
31. Pengelly LD, Rebuck AS, Campbell EJM. Loaded Breathing. Don Mills, Ontario, Longman, 1974.
32. Hudgel DW, Martin RJ, Johnson B. Mechanics of the respiratory system breathing pattern and lung volumes during sleep in normal man. *J Appl Physiol: Respir Environ Exercise Physiol* 1983; 56:133.

33. Berger AJ, Mitchell RA, Severinghous JW. Regulation of respiration. *N Engl J Med* 1977; 297:92, 138, 194.
34. Mitchell RA, Berger AJ. Neural regulation of respiration. *Am Rev Respir Dis* 1975; 111:208–224.
35. Magnussen G. Studies on the Respiration during Sleep. London, HK Lewis, 1944.
36. Ostergaard T. The excitability of the respiratory centre during sleep and during Evipan anaesthesia. *Acta Physiol Scand* 1944; 8:1–15.
37. Birchfield RI, Sicker HO, Heyman A. Alterations in respiratory function during natural sleep. *J Lab Clin Med* 1959; 54:216–227.
38. Reed DJ, Kellogg RH. Changes in respiratory response to CO_2 during natural sleep at sea level and at altitude. *J Appl Physiol* 1958; 13:325–330.
39. Bellville JW, Howland WS, Seed JC, et al. The effect of sleep on the respiratory response to carbon dioxide. *Anesthesiology* 1959; 20:628–634.
40. Phillipson EA, Kozar LF, Rebuck AS, et al. Ventilatory and waking responses to CO_2 in sleeping dogs. *Am Rev Respir Dis* 1977; 115:251–259.
41. Jouvet M. Paradoxical sleep—a study of its nature and mechanisms. *In* Progress in Brain Research, Sleep Mechanisms. Amsterdam, Elsevier, 1965, p 20.
42. Betrand F, Hugelin A. Respiratory synchronizing function of nucleus parabrachialis medelis: Pneumotaxic mechanisms. *J Neurophysiol* 1971; 34:189.
43. Pompeian O. The neurophysiological mechanisms of the postural and motor events during dysynchronized sleep. *In* SS Kety, EV Evants, HL Williams (eds). Sleep and Altered States of Consciousness. Baltimore, Williams & Wilkins, 1967, p 351.
44. White DP, Douglas NJ, Pickett CK, et al. Hypoxic and hypercapnic ventilatory responses decrease during sleep in adults. *Am Rev Respir Dis* 1982; 125(2):234.
45. Phillipson EA, Sullivan CE, Read DJC, et al. Ventilatory and waking responses to hypoxia in sleeping dogs. *J Appl Physiol* 1978; 44:512–520.
46. Douglas NJ, White DP, Weil JV, et al. Hypoxic ventilatory response decreases during sleep in man. *Am Rev Respir Dis* 1982; 125:286–289.
47. White DP, Douglas NJ, Pickett CK, et al. Hypoxic ventilatory response during sleep in normal premenopausal women. *Am Rev Respir Dis* 1982; 126:530–533.
48. Martin RJ, Ballard RD, Hudgel DW, et al. The effects of weight and chemosensitivity on respiratory sleep abnormalities: A family study. *Intl J Obes* 1986; 10:283–292.
49. Hugelin A, Bon Vallet M, Dell P. Activation reticulaire et corticale d'origine chemoceptive au cours de l'hypoxie. *Electroencephalogr Clin Neurophysiol* 1959; 11:325–340.
50. Bon Vallet M, Hugelin A, Dell P. Sensibilite comparee du systeme reticule activateur ascendent et du centre respiratoire aux gaz du sang et a l'adrenaline. *J Physiol (Paris)* 1955; 47:651–654.
51. Fink BR. Influence of cerebral activity in wakefulness on regulation of breathing. *J Appl Physiol* 1961; 16:15–20.

52. Sullivan CE, Murphy E, Kozar LF, et al. Waking and ventilatory responses to laryngeal stimulation in sleeping dogs. *J Appl Physiol* 1978; 45:681–689.
53. Hudgel DW, Kellum R, Martin RJ, et al. Depressed arousal response to airflow obstruction—a possible factor in near fatal nocturnal asthma. *Am Rev Respir Dis* 1982; 125(2):202.
54. Robin IG. Snoring. *Proc R Soc Med* 1968; 61:575–582.
55. Lugaresi E, Coccagna G, Farneti P, et al. Snoring. *Electroencephalogr Clin Neurophysiol* 1975; 39:59–64.
56. Lugaresi E, Cirignotta F, Coccagna G, et al. Some epidemiological data on snoring and cardiocirculatory disturbances. *Sleep* 1980; 3:221–224.
57. Khatri IM, Freis ED. Hemodynamic changes during sleep. *J Appl Physiol* 1967; 22:867–873.
58. Snyder F, Hobson JA, Morrison DF, et al. Changes in respiration, heart rate and systolic blood pressure in human sleep. *J Appl Physiol* 1964; 29:417–422.
59. Umemura S, Tochikubo O, Noda K, et al. Changes in blood pressure and plasma norepinephrine during sleep in essential hypertension. *Jpn Circ J* 1987; 51:1250–1256.
60. Miller JC, Horvath SM. Cardiac output during human sleep. *Aviat Space Environ Med* 1976; 47:1046–1051.
61. Smolensky M, Halberg F, Sargent F II. Chronobiology of the life sequence. *In* S Itoh, K Ogata, H Yoshimura (eds). Advances in Climatic Physiology. New York, Springer-Verlag, 1971.
62. Williams RL, Karacan I, Hursch CJ. Present-day EEG methods. *In* Electroencephalography of Human Sleep: Clinical Application. New York, John Wiley & Sons, 1974, pp 10–12.
63. Rechtschaffen A, Verdone P. Amount of dreaming: Effect of incentive, adaptation to laboratory, and individual differences. *Percept Mot Skills* 1964; 19:947–958.
64. Agnew HW Jr, Webb WB, Williams RL. The first night effect: An EEG study of sleep. *Psychophysiology* 1966; 2:263–266.
65. Williams RL, Karacan I, Hursch CJ. Normal sleep. *In* Electroencephalography of Human Sleep: Clinical Application. New York, John Wiley & Sons, 1974, pp 23–24, 26–68.
66. Rechtschaffen A, Kales A. A Manual of Standardized Terminology, Techniques, and Scoring System for Sleep Stages of Human Subjects. U.S. Department of Health, Education and Welfare, Public Health Service, National Institutes of Health, National Institute of Neurology Disease and Stroke, Neurological Information Network. Bethesda, Maryland, 1968, pp 1–12.
67. Roftwarg HP. Diagnostic classification of sleep and arousal disorders. *Sleep* 1979; 2:1–154.
68. Chaudhary BA, Burk NK. Ear oximetry in clinical practice. *Am Rev Respir Dis* 1978; 117:173–175.
69. Douglas NJ, Brash HM, Wrath PK, et al. Accuracy, sensitivity to carboxyhemoglobin and speed of response of the Hewlett-Packard 47201A ear oximeter. *Am Rev Respir Dis* 1979; 119:311–313.
70. Saunders NA, Powles ACP, Rebuck AS. Ear oximetry: Accuracy and

practicability in the assessment of arterial oxygenation. *Am Rev Respir Dis* 1976; 113:745–749.
71. McDowell JW, Thiede WH. Usefulness of the transcutaneous PO_2 monitor during exercise testing in adults. *Chest* 1980; 78:853–855.
72. Tremper KK, Waxman K, Shoemaker WC. Effects of hypoxia and shock on transcutaneous PO_2 values in dogs. *Crit Care Med* 1979; 7:526–531.
73. Tremper KK, Waxman K, Bowman R, et al. Continuous transcutaneous oxygen monitoring during respiratory failure, cardiac decompensation, cardiac arrest and CPR. *Crit Care Med* 1980; 8:377–381.
74. Hansen TN, Tooley WH. Skin surface carbon dioxide tension in sick infants. *Pediatrics* 1979; 64:942–945.
75. Tremper KK, Mentelos RA, Shoemaker WC. Effect of hypercarbia and shock on transcutaneous carbon dioxide at different electrode temperatures. *Crit Care Med* 1980; 8:608–612.
76. McLellan PA, Goldstein RS, Rancharan V, et al. Transcutaneous carbon dioxide monitoring. *Am Rev Respir Dis* 1981; 124:199–201.
77. Cohn MA, Watson H, Weisshart R, et al. A transducer for non-invasive monitoring of respiration. *In* ED Stott, EB Raftery, P Sleigh, et al. (eds). ISAM Proceedings of the Second International Symposium on Ambulatory Monitoring. London, Academic Press, 1975, pp 119–128.
78. Sharp JT, Druz WS, Foster JR, et al. Use of the respiratory magnetometer in diagnosis and classification of sleep apnea. *Chest* 1980; 77:350–353.
79. Martin RJ, Sanders MH, Gray BA, et al. Acute and long-term ventilatory effects of hyperoxia in the adult sleep apnea syndrome. *Am Rev Respir Dis* 1982; 125:175–180.

3

Ventilation and the Control of Respiration during Sleep: Normal Mechanisms, Pathologic Nocturnal Hypoventilation, and Central Sleep Apnea

David P. White, M.D.

It has become increasingly clear to individuals interested in the control of breathing that sleep is the time when ventilation reaches its lowest level[1–3] and the respiratory pattern becomes the most aberrant.[4,5] To understand why this occurs one must have some knowledge of the normal mechanisms that control ventilation during wakefulness and add to this information concerning the expected influence of sleep on these mechanisms. In addition, abnormalities in the control of breathing may develop, leading to further disordered breathing during sleep in some individuals.[6–8] It is the purpose of this chapter to outline how ventilation is controlled during wakefulness, how sleep influences these mechanisms, and, thus, what might be considered normal ventilation during sleep. In addition, abnormal respiration during sleep, specifically hypoventilation and central sleep apnea, will be addressed within the context of the previously outlined information. This should provide a framework in which to

Martin RJ: Cardiorespiratory Disorders During Sleep, 2nd Edition. Futura Publishing Company, Inc., Mount Kisco, NY, © 1990.

understand both why ventilation changes from wakefulness to sleep in normals and why respiration may become quite unstable under pathologic conditions.

Normal Ventilation and Ventilatory Control during Wakefulness

It is quite clear that during wakefulness ventilation is very precisely controlled, thus protecting arterial chemistry (Po_2 and Pco_2).[9–12] This stability is present despite wide variability in the metabolic demands of the body [oxygen consumption ($\dot{V}o_2$) and carbon dioxide production ($\dot{V}o_2$)] and considerable variability in the work of breathing. A normal individual when presented with a high metabolic rate (exercise)[9] or markedly increased work of breathing (inspiratory resistive loading)[13] will adjust the quantity and pattern of ventilation to maintain arterial homeostasis within narrow limits. To accomplish this a variety of mechanisms are employed, which, when grouped, are referred to as the metabolic or autonomic controllers of ventilation. Three such mechanisms will be addressed in a somewhat simplified manner here and are as follows: (1) arterial chemoreceptors, (2) metabolism and its influence on ventilation, and (3) intrapulmonary receptors.

Autonomic Ventilatory Control

Arterial Chemoreceptors

It is well known that rising Pco_2[12] or falling Po_2[11] will elicit a brisk ventilatory response in an attempt to correct arterial blood chemistry. Hypoxia is sensed at the carotid body[14] and hypercapnia (or rising hydrogen ion concentration) at two sites, the carotid body[15] and the medullary chemoreceptor.[16] Normal responses are demonstrated in Figure 1. The hypoxic ventilatory response represents a hyperbolic relationship with respiration increasing rapidly only after the Po_2 falls below approximately 60 mm Hg.[11] The hypercapnic ventilatory response, on the other hand, is linear between resting and elevated Pco_2 levels.[12] However, how individuals respond to a reduced Pco_2

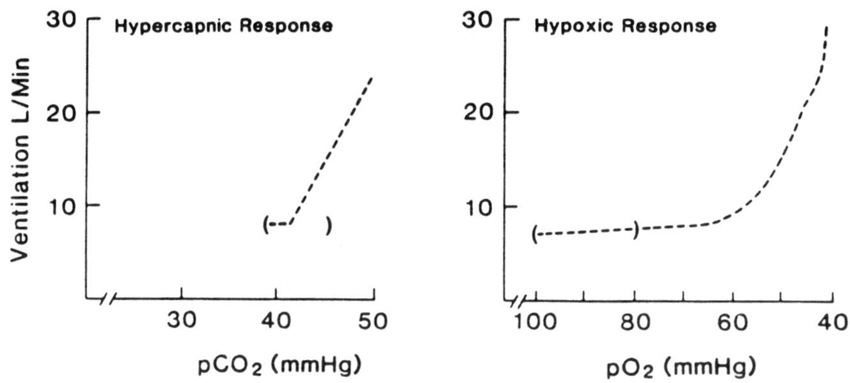

Figure 1. Schematic representation of normal hypercapnic and hypoxic ventilatory responses. Parentheses enclose normal ranges for Pco_2 and Po_2. (From: Clin Chest Med 1985;6 (4):626, with permission.)

(below normocapnic levels) is debatable and may be important during sleep as reduced Pco_2 levels are believed to inhibit ventilation.[17]

Although these chemoresponses clearly play a role in stimulating ventilation should hypoxia or hypercapnia develop, how important they are in maintaining eupneic ventilation is debatable. It seems clear that under normal conditions beat-to-beat and certainly breath-to-breath changes in extracellular fluid pH occur at the medullary chemoreceptor[18] and could influence respiratory center output within the eupneic range. In addition, the observation that reducing Pco_2 below the resting level inhibits ventilation[17] also suggests that Pco_2 may play an important role in maintaining ventilation in the unstimulated state. On the other hand, small changes in Po_2 within the normal range seem to have little effect on ventilation,[11] which suggests that carotid body output may not be essential in maintaining resting respiration. In addition, administering 100% O_2 or resecting the carotid sinus nerve[19] generally leads to little, if any, fall in ventilation, indicating little role for the carotid body in this control process.

Metabolism and Ventilation

Due to the fact that a close correlation between metabolic rate (particularly $\dot{V}co_2$) and ventilation has been observed under a number of conditions,[9,10] it has been postulated that CO_2 production or CO_2 delivery may independently influence respiration. This hypoth-

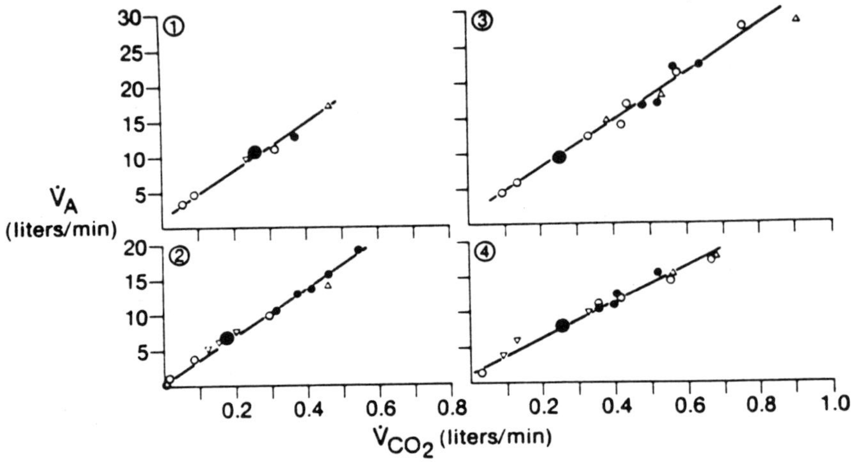

Figure 2. Response of alveolar ventilation ($\dot{V}A$) to changes in the rate of CO_2 production ($\dot{V}co_2$), induced by exercise alone (●); venous CO_2 loading or unloading alone (○); venous CO_2 unloading plus exercise (▽); venous CO_2 loading plus exercise (Δ). Large solid circle represents control value. Each panel represents a different sheep. (From: J Appl Physiol 1981;68:770, with permission.)

esis has centered around the observation that rising $\dot{V}co_2$ and alveolar ventilation are tightly linked during exercise (Fig. 2) at a time when no detectable change in arterial Po_2 or Pco_2 can be discerned.[9] In addition, removing metabolically produced CO_2 by extracorporeal means has been demonstrated to reduce ventilation to the point of apnea in awake sheep,[10] despite stable arterial chemistry. However, how $\dot{V}co_2$ or CO_2 delivery is detected physiologically remains obscure and is the subject of considerable debate. It would seem, therefore, that rising or falling metabolism can clearly affect ventilation. Whether this influence on respiration is primarily a product of changing $\dot{V}co_2$, a result of subtle changes in arterial Pco_2, or the product of yet to be defined CNS mechanisms remains unclear. However, changing metabolism clearly influences the level of ventilation, which may be important during sleep when metabolic rate falls.[20]

Intrapulmonary Receptors

A variety of receptors or reflexes that can influence ventilation and respiratory pattern have been identified in the airways and pulmonary parenchyma[21] and will be addressed here in a highly simplified manner. Although each can have a clear effect on breathing, their importance in man, particularly during eupneic ventilation, remains unclear. The reflex with which we are most familiar originates from the stretch receptor classically described by Hering and Breuer.[22] With rising lung inflation, inhibitory vagal afferent output increases, and this plays a role in terminating inspiration. The firing frequency from these receptors may also influence expiratory duration or TE. There are also irritant (rapidly adapting) receptors in the lung, which respond to endogenous chemicals, increasing lung inflation, exogenous irritants, and probably bronchoconstriction.[23,24] Finally pulmonary C fibers (previously called J receptors) have been identified that seem to respond to increasing pulmonary congestion and a variety of endogenous chemicals, yielding a rapid shallow pattern of ventilation.[25]

These intrapulmonary receptors are likely to play an important role in the regularization of respiratory pattern and tidal volume, particularly in animals.[21] In addition, under pathologic conditions such as asthma (bronchoconstriction), pulmonary congestion (heart failure), or inflammation (interstitial lung disease), the action of these receptors may influence respiration in a substantial way. However, recent studies in patients having undergone heart–lung transplantation and thus complete vagal denervation indicate that ventilatory volume and pattern are well controlled in the absence of intrapulmonary afferent input, at least under resting and exercise conditions.[26] This again suggests that at least in man intrapulmonary receptors probably play a relatively minor role in controlling ventilation.

The collective input from chemoreceptors and intrapulmonary receptors with some probable influence from metabolic sensors make up the principal autonomic controllers of respiration. It is beyond the scope of this chapter to address how the various afferent signals described above are integrated in the brain stem to yield a regular, rhythmic respiratory pattern with reasonably consistent tidal volume and ventilatory timing during wakefulness.[27] This is an exceedingly complex and poorly understood area and will not be addressed here. Suffice it to say that each afferent signal can independently influence ventilation, and collectively the output from these receptors probably is the primary stimulus to respiration. As a result, elimination of all afferent traffic is likely to yield apnea if behavioral influences (to be described below) are not present.[10,17,28]

Behavioral Influences on Respiration

Although commonly difficult to document, it is apparent that there are additional mechanisms to those described above that influence ventilation during wakefulness. These seem best categorized into two groups as originally outlined by Eliot Phillipson.[29] True "behavioral" influences on respiration relate to phonation, crying, or swallowing, which can clearly override autonomic control systems[30,31] and frequently lead to greater levels of ventilation than are strictly necessary to meet the metabolic demands of the body. On the other hand, the waking state seems to also exert a tonic stimulus to respiration over and above the previously described metabolic control mechanisms. This additional drive to breathe has been called the "wakefulness stimulus."[29]

Although the origin of this wakeful stimulus remains poorly understood, it has been hypothesized to result from either the activity of the descending reticular activating system[29,32–34] or be a product of tonic input from what are generally considered nonrespiratory sensors such as sight or hearing. Regardless of its source, it seems clear that ventilation will generally persist during wakefulness in man and animals even after near complete removal of metabolic stimulation,[28,35] particularly if behavioral events are occurring. These "wakeful" and "behavioral" stimuli to breathing, although poorly described, are likely important, particularly as we try to understand state or sleep influences on respiration.

Sleep and the Control of Ventilation

To grasp how respiration is likely to be affected by sleep, one must understand how sleep influences each of the mechanisms described above. Such effects on the respiratory controllers should explain how the sleeping state influences not only the quantity and timing of ventilation, but also the pattern or rhythmicity of respiration. However, before this can be accomplished, one must have some knowledge of sleep itself, particularly sleep staging as sleep is not a homogeneous state.

Sleep in man is currently organized using the system of Rechtschaffen and Kales[36], into four non-REM stages and REM sleep. This is accomplished by simultaneously recording the electroencephalogram (EEG), the electromyogram (EMG), and the electrooculogram (EOG). As a normal adult goes to sleep, he or she will systematically progress through the four non-REM sleep stages (numbered 1 to 4) with each representing a progressively "deeper" stage of sleep. Thus stages 1 and 2 represent fairly light sleep or the transition from wakefulness to sleep, while stages 3 and 4 (or slow-wave sleep) generally represent deeper, more stable sleep stages. This is generally followed by a period of REM sleep as originally described by Aserinsky and Kleitman[37], during which dreaming is common. It should be stated that REM sleep is also not a homogeneous state but is generally divided into "phasic" REM, during which eye movements are frequent, and "tonic" REM, when eye movements are rare or absent. This cycle of non-REM and REM sleep occurs repetitively during the night with a cycle length of approximately 90 minutes. As the night passes, the REM periods become longer and stage 3 and 4 sleep less common.

How respiratory control mechanisms are influenced by a particular sleep stage will determine the pattern and quantity of ventilation in that stage, which may be distinctly different from other stages. As the various non-REM sleep stages are more similar than different in terms of respiratory control, they will be grouped together in this discussion and only separated where distinct differences are apparent. REM sleep, which is consistently different from non-REM, will be addressed separately.

Sleep and Arterial Chemoresponses

Hypoxia

Although not carefully studied in man until the last 5–6 years, there are now convincing and fairly consistent data indicating that the ventilatory response to hypoxia is diminished during non-REM sleep[38–41] and probably further reduced during REM sleep[38,39,41] (Fig. 3). This observation differs from earlier studies that suggested a maintenance of hypoxic sensitivity during sleep.[42] In the earlier studies, however, current sleep staging techniques were not used (thus relying on behavioral criteria) and in a least one previous report, the Po_2 was not reduced to the level needed to adequately assess this response.[42] Despite these limitations, it was standard dogma until fairly recently that hypoxic sensitivity was well maintained during sleep.

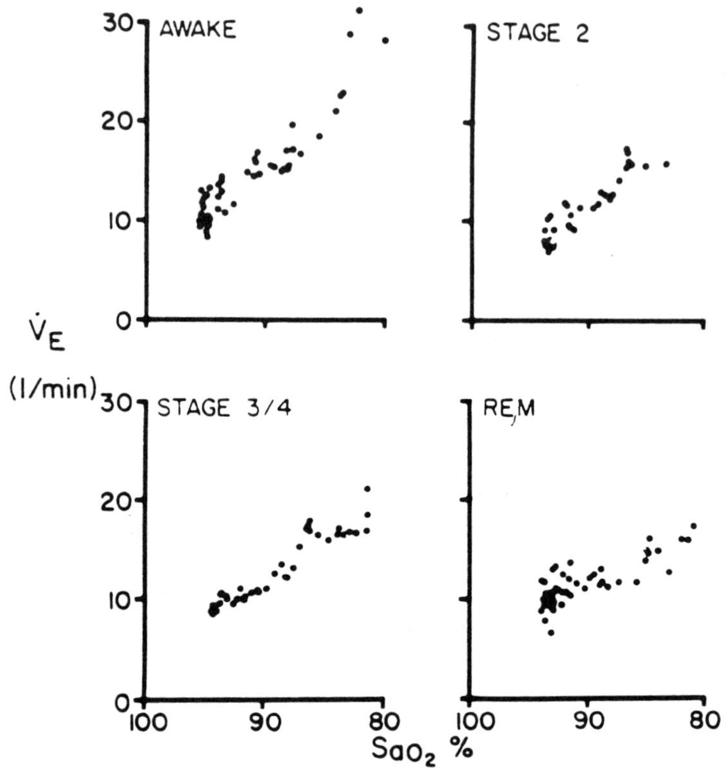

Figure 3. Representative hypoxic ventilatory response data showing decreased HVR during sleep, most marked during REM sleep (Sa_{O_2} = hemoglobin saturation; $\dot{V}_E$ = expired ventilation). (From: reference 39, with permission.)

Some discrepancies do exist in the current literature on this topic, with not all investigators finding a clear fall in this ventilatory response during sleep.[43] These differences probably relate first to variability in the gender of the subjects studied and second to whether isocapnia was maintained during hypoxia. Women seem to have a lower ventilatory response to hypoxia during wakefulness[41,44] and only a minimal fall in this response during non-REM sleep.[41] However, clear decrements in hypoxic sensitivity are evident in both males and females during REM sleep.[39,41] Thus, the mix of men and women could influence the results of non-REM studies. Second, failure to maintain isocapnia during hypoxic testing markedly blunts the response during both wakefulness and sleep, thus making differentiation between the two states difficult. One study in goats found clear differences in the hypoxic response between wakefulness and sleep when isocapnia was maintained and no difference when CO_2 was allowed to fall.[45] Thus one could conclude that the ventilatory response to isocapnic hypoxia is reduced about 30%–50% during non-REM sleep and 50%–75% during REM sleep with this decrement being more pronounced in men than women.

These observations should, however, be viewed with one potentially confounding variable in mind. The resistance to airflow in the upper airway increases during virtually all stages of sleep in almost all subjects studied.[46–48] As a result, a sleeping subject has a greater "work of breathing" prior to chemoresponse testing due to this partial upper airway collapse. As will be discussed later in this chapter, there is convincing evidence that sleep considerably reduces the ability to compensate for resistive loading.[49,50] As a result, the reduced ventilatory response to hypoxia (and hypercapnia as will be discussed below) could, in part, result from the high upper airway resistance present during sleep and not be totally a product of diminished chemosensitivity. In support of this concept is the observation that the occlusion pressure (P.1) response to hypercapnia (a purer measure of respiratory "drive") is well maintained during non-REM sleep despite diminished ventilatory responses.[51] Although never tested, one might assume this same principal applies to the hypoxic response. It therefore seems reasonable to conclude that the ability to respond to falling Po_2 is reduced during sleep, particularly REM sleep in man. Whether this is purely a product of falling chemosensitivity or results in part from elevated upper airway resistance remains unclear.

Animal data on the influence of sleep on the hypoxic response frequently differ from what is observed in man. For instance, Phillipson et al.[52] reported no change in the ventilatory response to hypoxia in either non-REM or REM sleep in tracheostomized dogs. However, Santiago et al.[45] noted a reduced response to isocapnic hypoxia in sleeping goats. Why such species differences exist is open to debate; however, in this chapter, comments will be confined to observations in man when adequate data are available.

Hypercapnia

There are two important variables in assessing the hypercapnic ventilatory response. First, the slope of the linear relationship between ventilation and Pco_2 is always reported. Second, the position of this curve (or response) may also be important as shifts in the response may allow higher or lower Pco_2 levels to occur without stimulating ventilation. Current studies suggest that both the slope and the position of the hypercapnic ventilatory response may be influenced by sleep.[2,3,53–55]

During non-REM sleep, a number of studies[2,3,53,54] indicate a substantial fall occurs in the slope of the hypercapnic ventilatory response (Fig. 4). Although the quantity of this decrement varies between studies, most report a 20%–50% reduction. This fall in the hypercapnic response induced by non-REM sleep, although commonly reported, has not always been observed, as several investigators report similar values during wakefulness and sleep.[40,56] However, most studies failing to observe a reduction in this response either obtained fairly small quantities of data[40] or produced only modest increments in Pco_2,[56] both of which may have influenced their results. The preponderance of data clearly indicate a fall in this response during non-REM sleep.

Data during REM sleep have proved more difficult to obtain, with only two investigators reporting substantial data.[53,55] In one, this response was clearly lower during REM sleep than during either wakefulness or non-REM sleep.[53] In the other, the response tended to be lowest during REM sleep but was not statistically lower than occurred in non-REM sleep.[55] It would seem, therefore, that the slope of the hypercapnic response falls during non-REM sleep but probably reaches its lowest level during REM sleep with similar results being obtained in both men and women.

How sleep influences the position of the hypercapnic ventilatory response is less clear and is probably a result of the poor methods currently available to define it. Using the intercept of the CO_2 response on the x or Pco_2 axis (generally called "B") seems inadequate as this value is clearly affected by both the slope and position of the curve. Despite this limitation, several investigators have observed non-REM sleep to shift the hypercapnic response to the right whether or not slope changes were observed.[57,58] In addition, at least one study,[53] although failing to observe a change in the intercept, clearly observed a shift in the position of the CO_2 response line away from the resting ventilation set point (Fig. 5), suggesting that greater increments in Pco_2 would be needed to stimulate ventilation during non-REM sleep than are commonly observed during wakefulness. Data during REM sleep are too sparse and variable to clearly define the position of this

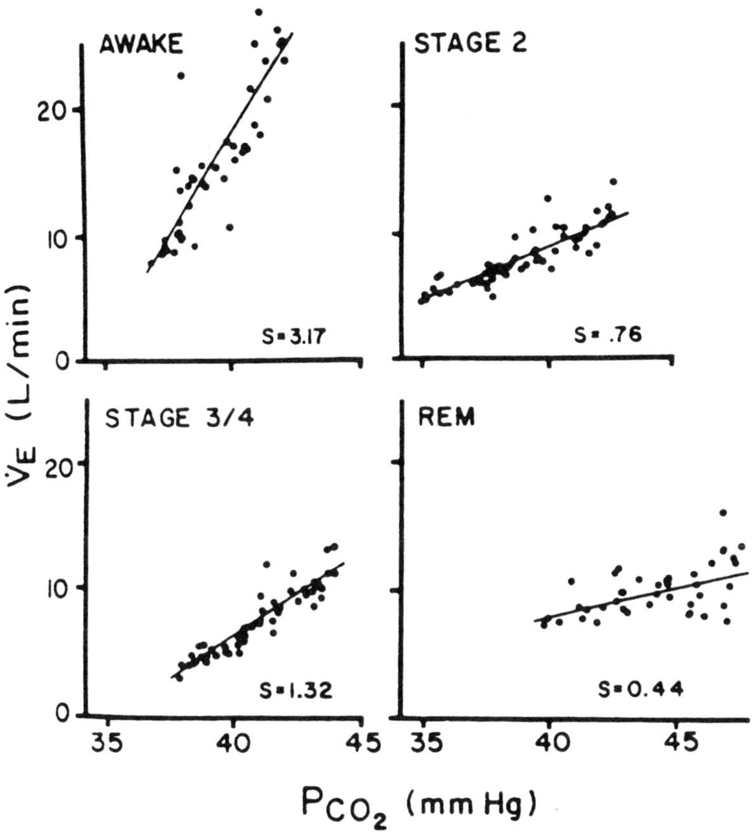

Figure 4. Representative hypercapnic ventilatory response data showing decreased hypercapnic ventilatory response in sleep most marked during REM sleep. (From: reference 53, with permission.)

response, making shifts difficult to discern. It would seem, therefore, that sleep induces some shift in the CO_2 response curve to the right or to higher Pco_2 values. Whether the position of this response differs between sleep stages remains unresolved.

The importance of Pco_2 as a stimulus to ventilation during sleep cannot be overestimated. Both recent[17] and older studies[59] indicate the presence of a hypocapnic "apnea threshold" during sleep that is likely absent during wakefulness. This apnea threshold is the Pco_2 level at or below which ventilation ceases and an apnea ensues. Each individual seems to have a consistent apnea threshold during non-REM sleep that is remarkably close to the waking P_{CO_2} level.[59] As will be discussed later in the chapter, P_{CO_2} generally rises about 2–6 mm Hg when an individual goes to sleep. Simply reducing this sleeping P_{CO_2} by passive hyperventilation back to the waking level or slightly below it will lead to an apnea in that individual (Fig. 6). Thus P_{CO_2} may be critically important in the maintenance of rhythmic ventilation during sleep. During wakefulness, apnea following hyperventilation (whether active or passive) is highly inconsistent,[60,61] again suggesting that behavioral or "wakeful" stimuli importantly influence

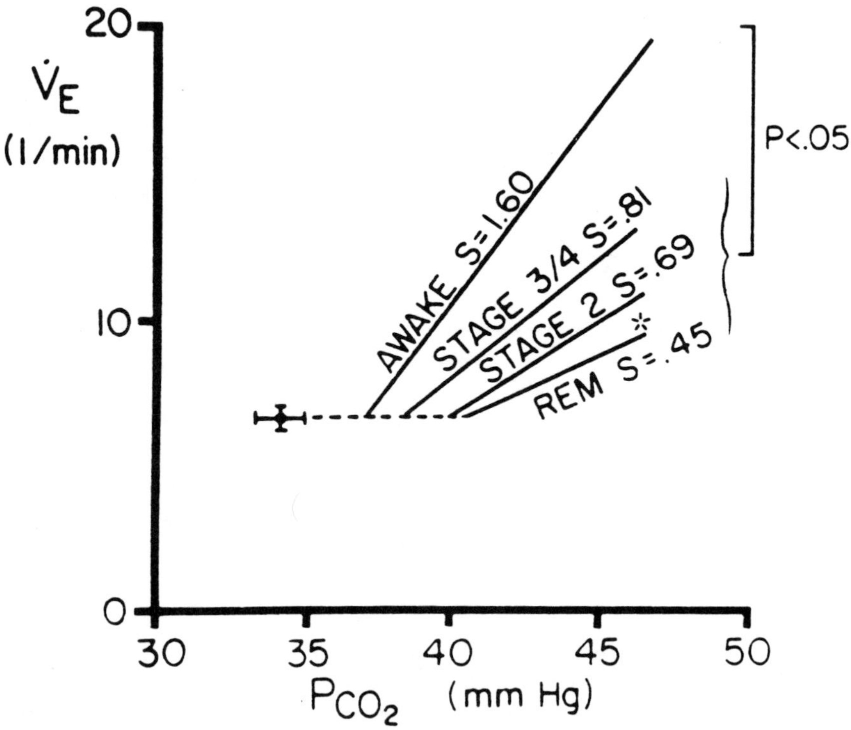

Figure 5. Mean minute ventilation/$P_{ET}CO_2$ relationship for all 12 subjects indicating the mean ± SEM resting minute ventilation/CO_2 point in the awake state. The hypercapnic ventilatory response is reduced in stage 2 and stage 3/4 compared with that in wakefulness and is further decreased in REM sleep. $\dot{V}_E$ = expired ventilation; *$P < 0.05$ REM different from stage 2 and 3/4 sleep. (From: reference 53, with permission.)

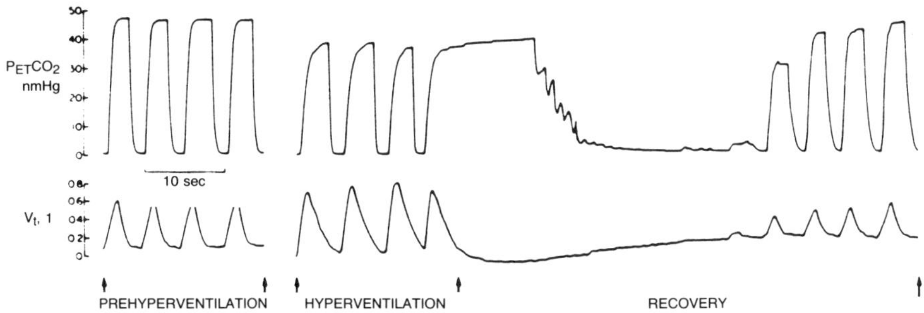

Figure 6. Posthyperventilation apnea following 3 minutes of passive, positive pressure hyperventilation during hyperoxic non-REM sleep. O_2 saturation was 100% in prehyperventilation, hyperventilation, and recovery periods. (From: J Appl Physiol 1983;55:816, with permission.)

respiration during wakefulness even when metabolic stimuli are abolished.

Metabolic Rate and Ventilation During Sleep

As stated previously, during wakefulness the level of ventilation is tightly linked to metabolic rate, particularly $\dot{V}CO_2$. If the metabolic rate changes during sleep, this could have clear effects on ventilation. The influence of sleep on metabolic rate has been the subject of considerable investigation, with the majority of studies indicating a clear decrement in $\dot{V}O_2$ and $\dot{V}CO_2$ during sleep.[62–64] Whether metabolism is higher during REM than non-REM sleep varies, with proponents on both sides.[62,63] However, all sleeping states seem to yield a lower metabolic rate than wakefulness. Time of night also appears to have some effect on sleeping $\dot{V}O_2$ and $\dot{V}CO_2$, with levels falling fairly promptly following sleep onset and continuing to drop slowly through the night[62] until about 4–5 AM when levels rise slowly until arousal (Fig. 7).

Ventilation tends to follow metabolic rate changes during sleep.[62] As shown in Figure 8 (from the only study to my knowledge addressing this issue) the correlation between expired ventilation and $\dot{V}CO_2$ was quite close during all phases of sleep. It would seem, therefore, that the falling metabolism encountered during sleep is at least in part responsible for the simultaneously encountered

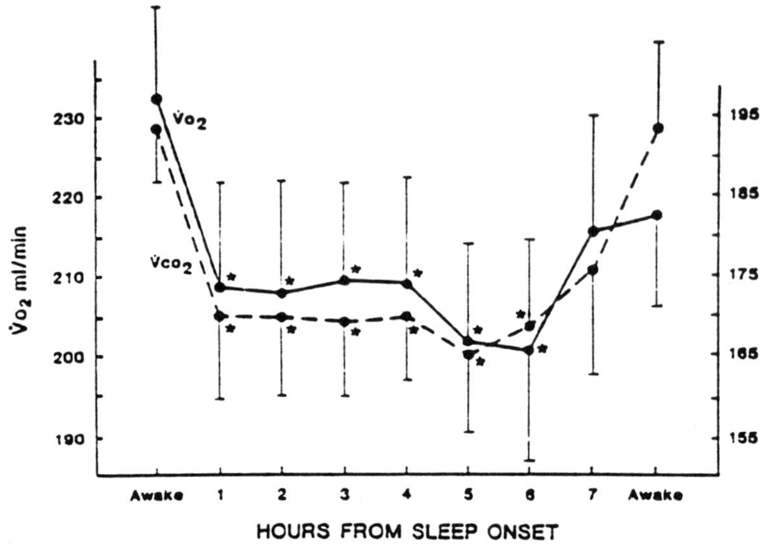

Figure 7. Effect of time (hours from sleep onset) on O_2 consumption ($\dot{V}O_2$) and CO_2 production ($\dot{V}CO_2$) is shown. $\dot{V}O_2$ and $\dot{V}CO_2$ decreased rapidly after sleep onset, remained fairly constant through the night, and began to rise toward morning. **P*< 0.05 different from mean awake value (analysis of variance). (From: reference 62, with permission.)

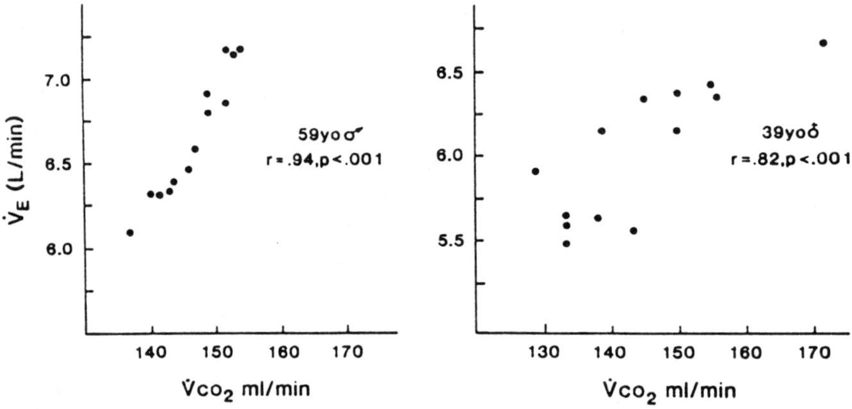

Figure 8. Correlation between ventilation ($\dot{V}_E$) and CO_2 production ($\dot{V}CO_2$) during sleep in two individuals is shown. Points are mean values for a single recording period (3–25 minutes) in that individual. All stages of sleep are included for each subject. Ventilation correlates closely with $\dot{V}CO_2$ during sleep. (From: reference 62, with permission.)

decrement in ventilation that will be addressed at length later. However, falling CO_2 production cannot be the total explanation for decrements in ventilation during sleep as P_{CO_2} rises during the night,[1–3,54] indicating greater falls in alveolar ventilation than $\dot{V}_{CO_2}$. Possible explanations for the discrepancy will be addressed later in the chapter.

Sleep and Intrapulmonary Receptors

Minimal information is currently available in man regarding the influence of sleep on intrapulmonary receptor mechanisms. An exception, however, are studies of cough or irritant receptors. During wakefulness the instillation of irritants into the airway generally leads to cough, assumedly through irritant receptor mechanisms. Studies in both normal men[65] and individuals with chronic bronchitis and emphysema[66] indicate that this cough reflex is suppressed during sleep and that frequently arousal is needed for coughing to occur. This suggests a down-regulation of this reflex during sleep. Similar observations have been made in animals.

On the other hand, a variety of studies in animals suggest that pulmonary stretch reflexes remain active during sleep, particularly non-REM sleep. In both opossums[67] and dogs,[68] sustained lung inflation can lead to apnea during slow-wave sleep, indicating intact reflexes. The data for REM sleep are less clear, but suggest that the reflex is intact and active during tonic REM sleep.[69] Studies of complete vagal afferent blockade on unstimulated respiration during sleep in animals have also been completed using either vagal cooling or vagotomy. Vagal blockade[70,71] generally leads to a slowing of respiratory rate with larger tidal volume during non-REM or slow-wave sleep (Fig. 9). During REM sleep[71] this response is somewhat variable but is likely still present (Fig. 9). These studies suggest that in animals intrapulmonary reflexes continue to be active during sleep and are an important influence on respiratory pattern. An exception to this may be irritant receptors, which are clearly less active during sleep.[68] In addition, phasic REM sleep seems to be a state during which respiration is minimally influenced by standard metabolic stimuli.[69] Whether these same principals apply to man is debatable as intrapulmonary reflexes generally have less influence on respiration in humans than animals.

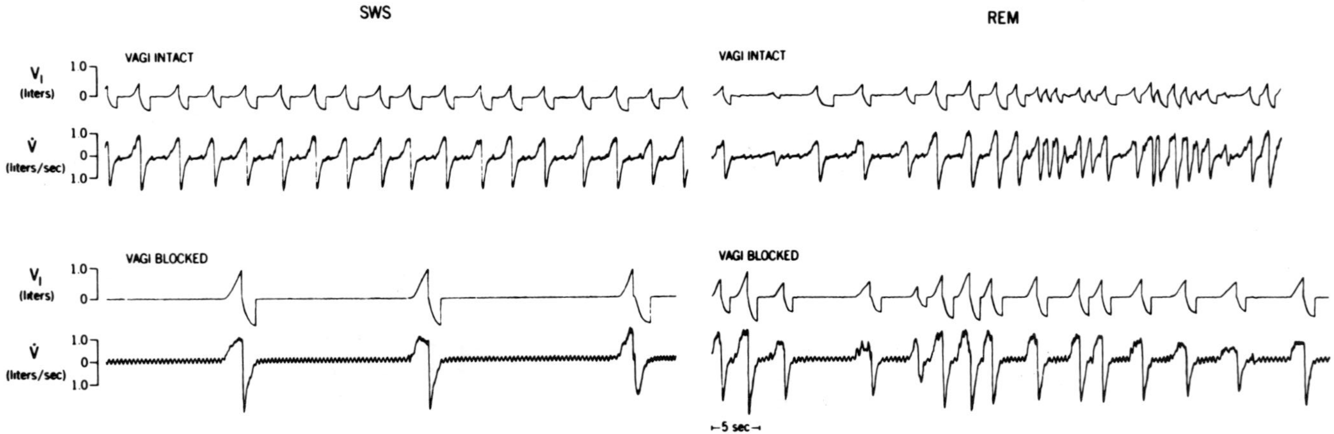

Figure 9. Recorder tracings in sleeping dog demonstrating effects of cervical blockade on pattern of breathing in slow-wave (SWS) and REM sleep V_I, inspired tidal volume (above zero line); $\dot{V}$, rate of airflow (inspiration upwards). Note vagal blockade failed to abolish irregularity of breathing pattern during REM sleep. (From: reference 70, with permission.)

Sleep: Loss of the "Wakefulness" Stimulus and Behavioral Influences on Respiration

Although the wakefulness stimulus to respiration remains a somewhat vague concept, it seems clear that the reticular activating system (the primary source of arousal) can influence respiration.[32–34] Animal studies, primarily in the cat, indicate that electrical stimulation of the brain-stem reticular formation has clear effects on respiration, generally an increase in phrenic nerve activity, which occurs independently of the afferent mechanisms discussed above.[32–34] It thus seems likely that the state of wakefulness or arousal can influence respiration, probably through reticular formation mechanisms. Thus loss of this tonic stimulus, as is likely to occur during sleep, may lead to a reduced drive to breath and a quantitative fall in ventilation.

Behavioral influences on respiration also appear to be markedly reduced or absent during sleep, particularly non-REM sleep. Clearly phonation, laughing, or crying, events that may override normal metabolic control mechanisms during wakefulness, are absent during sleep. Ventilation during non-REM sleep therefore becomes nearly totally dependent on metabolic control mechanisms as both the tonic influence of the wakefulness stimulus (reticular systems) and intermittent effects of behavioral events are abolished.[29] Thus cortical and reticular influences on breathing during non-REM sleep are absent.

During REM sleep, this situation changes. Studies described above indicate that chemoreceptor responses (hypoxia and hypercapnia) reach their lowest level during REM sleep[38,39,41,53] at a time when intrapulmonary receptors seem to have little effect on respiration.[69] As a result, metabolic control mechanisms seem to have little influence on respiration during REM sleep. This is particularly true of phasic REM sleep when standard autonomic stimuli have minimal, if any, effect on ventilation.[69] Control mechanisms during tonic REM sleep may be closer to those observed during non-REM sleep, although data in the two REM states are incomplete.

It would seem, therefore, that three clear states are emerging: wakefulness, non-REM, and REM sleep. During wakefulness metabolic control systems are clearly important in the maintenance of ventilation. However, these control mechanisms are frequently superseded by wakeful or behavioral events. During non-REM sleep, when all behavioral and wakeful stimuli are abolished, respiration becomes strictly controlled by metabolic mechanisms. These autonomic control systems may be down-regulated during non-REM sleep, which is certainly the case for the chemoresponses, but the preeminence of these mechanisms in controlling ventilation in this particular state seems clear. During REM sleep neither wakeful stimuli nor metabolic control systems are of apparent importance in respiratory events. What controls ventilation during REM sleep, particularly phasic REM sleep, is unclear. However, the irregular pattern of breathing that is characteristic of this state has led to the postulate that behavioral mechanisms have reemerged as important controls of respiration.[29] In support of this hypothesis is the observation that respiratory neurons during REM sleep have a firing frequency that relates more directly to nonrespiratory neural events such as PGO (pontine-geniculo-occipital) waves, than to standard respiratory stimuli.[72]

In support of this basic outline of sleep influences on respiratory control mechanisms is a series of protocols in dogs conducted by Phillipson, Sullivan, and colleagues.[69,70,73] These studies demonstrated that ventilation during non-REM sleep could be markedly diminished if all afferent stimuli were abolished. This was accomplished by combining vagal cooling (intrapulmonary receptors) plus metabolic alkalosis (CO_2 response) and hyperoxia (O_2 response). As shown in Figure 10, under these conditions, there was a marked slowing of ventilation with frank respiratory pauses, which strongly supports the importance of autonomic control systems during non-REM sleep. In contrast, during REM sleep neither vagal blockade (Fig. 9) nor CO_2 rebreathing (Fig. 11) could regularize or particularly stimulate ventilation.[69,70,73] Breathing during REM sleep therefore seems to proceed rather independently of these control systems.

Normal Ventilation during Sleep

Quantitative Changes from Wakefulness to Non-REM Sleep

Considerable data have accumulated over the last 5–10 years regarding sleep influences on quantitative measures of ventilation in normals.[1,2,17,46,54,74] In assessing these data, one must realize that "normals" are often difficult to define and that the apparatus needed to measure respiration can significantly influence the variables being

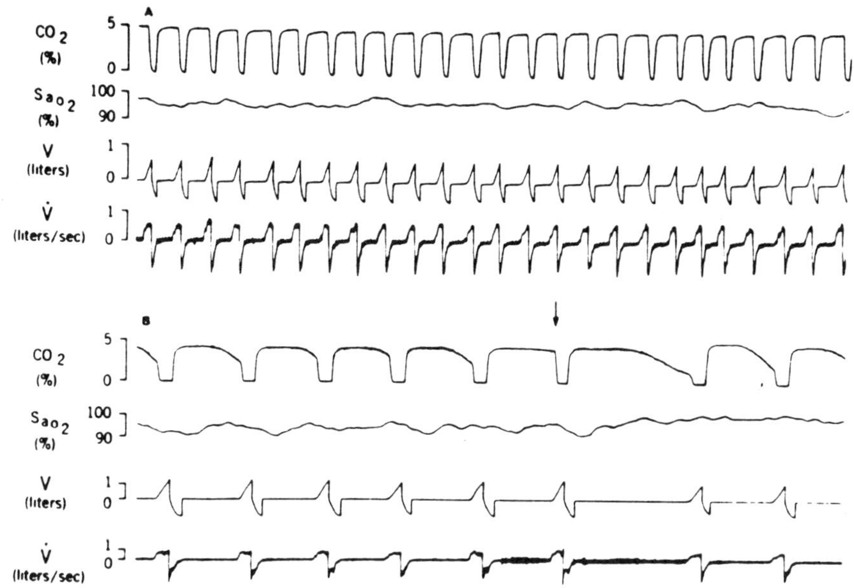

Figure 10. Recorder tracing from dog 1 showing typical examples of breathing pattern during slow wave sleep (SWS) with vagi intact (A), and with vagi cold-blocked (B). CO_2, concentration of CO_2 in tracheal gas; Sa_{O_2}, arterial oxygen saturation measured with an ear oximeter; V, inspired volume (expired volume, below zero line); V̇, airflow rate (inspiration upward); note the change in gain with both V and V̇ during vagal block. At arrow the dog inhaled one breath of 100% O_2. (From: reference 73, with permission.)

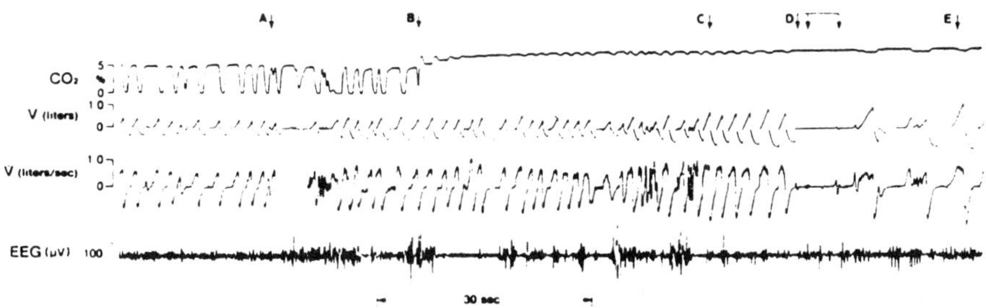

Figure 11. Recorder tracing in sleeping dog showing persistance of irregular pattern of breathing during REM sleep despite progressive hypercapnia. CO_2, concentration of CO_2 in tracheal gas; V, inspired volume (above zero line); V̇ rate of airflow (inspiration upwards); EEG, electroencephalogram. A, onset of phasic rapid-eye-movement sleep; B, onset of CO_2 rebreathing; C, cessation of generalized muscular twitching; D, dog swallowing; E, arousal. (From: reference 69, with permission.)

assessed.[75] With these limitations in mind, it seems clear that ventilation falls in the transition from wakefulness to non-REM sleep. A variety of investigators, using current sleep-staging techniques, have demonstrated a consist, reproducible fall in minute ventilation from wakefulness to stable non-REM sleep.[1,2,17,46,54,74] Although, as stated previously, non-REM sleep is not a completely homogeneous state, the majority of these studies were completed in stage 2 or stage 3–4 sleep with no clear ventilatory differences between these stages being evident. How great a decrement in ventilation was encountered varied somewhat between studies, but was generally 0.5–1.5 L/min.

The change in respiratory pattern responsible for this decrement in ventilation is less clear. The majority of studies indicate that a reduced tidal volume occurs during non-REM sleep[1,2,17,46,54] and is the cause of falling minute ventilation, although this has not always been observed.[74] The frequency response to non-REM sleep is highly variable from one study to the next with some reporting clear decrements[54,74] in respiratory rate and others modest increases.[1,2,17,46] This variability is likely a product of multiple factors such as stability and depth of the sleep state, type of monitoring equipment used to measure ventilation (face mask versus inductive plethysmography), and individual variability in adaptation to this equipment during wakefulness. Despite these limitations, it seems clear that minute ventilation falls from wakefulness to stable non-REM sleep and that this decrement is primarily a product of falling tidal volume.

As one might expect, this fall in ventilation is associated with changes in arterial blood gas tensions. As published reports vary somewhat in how much ventilation falls during sleep, the magnitude of the influence of sleep on Pco_2 and Po_2 also varies. Most studies report a rise in Pco_2 of 2–7 mm Hg[1–3,51,53,54] and a fall in Po_2 of 3–10 mm Hg.[13,76] These are modest changes and are what might be expected from the previously described fall in minute ventilation.

The events responsible for this decrement in ventilation during sleep are not completely understood, which likely reflects the importance of multiple etiologic factors. As stated previously, both $\dot{V}o_2$ and $\dot{V}co_2$ fall during sleep,[62–64] which may in part explain the observed reduction in sleeping ventilation. However, falling $\dot{V}co_2$ cannot totally account for these sleep-induced respiratory changes as Pco_2 rises during the night.[1–3,51,53,54] Thus alveolar ventilation is falling more than metabolic rate. Three mechanisms likely interact in producing this disproportionate reduction in ventilation.

First, the "wakefulness" stimulus is lost with sleep onset. Although poorly understood, the brain-stem reticular formation probably exerts a tonic influence on respiration[32–34] over and above standard metabolic control mechanisms. With the loss of this stimulus, ventilation is likely to fall. Second, the chemoresponses are reduced during non-REM sleep,[38–41,53,54] not only in terms of the slope of these responses, but also, in the case of the CO_2 stimulus, there is a shift in the position of the response. This likely indicates a down-regulation of central respiratory control mechanisms such that higher Pco_2 levels are tolerated without an increment in respiratory muscle stimulation. Thus Pco_2 rises. Finally, a multitude of studies indicate that airway resistance increases as an individual moves from wakefulness to non-REM sleep.[46–48] This seems to be a product of a sleep-induced fall in the activity of the pharyngeal dilator muscles with partial pharyngeal collapse. There is also fairly convincing evidence, as stated above, that normal men have a reduced ability to compensate for flow resistive loads during sleep.[49,50] Thus rising pharyngeal resistance during sleep with an associated inability to completely compensate for this load may lead to hypoventilation.

These three sleep-induced events (loss of the wakefulness stimulus, reduced chemoresponsiveness, and elevated pharyngeal resistance) alone or in combination seem likely to explain the previously described fall in ventilation noted with the loss of wakefulness. The relative importance of each probably varies from one individual to the next with the severity of nocturnal hypoventilation likely reflecting the magnitude of the sleep influence on each control mechanism.

REM Sleep

Fewer data are currently available regarding the influence of REM sleep on quantitative measures of respiration due to the relatively short duration of this stage of sleep and the fact that the instrumentation needed to monitor respiration frequently disrupts sleep, thereby precluding sustained periods of REM sleep. Despite these limitations, at least five investigators have quantitated respiration during REM sleep, and each reports at least some fall in minute ventilation when compared to wakefulness.[1,46,74,77,78] This decrement varies from nominally detectable to about 1.6 L/min, depending on the study.

Whether ventilation during REM sleep differs from that encountered during non-REM sleep is less clear. Various investigators find

REM ventilation to be less than,[1] the same,[46,77] or greater than[74,78] that encountered during non-REM sleep. This discrepancy probably relates primarily to the heterogeneity of REM sleep. As stated previously, REM sleep is currently divided into phasic REM, during which eye movements are frequent, and tonic REM, when such eye movements are absent. Recent investigation indicates that eye movements are associated with the inhibition of ventilation with a fairly close negative correlation existing between the frequency of eye movements and minute ventilation.[79] Thus the previously described variability in measures of ventilation during REM sleep may reflect the type of REM sleep present when ventilation was quantitated. It would seem, therefore, that ventilation during REM sleep is probably similar quantitatively to that encountered during non-REM although quite a bit more variable depending on the presence or absence of eye movements.

The influence of REM sleep on tidal volume and frequency is even more controversial than was described above for non-REM sleep. Most studies report a fall in tidal volume during REM sleep when compared to wakefulness.[1,46,77] However the data regarding respiratory frequency during REM sleep are highly variable with no clear consensus emerging. These discrepancies likely reflect the differences between tonic and phasic REM sleep. Blood gas changes during REM sleep in normals are probably similar to those encountered during non-REM sleep, although erratic ventilation with frequent small tidal volumes makes accurate end-tidal gas determinations hard to obtain. Thus meaningful conclusions are difficult to reach.

The explanations for the fall in ventilation during REM sleep when compared to wakefulness are probably similar to those previously described during non-REM sleep. Loss of the wakefulness stimulus, falling metabolic rate, very reduced chemoresponsiveness, and elevated upper airway resistance all seem likely to contribute. However, the mechanism by which rapid eye movements are associated with transient inhibition of respiratory muscle activity is unclear. Animal data indicate that eye movements during phasic REM sleep are temporally associated with either inhibition or excitation of the diaphragmatic EMG.[80] Similar events seem likely in man, although inhibition seems to be the predominant influence of such eye movements. Why this occurs either teleologically or functionally remains obscure. Finally, ventilation during REM sleep, as stated previously, seems to be much less influenced by metabolic events than occurs at any other time, which may help explain the erratic respiration characteristic of this state.

Sleep-induced Changes in Respiratory Rhythmicity

Non-REM Sleep

Ventilatory pattern or rhythmicity during wakefulness is frequently difficult to assess due to behavioral influences on respiration. Talking, excitement, swallowing, etc., can interrupt or stimulate ventilation. However, in the quiet, unstimulated state, most investigators believe respiration to be reasonably regular during wakefulness with a recurring tidal volume and stable frequency. However, this commonly changes during sleep.

In the transition from wakefulness to sleep ventilation frequently oscillates (Fig. 12) with tidal volume rhythmically waxing and waning between large breaths and small.[2–5,57,81] Depending on the amplitude of this oscillation, frank apneas may occur at the nadir of the cycle. This ventilatory pattern frequently resembles Cheyne-Stokes breathing. This irregular respiratory pattern does not occur in all subjects, but is a common occurrence at sleep onset.

The explanation for this oscillating ventilatory pattern at sleep onset probably relates to the instability of sleep in the early transition between wakefulness and sleep (stage 1) and the shift in respiratory control mechanisms that occurs with loss of arousal. With the transition from wakefulness to stage 1 sleep, the wakefulness stimulus is lost and the chemoresponses are down-regulated as discussed previously. Thus ventilation falls rapidly and P_{CO_2} rises. If sleep persists at this time, ventilation is likely to stabilize without oscillation. More commonly, however, a transient arousal occurs or at least an increase in alpha activity on the EEG can be detected, indicating a lightening of sleep. The individual therefore shifts back to wakeful control mechanisms that stimulate ventilation and lead to a series of large breaths.[31] As a result ventilation waxes and wanes between transient hyperpnea with arousal and hypopnea or apnea with the onset of sleep. Such waxing and waning of ventilation is likely to persist until stable sleep is achieved, usually stage 2, 3, or 4.

At this juncture, during stable non-REM sleep, ventilation reverts to metabolic control mechanisms and the respiratory pattern

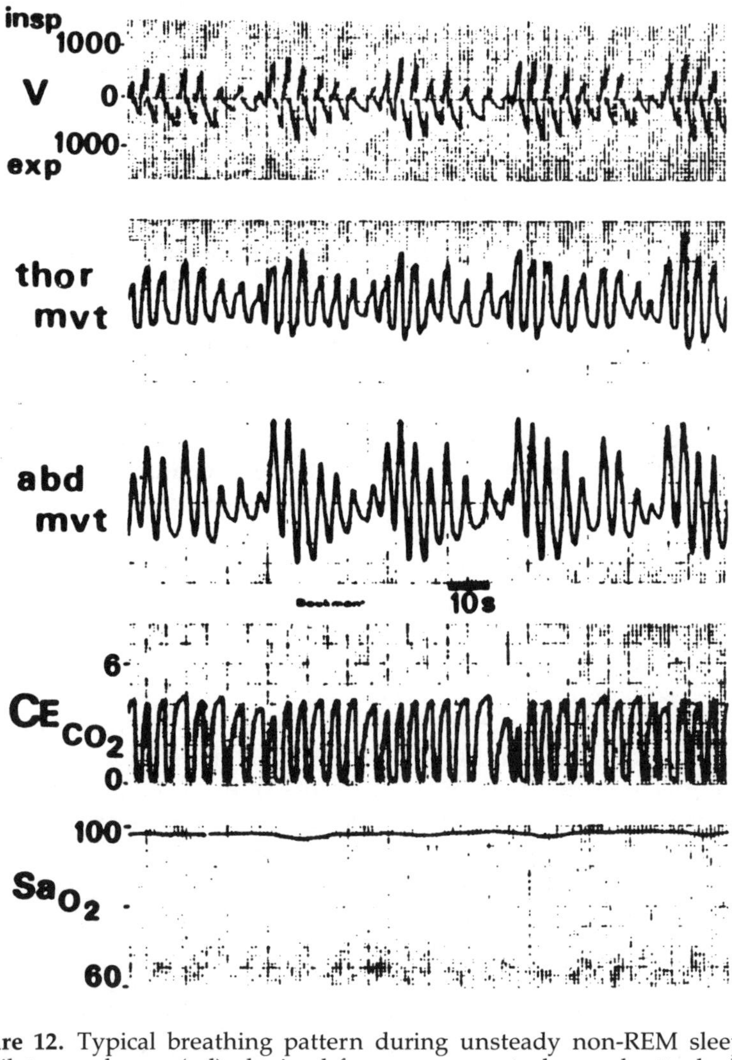

Figure 12. Typical breathing pattern during unsteady non-REM sleep. V, ventilatory volumes (ml) obtained from a pneumotachograph attached to a face mask; insp, inspiration; exp, expiration; thor mvt, abd mvt, thoracic and abdominal movements; CE_{CO_2}, CO_2 concentration (percent) in the face mask; SA_{O_2}, oxygen saturation (percent). (From: Clin Chest Med 1985;6:578, with permission.)

generally becomes exceedingly rhythmic (Fig. 13). As long as the sleep stage is stable and behavioral events are virtually abolished, there is nothing to disrupt this regular pattern with repetitive breaths of similar amplitude and frequency.

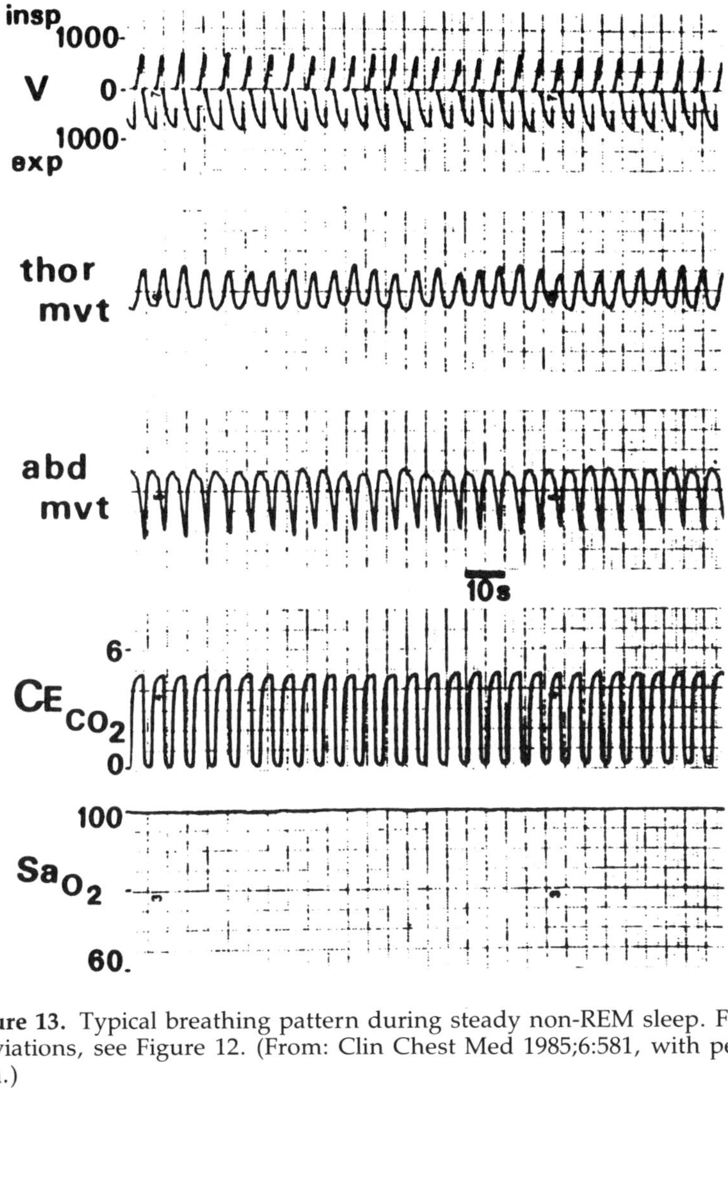

Figure 13. Typical breathing pattern during steady non-REM sleep. For abbreviations, see Figure 12. (From: Clin Chest Med 1985;6:581, with permission.)

REM Sleep

The pattern of respiration during REM sleep, as stated previously, is exceedingly irregular, particularly during phasic REM (Fig. 14). This irregular ventilation does not appear to be random but is related to the eye movements associated with this sleep stage.[79] Dur-

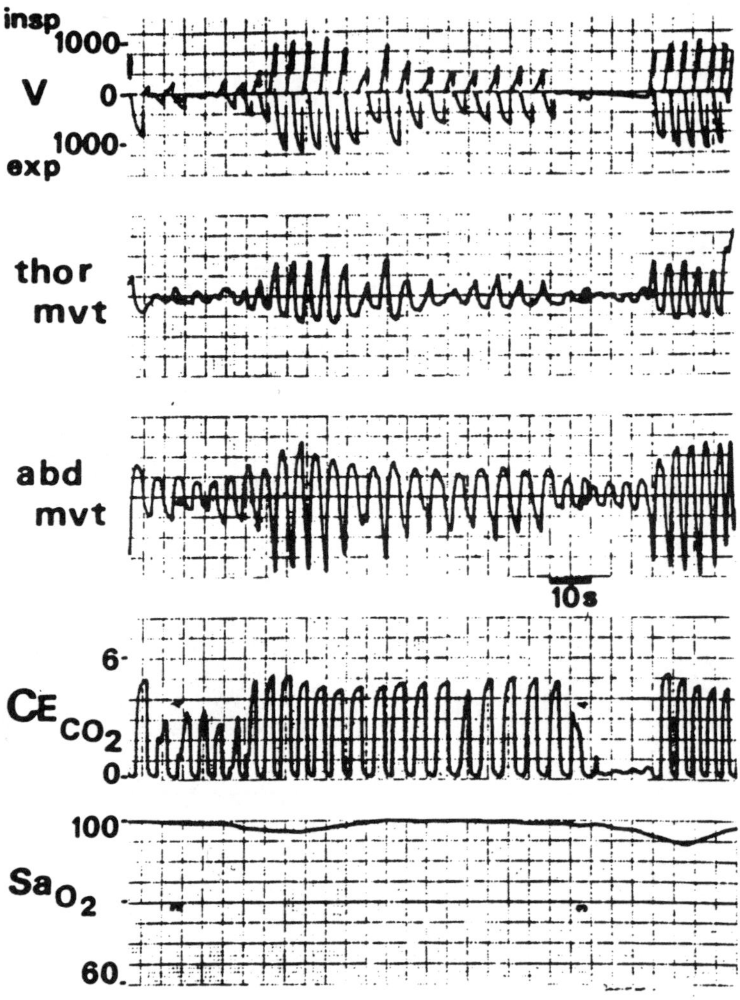

Figure 14. Typical breathing pattern during REM sleep. For abbreviations, see Figure 12. (From: Clin Chest Med 1985;6:584, with permission.)

ing actual rapid eye movements, diaphagmatic activity is commonly inhibited leading to small breaths.[80,82] When these eye movements are absent, ventilation increases, probably to recover from the previous period of hypoventilation or apnea. As a result respiration may be regular during periods of tonic REM sleep when eye movements are absent or chaotic during phasic REM when eye movements are frequent. Why eye movements are temporally associated with changes in respiratory muscle activity and thus ventilatory pattern is unclear. It seems that a variety of neurologic events such as eye movements, PGO waves, and muscle inhibition are part of REM sleep. Further investigation will be necessary before we understand both the importance of REM sleep and the mechanisms producing it.

As stated previously, metabolic control mechanisms seem to have little influence on respiratory pattern during phasic REM sleep. However, quantitative measures of ventilation during REM sleep are quite similar to those encountered during non-REM sleep. Thus the respiratory needs of the body are likely being met, if not transiently during eye movements, at least over more sustained periods of REM sleep.

Ventilatory Protection during Sleep

As addressed at the beginning of this chapter, ventilation and arterial blood gas homeostasis are carefully protected during wakefulness despite large changes in metabolic rate, inspired oxygen concentration, and the work of breathing. As should now be clear, this ability to protect ventilation changes considerably with the onset of sleep. Chemoresponses, as outlined, are considerably reduced during non-REM sleep and fall further during REM sleep.[38,39,41,53,55] Thus protection against changes in inspired O_2 or rising Pco_2 are diminished.

Current data also suggest that man's ability to compensate for increased work of breathing is diminished during sleep.[49,50] This has been tested primarily by the addition of resistive loads to inspiration during sleep while monitoring changes in ventilation. Several studies[49,50] indicate a large initial fall in ventilation occurs following the application of inspiratory loads during non-REM sleep (Fig. 15). Over time there is some recovery,[49] but minute ventilation never reaches preload levels, at least over the time period studied. This differs considerably from what has been observed during wakefulness when ventilation is well maintained despite the addition of large inspiratory resistors.[49] As the mechanisms necessary for load compensation dur-

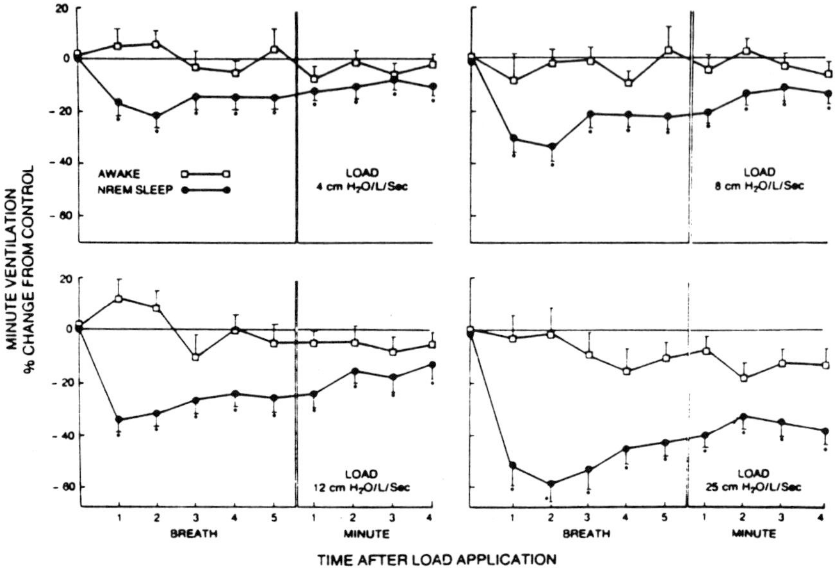

Figure 15. Mean (±SE) values for all subjects for minute ventilation expressed as percent change from control over the first five consecutive breaths and minutes 1–4 after application of each resistive load during wakefulness and non-REM (NREM) sleep. Note that minute ventilation was well maintained after resistive load application during wakefulness but decreased significantly from control values at all points after resistive load application during non-REM sleep. *$P < 0.05$ different from control. (From: reference 50, with permission.)

ing wakefulness are poorly understood, how sleep influences these mechanisms is even less well known. However, it does seem that suprapontine events may be important in load compensation as arousal or wakefulness is necessary for such compensation to occur.[49,50,83]

Thus it would seem that ventilation is more fragile or less well protected during sleep. As a result, any change in arterial blood gases or the work of breathing could lead to problems during sleep while compensation for such events might well be adequate during wakefulness.

Pathologic Nocturnal Hypoventilation

From what has been described above, it should be clear that virtually everyone hypoventilates to some extent during sleep and that this fall in ventilation is associated with a modest rise in PCO_2 and fall in PO_2. However, for a variety of reasons some individuals hypoventilate more than might be considered "normal," and this can lead to larger increments in PCO_2 and often important decrements in PO_2. Although there are likely to be many reasons for nocturnal hypoventilation, the majority will fall into one of three groups: (1) increased work of breathing, (2) diminished respiratory muscle strength, and (3) abnormal control of breathing mechanisms.

Nocturnal Hypoventilation Secondary to Increased Work of Breathing

Virtually any disease process that adversely affects the respiratory airways (upper or lower), the lung parenchyma, or the chest wall can lead to either increased airflow resistance or decreased lung compliance, both of which increase the work of breathing. As was stated above, a variety of compensatory mechanisms are active during wakefulness to prevent hypoventilation under these circumstances. However, during sleep these mechanisms are often less effective, which can lead to inadequate levels of ventilation.

Increased Upper Airway Resistance

As will be described in detail elsewhere in this book, upper airway resistance increases during sleep in virtually all groups studied.[46–48] This "normal" increment in pharyngeal resistance may in part be responsible for the decrement in ventilation seen during sleep in the general population. However, in some individuals, the sleep-induced rise in pharyngeal resistance is quite large and can lead to considerable hypoventilation.

If we consider the results of studies by Hudgel et al.[46] and Wiegand et al.[48] as representative of the normal rise in supraglottic resistance during sleep, then upper airway resistance in normal men probably climbs from a mean of about 3–4 cm H_2O/L/s during wakefulness to a mean of 8–12 cm H_2O/L/s during non-REM sleep. Several groups have been identified in whom higher pharyngeal resistance is encountered during sleep. The most common and prominent such group is snorers.[47] Snoring probably results from vibration of the soft palate, uvula, and other pharyngeal tissue but also indicates a somewhat compromised pharyngeal airway during sleep. Studies by Skatrud and Dempsey[47] reported a maximum total pulmonary resistance of 57.8 ± 21.9 cm H_2O/L/s during non-REM sleep in snorers and a value of only 10.2 ± 2.0 cm H_2O/L/s in nonsnorers.[47] This was associated with a greater sleep-induced fall in tidal volume in snorers than nonsnorers. Other reports also suggest snorers hypoventilate more during sleep than do nonsnorers.[51,84] As a result high pharyngeal resistance leads to a reduction in ventilation during sleep, probably in a similar manner to the hypoventilation described above following the addition of an external inspiratory resistive load.

There are probably other groups in whom pharyngeal resistance is high during sleep. Sleep apnea patients obviously have complete pharyngeal occlusion during sleep, which leads to recurrent apnea and subsequent arousal.[85] As ventilation is commonly cycling between apnea and hyperpnea in these individuals, it is difficult to determine the effect of sleep on stable ventilation. Other individuals exhibit a syndrome quite similar to obstructive sleep apnea, but never actually completely occlude the upper airway during sleep. This has been called, by one group of investigators,[86] the "sleep hypopnea syndrome." These individuals have cycling hypopneas probably associated with very high upper airway resistance, which leads to hypoxia, hypercapnia, and subsequently arousal. These individuals demonstrate once again that the ability to compensate for high airflow resistance is compromised during sleep and that hypoventilation will occur under these circumstances. This can be mild sustained hypoventilation, as occurs in snorers, or transient large decrements in ventilation followed by arousal, as occurs in individuals with sleep hypopneas.

Increased Lower Airway Resistance

There are two groups of patients well known to have elevated lower airflow resistance during wakefulness and probably during sleep. These are asthmatics with presumably reversible obstructive airway disease and patients with chronic obstructive pulmonary disease, which is obviously less reversible. One would expect these individuals to hypoventilate more during sleep than normals for the reasons outlined above. However, this is not always the case.

Some asthmatics are known to develop progressive bronchoconstriction during sleep leading to subsequent arousal with wheezing and shortness of breath.[87] This nocturnal asthma is an exceedingly common phenomenon.[87] Several reports indicate that total pulmonary resistance increases during sleep in asthmatics presumably secondary to bronchial smooth muscle constriction,[88] although other explanations are possible. However, what little data are available indicate that asthmatics do not hypoventilate more than normal during sleep[89,90] and that nocturnal hypoxia and hypercapnia are uncommon.[91,92] One study actually reports producing considerable bronchoconstriction during sleep with methacholine in a group of asthmatics, yet observed ventilation to be well maintained.[89] Why man would compensate completely for the increased work of breathing associated with bronchoconstriction yet do so poorly with increased pharyngeal resistance or added resistive loads is difficult to understand. One might argue that bronchoconstriction produces primarily expiratory airflow resistance that is dealt with adequately during sleep while pharyngeal collapse leads to inspiratory obstruction with poor compensation. Alternatively, the events associated with bronchoconstriction may actually stimulate respiration through vagal afferent pathways leading to a maintenance of ventilation. However, further studies will be needed to document the validity of either hypothesis. For now we must simply conclude that nocturnal asthma does not lead to important hypoventilation during sleep.

Breathing during sleep in patients with chronic obstructive pulmonary disease is another story, however. Considerable data indicate that potentially severe hypoxemia may develop during REM sleep in patients with this disorder.[93,94] What causes this fall in arterial oxygen saturation in patients with chronic obstructive lung disease is openly debated. It seems clear that some hypoventilation occurs in these patients during these REM-related hypoxemic episodes as the P_{CO_2} rises.[95] However, this rise in P_{CO_2} is considerably less than the simultaneous fall in P_{O_2}, leading other investigators to postulate that ventilation perfusion mismatching is occurring and contributing to the hypoxemia.[96] Indeed there are some data suggesting that an increased shunt fraction develops during REM sleep in these patients.[97] Finally, falling functional residual capacity (FRC) may also be contributing to the hypoxemia.[98] It would seem, therefore, that some decrement in minute ventilation does occur during sleep in these patients, particularly during REM sleep. However, there is no evidence of a large reduction in ventilation during either non-REM or REM sleep, which suggests that load compensation for increased airway resistance is reasonably good in these individuals. Therefore patients with chronic obstructive lung disease, like the asthmatics, seem to deal with an increased work of breathing during sleep better than would be predicted based on studies using external resistors.

It should be added that many investigators believe that the sleep-induced fall in arterial oxygen saturation in patients with chronic obstructive lung disease and several other disorders to be discussed below is simply the product of a normal sleep-induced decrement in ventilation occurring in individuals with lower arterial oxygen saturation.[99] This hypothesis assumes that similar decrements in Po_2 will occur in individuals with normal and abnormal pulmonary function, but that arterial oxygen saturation will fall further in patients with resting hypoxemia due to their position on the oxyhemoglobin dissociation curve. Thus we should be able to predict the level of desaturation that will occur in a given individual during sleep, and indeed this is frequently the case.[99] Therefore, quantitatively small decrements in ventilation may have important effects on arterial oxygen saturation in individuals with waking hypoxemia.

Why hypoxemia in these patients is more common during REM than non-REM sleep is not completely clear. As stated previously, ventilation during REM sleep in normals is probably not lower than is encountered during non-REM sleep, although there is some debate about this.[1,46,74,77,78] However, a number of investigators have demonstrated some inhibition of intercostal muscle activity during REM sleep in humans,[100,101] and certainly the rib cage contribution to ventilation diminishes.[74,101] If patients with chronic obstructive lung disease are more dependent on intercostal muscle activity than normal, REM-induced decrements in the activity of these muscles could lead to hypoventilation. A reduction in the activity of these muscles could also yield reduced lung volumes (FRC) and subsequent hypoxemia. As will be discussed later in this chapter, REM-related hypoxemia is a common occurrence in a variety of respiratory disorders and in each disorder may relate to loss of intercostal or diaphragmatic muscle activity with hypoventilation, reduced lung volumes, or both.

Chest Wall Deformity

Only a few patients with chest wall deformity, primarily kyphoscoliosis, have been studied during sleep to date. However, what data are available indicate that arterial oxygen desaturation does occur commonly in these individuals, particularly during REM sleep.[102] Although frank apneas were observed in many of these patients, some degree of arterial oxygen desaturation was noted during non-apneic periods and in patients without apneas at all. The same factors contributing to hypoxemia described about for patients with obstructive lung disease (hypoventilation, ventilation–perfusion mismatching, and falling functional residual capacity) may also apply here, although this has not been studied. Abnormalities in the control of breathing (reduced hypoxic and hypercapnic ventilatory responses) which have been observed in many of these patients may also be contributing to this hypoventilation. Therefore, once again, increased work of breathing is associated with hypoxemia during sleep, particularly REM sleep. However, there is no clear evidence at this time that this hypoxemia is primarily related to sleep-induced hypoventilation resulting from poor compensatory mechanisms.

Interstitial Lung Disease

Patients with interstitial lung disease are a group with clearly increased work of breathing due to reduced lung compliance. One might therefore expect such individuals to have both hypoventilation during sleep due to poor respiration compensation and arterial oxygen desaturation during REM due to similar sleep-induced events as were described for patients with chronic obstructive pulmonary disease (COPD) and kyphoscoliosis. However, this is generally not the case. Although patients with interstitial lung disease have rapid shallow breathing and are frequently somewhat desaturated during wakefulness, breathing abnormalities are quite uncommon during sleep.[103–105] In one report in which 11 patients were studied, very few apneas were observed, arterial oxygen saturation was well maintained at waking levels during non-REM sleep, and during REM sleep mean oxygen saturation fell only 2.8%.[104] It would seem therefore that minimal if any pathologic hypoventilation is occurring during sleep in this group. The REM-related desaturation may well reflect mild hypoventilation in an individual with waking hypoxemia as the mean Sa_{O_2} was only 89.2% prior to sleep onset.[104] In addition, decreased intercostal muscle activity may also contribute.

In conclusion, increased work of breathing has a variable effect on respiration during sleep. With externally applied resistors or substantial pharyngeal collapse during sleep, hypoventilation is common, even during non-REM sleep. However, with lung disease there are currently no data indicating that important hypoventilation is a problem. There may be some fall in ventilation during REM sleep in patients with COPD or kyphoscoliosis, but it is likely modest and probably only part of the explanation for the hypoxemia encountered during that sleep stage.

Nocturnal Hypoventilation Secondary to Diminished Respiratory Muscle Strength

A number of reports indicate that breathing abnormalities occur during sleep in patients with respiratory muscle weakness.[106–109] The patients studied generally have either muscular dystrophy or the sequelae of poliomyelitis. Although these reports indicate that a large number of these patients have both central and obstructive apneas during sleep, additional data indicate that some degree of hypoventilation is also occurring, particularly during REM sleep.[106,107] In a muscular dystrophy patient studied carefully by Shatrud et al., arterial oxygen saturation was 5% lower during slow-wave sleep than was encountered during wakefulness despite rhythmic ventilation (Fig. 16).[107] During REM sleep transient periods of hypoventilation with severe hypoxemia were encountered without evidence of upper airway obstruction. Thus both sustained periods of reduced ventilation and transient epiodes of hypoventilation occurred in this individual.

A variety of studies indicate that REM-related arterial oxygen desaturation is common in patients with muscular dystrophy.[106,107] Although, as stated above, apneas are frequent in these patients, much of the desaturation does not occur in temporal association with apnea and is believed to be a product of sustained hypoventilation, although minute ventilation has never actually been measured during sleep in these individuals. It seems likely, once again, that a variety of mechanisms are important. REM-related decrements in the activity of intercostal muscles may be critical here as the intercostal muscles assume an increasing role in supporting ventilation as the diaphragms weakens. Thus hypoventilation could well result. This reduced muscle activity may also cause a fall in lung volume that may contribute to the hypoxemia. The ventilation–perfusion mismatching encountered in COPD patients seems less likely here since most of these individuals have normal lung parenchyma. Finally, several investigators have postulated that control of breathing abnormalities may develop in many of these patients and could contribute to both the apneas and the hypoventilation seen during sleep.[106,110] Such a theory is hard to test as ventilatory responses to hypoxia and hyper-

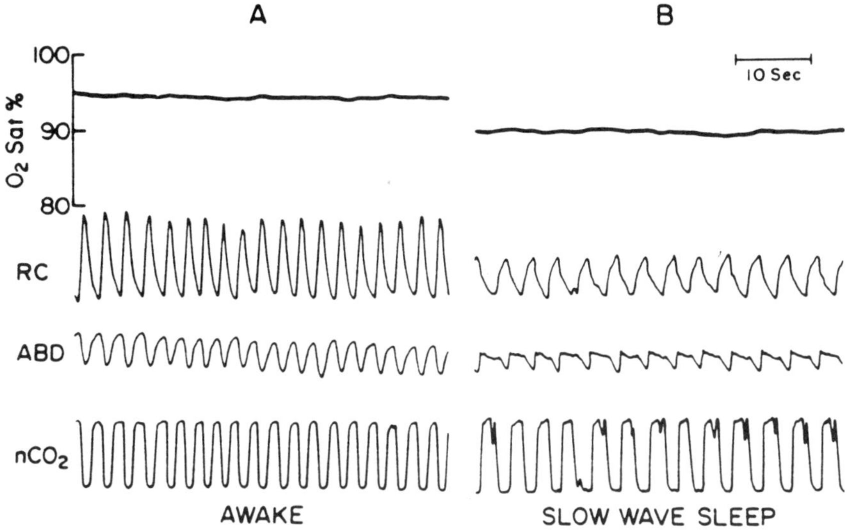

Figure 16. Comparison of oxygen saturation, magnetometry, and nasal flow during wakefulness (panel A) and slow-wave sleep (panel B). Rib cage and abdominal excursions are in arbitrary units. The nCO_2 represents nasal CO_2 concentration, which is presented as a qualitative index of flow at the nose. (From: reference 107, with permission.)

capnia are difficult to interpret in an individual with muscle weakness. However, this possibility cannot be discounted. Once again, a variety of factors may contribute to this desaturation, but some level of hypoventilation seems likely to be important.

Therefore, in any patient with important respiratory muscle weakness, sleep-induced decrements in arterial oxygen saturation must be considered despite normal waking arterial blood gases. As many of these patients can become hypersomnolent as their disease progress (a probable product of respiratory-induced sleep disruption), a sleep evaluation is likely to be fruitful.

Nocturnal Hypoventilation Secondary to Abnormal Control of Breathing Mechanisms

To state that an individual has a "control of breathing abnormality" is difficult as there are very few quantifiable variables to assess these mechanisms. However, generally the hypoxic and hypercapnic ventilatory responses are measured and, if these are found to be quite low (little response to these chemical stimuli), a problem with the control of breathing is identified. There is, however, a considerable range of normal values in these responses in individuals who breathe quite normally, making it, once again, difficult to define abnormal.[111] For the purpose of this discussion, we will consider anyone with a very reduced response to hypoxia and hypercapnia (generally associated with waking hypercapnia), in whom severe lung disease is absent, to have a control of breathing problem. Such problems may also exist in patients with parenchymal lung disease such as the "blue bloater" with obstructive lung disease or the patient with respiratory muscle disease such as muscular dystrophy[110] as described above. However, control of breathing abnormalities are often more difficult to define in these individuals.

Examples of "pure" control of breathing abnormalities would be central alveolar hypoventilation[6] and the obesity–hypoventilation syndrome (Pickwickian syndrome[7,8]). In the former, the patients have no parenchymal lung disease yet generally have waking hypercapnia and often hypoxemia, which can lead to pulmonary hypertension and cor pulmonale. In the latter, the patients are obese, which may increase the work of breathing, yet again have no parenchymal lung disease.[112] However, these patients generally hypoventilate with hypoxia, hypercapnia, and the expected sequelae of these chronic blood gas abnormalities.

Breathing during sleep in individuals with the two disorders mentioned above has not been thoroughly described. It is clear that breathing abnormalities are abundant in these individuals with both central and obstructive apneas being commonly reported.[6,7] However, hypoxemia and hypercapnia are generally observed apart from frank apneas, suggesting that important sustained decrements in ventilation may also be occurring. In patients with the obesity–hypoventilation syndrome, this may result from a combination of high phyaryngeal resistance during sleep that probably occurs in most obese individuals[113] plus control of breathing abnormalities. That upper airway obstruction is not the whole explanation for nocturnal disordered breathing in these patients is evident as tracheostomy does not always completely resolve either waking hypercapnia or sleeping hypoventilation and central apneas. However, many such patients improve considerably with relief of upper airway obstruction.[114] In patients with central alveolar hypoventilation there are few mechanisms implicated as a cause of breathing problems during sleep other than "control" disorders.

Why reduced or absent hypoxic and/or hypercapnic ventilatory responses would lead to apneas and hypoventilation during sleep is not completely clear. It is also not totally surprising based on what has been stated earlier in the chapter about the control of breathing. During non-REM sleep respiration is controlled almost completely by metabolic or autonomic systems of which the chemoresponses (hypoxic and hypercapnic responses) play a prominent role. If this stimulus to respiration is absent during sleep, as is likely the case, then one might expect considerable hypoventilation or even apnea to occur. During wakefulness, when behavioral and wakeful stimulation of ventilation are present, this absence of chemoresponsiveness may be less critical.

These are a variety of additional respiratory disorders in which abnormalities in the control of breathing have been implicated as a contributing factor to waking and sleeping hypoventilation. Many investigators believe that the classically described "blue bloater" is an individual with obstructive lung disease and deficient chemoresponses thus yielding waking hypoxia and hypercapnia. During sleep it is clear that blue bloaters frequently have greater arterial oxygen desaturation than "pink puffers" in whom chemoresponses appear to be closer to normal.[93,94,99] Whether this desaturation is a product of greater hypoventilation during sleep in the blue bloater than the pink puffer or relates more to the fact that blue bloaters are more hypoxic during wakefulness and are thus on a steeper portion of the oxyhemoglobin dissociation curve is debatable. However, many believe that reduced hypoxic and hypercapnic responses in this group lead to greater hypoventilation during both wakefulness and sleep.

Similar principles may apply to patients with respiratory muscle disease (such as muscular dystrophy) or chest wall deformity (such as kyphoscoliosis). Many of these individuals, when tested, have severe respiratory impairment, waking hypercapnia, and reduced responses to hypoxia and hypercapnia.[102,110] Although these patients may not have a "primary" control of breathing disorder, chronic hypoxia and hypercapnia may blunt these responses leading to an "acquired" disorder.[115] This reduced chemoresponsiveness may then contribute to further hypoventilation during sleep, as described above. Therefore the combination of increased work of breathing and reduced chemoresponsives may significantly influence ventilation during sleep in patients with parenchymal lung disease or chest wall abnormalities.

In conclusion, it seems that some degree of hypoventilation occurs in all individuals when they go to sleep and is generally associated with mild hypoxia and hypercapnia. In patients with increased work of breathing due to either high upper airway resistance, parenchymal lung disease, or chest wall deformity, greater decrements in ventilation probably occur during sleep, particularly during REM sleep, although minute ventilation has rarely been quantitated in these individuals. Whether this fall in ventilation is secondary to poor compensation for their increased work of breathing, results from diminishing intercostal muscle activity during REM sleep, or reflects generalized muscle weakness plus poor control of breathing mechanisms remains to be established. However, hypoventilation during sleep is likely to occur commonly in individuals with respiratory disorders that may only minimally influence arterial blood gases during wakefulness. Therefore physicians should look carefully for such breathing abnormalities during sleep in patients demonstrating the sequelae of chronic hypoxia or hypercapnia in whom major blood gas abnormalities are not present during the day.

Central Sleep Apnea

As has been outlined above, quantitative decrements in the volume of ventilation occur in the transition from wakefulness to sleep in both normal individuals and in patients with a variety of pulmonary disorders. Similarly, the respiratory pattern, which is generally rhythmic in the unstimulated wakeful state, may become dysrhythmic with sleep onset in putative normals and in patients with a variety of pathological states. In this section, we will only briefly discuss the mechanisms by which central apneas may occur in normals as this has been outlined previously. We will then concentrate on the pathophysiologic states that lead to more frequent central apneas and address the impact of these apneas on the physiologic and neuropsychological functioning of the patient.

Currently a central apnea is defined as a 10-second or longer pause in respiration occurring during sleep that is associated with no respiratory effort. It obviously differs from the obstructive or mixed apnea discussed elsewhere by the absence of pharyngeal occlusion. The mechanisms leading to central apneas may also differ from those producing obstructive events, although most patients with frequent respiratory pauses during sleep will demonstrate all three types of apnea, suggesting some overlap in the etiology of these events.[116,117]

However, pure or even predominant central sleep apnea is reasonably uncommon and generally accounts for less than 10% of apnea patients encountered in the sleep laboratory.[116] These patients also represent a heterogeneous group with a variety of very different disorders leading to a common event: central apnea. As a result, central sleep apnea does not represent a single disorder, but is a manifestation of a number of pathologic processes.

As was described in some detail previously, central apneas occur commonly in normals during the transition from wakefulness to sleep. This probably reflects the recurrent switching from the wakeful to the sleeping respiratory control system prior to establishing stable sleep. These nonobstructive apneas are also frequently encountered during REM sleep. As central apneas occur commonly in normals, it is often difficult to define what is a pathological number of apneas or more apneas than one would expect to occur in an otherwise normal individual. A variety of investigators have studied the ventilatory pattern during sleep in normals and have commonly observed apneas.[2,4,5,118–120] A few even report that the majority of these apneas are of the central type,[119] although most do not distinguish between central and obstructive events. Despite these studies, it remains unclear what percentage of normal individuals have apneas, what type of apnea is most common, how many apneas must occur before sleep is substantially disrupted, or the severity of blood gas abnormalities associated with these apneas necessary to impact physiologically on the patient. Currently, more than five apneas per hour of sleep is considered abnormal. However, this is somewhat arbitrary as men have more apneas than women and older individuals more than younger ones. Therefore, in deciding if a pathologic condition exists, one must consider the symptoms and physiologic state of the patient rather than simply the number of apneas occurring on a single night in the sleep laboratory.

Clinical Consequences of Central Sleep Apnea

As with any disorder of respiration during sleep, the sequelae of the abnormal breathing relate primarily to the disruption of sleep and the impact of blood gas abnormalities on cardiovascular function. Although the acute effects of central apneas on cardiovascular function have only been assessed in a few subjects,[121] these changes appear to be quite similar to what is observed with obstructive apneas. Both pulmonary and systemic pressures rise transiently during these apneas and return to near waking values with a resumption of rhythmic breathing.[121] Although the pressures encountered during central apneas may be somewhat less than have been described during obstructive events, this probably reflects the longer duration and lower arterial oxygen saturation encountered during obstructive apneas rather than a true difference between apnea types in their influence on cardiovascular function.

Whether transient changes in pulmonary artery pressure occurring during sleep can lead to fixed pulmonary hypertension and subsequently cor pulmonale is open to debate. There is some evidence that mildly elevated pulmonary artery pressure may persist during the day in patients with severe obstructive sleep apnea.[122] However, there are few data indicating that cor pulmonale develops in individuals with isolated sleep apnea.[123] Most studies suggest that when waking hypoxemia or additional obstructive lung disease is combined with sleep apnea right ventricular dysfunction may then develop.[123] However, sleep apnea alone seldom produces this consequence. These observations, however, have been made in patients with obstructive sleep apnea. How they apply to central apnea is open to debate.

Sustained systemic hypertension seems to be another fairly common consequence, or at least accompaniment, of sleep apnea with this hypertension generally improving with treatment of the sleep disorder.[124] Once again, these observations have been made primarily in obstructive apnea patients. There seems little reason, however, to suspect that central apnea patients would be different.

The neuropsychologic consequences of central sleep apnea seem to be somewhat different than are encountered in obstructive sleep apnea, which is surprising.[116,117] Patients with obstructive sleep apnea generally complain of hypersomnolence with difficulty maintaining wakefulness during the day.[116,117] On the other hand, the few reports available indicate that central apnea patients more commonly complain of insomnia and difficulty falling asleep. The one study in which "sleepiness" was assessed in both central and obstructive apnea patients indicates that individuals with central apnea do have a much longer sleep latency (as assessed by multiple sleep latency testing) and therefore less somnolence than the obstructive apnea patients.[117] Why this is the case is confusing, although several explanations seem possible. Central apneas may lead to fewer arousals and less arterial oxygen desaturation than obstructive events, both of which (arousals and desaturation) have been implicated as a cause of hypersomnolence. Thus they may have less sleepiness during the day. On the other hand, any disorder, such as insomnia, that leads to an increase in the time spent in the transition between wakefulness and sleep could lead to more central apneas. If insomniacs have more spontaneous arousals during the night and, as a result, must "fall asleep" more often, the number of central apneas may increase as a result of the waxing and waning between wakeful and sleeping respiratory control systems as described above. Thus insomnia could lead to central apneas. This is pure speculation, however, and the explanation for the differing symptoms in central and obstructive apnea awaits further investigation.

Patients with either central or obstructive apneas often complain of depression, decreased libido or sexual dysfunction, plus generalized fatigue.[116,117,125] The sleep-related event that leads to these symptoms plus the hypersomnolence or insomnia described above is unknown. It would seem likely that these symptoms are related to either sleep disruption secondary to apnea-associated arousals or arterial blood gas abnormalities that occur during apneas. Studies have shown correlations between symptoms and measures of both sleep disruption and arterial oxygen desaturation. As a result it remains somewhat unclear what is leading to the neuropsychological dysfunction of sleep apnea. That it occurs, however, seems clear. How many apneas or how much sleep disordered breathing is required to produce such symptomatology also remains to be firmly established. This is a particularly difficult issue as some disordered breathing occurs in most normals which, as was addressed above, makes defining normal values somewhat of a problem. As a result, each physician is forced to make individual decisions regarding each patient. If many apneas are present and symptoms are prominent, a clear association seems likely and treatment is indicated. However, if relatively few apneas are observed, perhaps 5–10 per hour of sleep, and symptoms are vague, decisions regarding care of the patient are much more difficult and no clear guidelines are currently available.

Pathophysiology of Central Sleep Apnea

As stated above, central sleep apnea is not a disorder with a single etiology but is often a manifestation of a variety of pathologic conditions or occurs when no clear etiology can be discerned. Regardless of the etiology, a central apnea represents a total loss of the stimulus to breathe[126] with no respiratory muscle activity occurring during the pause (Fig. 17). As a result, as we attempt to understand

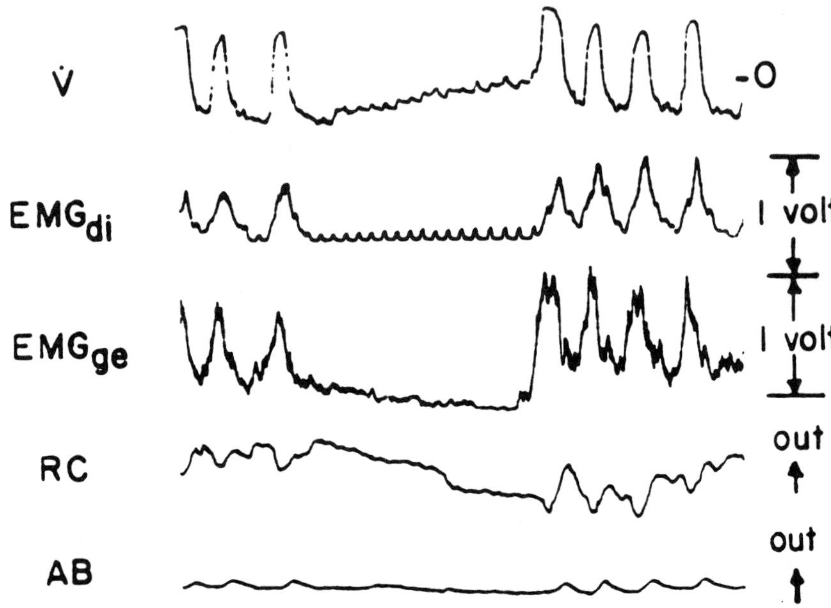

Figure 17. A representative central apnea. There is an abrupt and complete loss of both diaphragmatic (EMG_{di}) and genioglossal (EMG_{ge}) activity with sudden resumption of activity at the onset of breathing. Rig cage (RC) volume gradually decreases to the baseline expiratory value and even further. (From: reference 126, with permission.)

these respiratory pauses, we must evoke mechanisms that would temporarily abolish all respiratory center output or cause this respiratory activity to wax and wane. A variety of events could produce such a condition and will be addressed below.

Control of Breathing and Central Sleep Apnea

From what has been said above, it seems clear that during non-REM sleep ventilation is primarily, if not solely, controlled by metabolic mechanisms with the P_{CO_2} level being the single most important metabolic variable in this control system.[17] As a result, any process that either pushes the P_{CO_2} level below the apneic threshold or markedly diminishes or abolishes CO_2 sensitivity is likely to produce apneas.

There are a variety of mechanisms that can lead to a P_{CO_2} level transiently reduced below the apnea threshold. First, as stated previously, simply falling asleep may produce this situation. The waking Pco_2 level may be inadequate to stimulate ventilation during sleep.[17] Therefore as the individual shifts from the awake to the non-REM respiratory control system ventilation may cease until the Pco_2 rises to an adequate level. Thus central apnea may occur in normals.

Man at high altitude is another situation in which central apneas are commonly observed during sleep.[127] The presumed mechanism is as follows. The hypoxia encountered at altitude stimulates ventilation and thus leads to hypocapnia. If the hypoxic stimulus is adequate, Pco_2 may fall below a threshold value and apnea ensues. During the apnea, Pco_2 rises and Po_2 falls, both of which ultimately stimulate ventilation and an hyperpneic phase occurs. This hyperventilation corrects or improves oxygenation yet again leads to a diminished arterial Pco_2 level and apnea. Thus ventilation waxes and wanes between apnea and hyperpnea in an often rhythmic fashion. These same mechanisms are likely operative during wakefulness, and some investigators have observed ventilation to cycle in waking subjects. However, behavioral events and the wakeful stimulus are generally adequate to prevent apnea from commonly occurring while the individual is awake.

Not everyone at altitude has periodic ventilation even during sleep.[127,128] The single most important determinant of who does and does not have this cycling respiratory pattern seems to be the magnitude of the sleeping hypoxic ventilatory response.[127,128] Individuals with a high ventilatory response to hypoxia will have more hyperventilation at altitude, a lower Pco_2 level, and thus a greater likelihood of central apneas. Those with lower hypoxic drives hyperventilate less, have a higher Pco_2, and therefore less tendency to cycle. There is, therefore, considerable variability between individuals in the quantity of periodic breathing occurring at altitude.

The level of the ventilatory response to chemical stimuli (hypoxia and hypercapnia) has also been implicated as a cause or mediator of central sleep apnea apart from the altitude studies described above. High ventilatory responses to hypoxia and/or hypercapnia at sea level may lead to central apneas by mechanisms similar to those occurring at altitude.[130,131] Individuals with high chemosensitivity may, at baseline, have a lower Pco_2 level.[130] With a sigh or isolated large breath during sleep, Pco_2 may fall below the apnea threshold initiating the first respiratory pause. During this apnea, Pco_2 rises and Po_2 falls until ventilation is ultimately stimulated again. However, in an individual with a large response to these stimuli, ventilation may occur in excess of what is necessary to simply correct the Pco_2 level to a normal value. Thus hypocapnia is again produced with an ensuing apnea. Therefore ventilation waxes and wanes between apnea and hyperpnea. This respiratory instability is believed to occur primarily as a result of the shape[131] of the hypoxic ventilatory response (Fig. 1). As can be seen, this is a hyperbolic relationship with little simulation of ventilation occurring until the Po_2 falls below approximately 60 mm Hg. Thereafter respiration is progressively stimulated in a hyperbolic manner. As a result, in an individual with a high hypoxic response, ventilation may be strongly stimulated at the end of an apnea as the Po_2 falls. Thus hyperpnea ensues, leading to hypocapnia and the next apnea. High responses to rising Pco_2 may also be important in producing central apneas in a somewhat similar manner to that described above.[129] In conclusion it would seem that elevated chemoresponsiveness may lead to respiratory instability and thus be an independent risk factor for the development of cycling apneas.

On the other hand, extremely low responses to chemical stimuli may also predispose an individual to respiratory pauses during sleep.[6–8,130] As stated previously, metabolic controllers of respiration are quite important during sleep with chemoresponses playing a prominent role. If these responses are markedly reduced, there may be no drive to breathe during sleep. In individuals with central alveolar hypoventilation, for example, hypercapnia is common during wakefulness despite normal lung function.[6] These patients also have very low chemoresponsiveness and thus central apneas during sleep. Patients with the obesity–hypoventilation syndrome (Pickwickian syndrome) also have reduced responses to hypoxia[18] and hypercapnia and abnormal respiration during sleep. Although these patients commonly have obstructive apneas (probably secondary to the influence of obesity on the upper airway[113]), central events are also frequently observed. It would seem, therefore, that the extremes of chemoresponsiveness may adversely affect ventilation during sleep. High responses produce respiratory instability with cycling events while reduced chemosensitivity leads to a very diminished drive to breathe during sleep and thus central apneas.

It should be stated that the principles of respiratory control described above as they apply to the development of central sleep apnea are relevant primarily to events occurring during non-REM sleep during which ventilation is under metabolic control. However, central apneas are quite common during REM sleep also yet probably occur for different reasons. During REM sleep respiratory muscle activity is periodically inhibited for reasons that are currently unclear.[80,82,100,101] This inhibition tends to be associated with rapid eye movements in humans[79,82] and PGO (pontine-geniculo-occipital) waves in animals[72,132] and occurs as a results of hyperpolarization of the muscle. Although the cause and function of this muscular inhibition remains obscure, it seems clear that it can transiently inhibit ventilation to the point of apnea or certainly hypopnea. As a result, virtually all humans will have some respiratory instability during REM sleep as a result of these events.

The Upper Airway and Central Sleep Apnea

Although upper airway collapse is the principal event in the development of obstructive sleep apnea, abnormalities of both the nasal and pharyngeal airway may also lead to central apneas. Nasal obstruction, whether naturally occurring[133] or artificially produced,[134] is well known to produce apneas during sleep. Although current data suggest that most of these apneas are obstructive in nature,[135] central apneas have also been observed.[134] Why apneas of either type occur during partial or complete nasal obstruction is open to debate. It would seem that these apneas probably relate to: (1) loss of stimulation of receptors located in the nose, (2) high intrapharyngeal negative pressure due to partial nasal obstruction that could collapse the pharynx, or (3) simply the loss of the nose as a breathing route and inability to switch to oral ventilation during sleep. Recent data support the former two concepts. Nasal anesthesia during sleep has been shown to lead to central apneas,[136] suggesting a role for nasal receptors in the maintenance of rhythmic ventilation during sleep. In addition, the application of external resistive loads during wakefulness (simulating nasal congestion) can lead to partial pharyngeal collapse in normals,[137] a phenomenon that is more dramatic during sleep when pharyngeal dilator muscles are probably less active.[48] As a result, events occurring in the nose can influence the respiratory pattern during sleep, with both central and obstructive apneas being observed.

In addition, there are some data in both adults and infants that indicate that pharyngeal collapse[138] or pharyngeal receptor stimulation[139] may inhibit ventilation and thus lead to central apneas. One study reports elimination of central apneas with high levels of nasal continuous positive airway pressure (CPAP), suggesting that maintaining pharyngeal patency in these individuals will prevent the development of central apneas.[138] In addition, they observed oropharyngeal anesthesia abolished central apneas in these patients, again indicating a role for a pharyngeal receptor in their origin. Why such a receptor would be present in man is unclear, but inhibition of ventilation may prevent recurrent respiratory efforts against an occluded airway, thus ultimately allowing the airway to open. In infants, stimulation of upper airway reflexes by instilling small boluses of physiologic saline into the oropharynx frequently led to central apneas during sleep.[139] This is likely a protective mechanism to avoid aspiration. It would seem, therefore, that a variety of upper airway receptors may influence respiratory rhythmicity and lead to apnea during sleep.

Central Apneas in Congestive Heart Failure

Cheyne-Stokes ventilation is a common respiratory pattern in patients with severe left ventricular dysfunction. Recent data indicate that this cycling ventilatory pattern frequently persists during sleep with central apneas occurring at the nadir of the respiratory cycle.[140] In addition, at least one study suggests that respiratory dysrhythmias during sleep may be a poor prognostic sign in these patients with greater mortality occurring in patients with sleep disordered breathing and heart failure than in those without the sleep-related respiratory problem.[141]

Why this waxing and waning of ventilation occurs in patient with reduced left ventricular function is poorly understood. However, it is believed to relate to delayed or increased circulation time.[142] An increased circulation time can potentially produce unstable ventilation due to the delay that occurs between mechanical changes in ventilation (hyperpnea or hypopnea) and receptor stimulation due to changes in arterial blood gases. If an individual hypoventilates or has an apnea, a substantial period of time will pass before rising Pco_2 and falling Po_2 are detected at the appropriate receptor. At that time ventilation is stimulated for a disproportionately long period of time because the corrected blood gases are again not perceived at the receptor for an abnormally long time period. Thus ventilation can wax and wane, with frank apneas occurring commonly at the nadir of this cycle.

Whether this is the true explanation for Cheyne-Stokes respiration in patients with heart failure during wakefulness or sleep remains obscure. Clearly, cycling ventilation can be induced in animals with a several-fold increase in circulation time produced by simply diverting blood flow into long external circuits.[143] However, it seems unlikely that congestive heart failure produces a circulatory delay of this magnitude, thus making the final etiology of this respiratory pattern open to debate.

Neurologic Disorders and Central Sleep Apnea

It seems logical that any disease that can affect the neurologic mechanisms that control ventilation could lead to an abnormal respiratory pattern, particularly central apneas during non-REM sleep when respiration is controlled so completely by such mechanisms. Indeed, a variety of neurologic disorders have been associated with central sleep apnea. The most common ones are probably those producing autonomic dysfunction[144,145] such as the Shy-Drager syndrome, familial dysautonomia, or diabetes mellitus. All have been associated with the development of apneas during sleep with both central and obstructive events being observed. Additional neurologic disorders such as cervical cordotomy,[146] encephalitis,[147] or brain-stem infarction[148] have been associated with apneas during sleep.

Why a particular neurologic disorder leads to breathing abnormalities during sleep in unclear. Our lack of understanding of this process is a product of both the complexity of the neurologic mechanisms that control ventilation and the paucity of tests in man available to evaluate respiratory control systems. The only commonly available tests of ventilation control are the hypoxic and hypercapnic ventilatory responses described above. In patients with central sleep apnea and suspected neurologic disorders, these responses are often reduced. However, they are also commonly normal, making it somewhat difficult to evaluate their role in the development of respiratory disorders of sleep. In one patient with encephalitis, these chemoresponses were markedly reduced at the same time he was experiencing nocturnal hypoventilation and central apneas.[147] With the return of these response to normal levels, breathing during sleep markedly improved. This suggests an important role for chemoresponses in the development of nocturnal breathing problems. However, this relationship is only correlative and does not prove cause and effect.

The point that seems clear is that neurologic disorders may lead to apneas during sleep and respiratory control instability without our being able to document a discrete control of breathing problem (reduced hypoxic or hypercapnic response). On the other hand, control of breathing abnormalities may exist and lead to central sleep apnea without other overt neurologic manifestations. As a result, the relationship between neurologic disorders, the control of breathing, and central apnea remains somewhat obscure. However, that breathing abnormalities become more obvious during sleep in individuals with more diffuse neurologic disease or isolated abnormalities of respiratory control is not surprising. During wakefulness, "back-up" mechanisms such as behavioral influences on respiration may sustain breathing. During sleep, metabolic systems become primal, and if autonomic control mechanisms are not intact, apneas may occur.

Conclusions

In conclusion, it seems that central apneas are events that occur commonly in normals and may, in these individuals, produce few or no adverse effects. On the other hand, frequent central apneas that disrupt sleep and lead to severe blood gas abnormalities are likely pathologic, with important adverse effects on the afflicted patient. As a result, individuals with central sleep apnea should be evaluated not only for the presence of apneas, but also for evidence of sequelae of these apneas before deciding if the process is pathologic.

The etiology of central apneas probably varies dramatically from one individual to the next, with the disorder representing a common manifestation of a variety of pathologic process rather than a discrete entity. As a result, in searching for the cause of central sleep apnea in a given patient, many possibilities must be considered as discussed above. However, frequently no clear etiology will emerge.

References

1. Douglas J, White DP, Pickett CK, et al. Respiration during sleep in normal man. *Thorax* 1982; 37:840–844.
2. Bulow K. Respiration and wakefulness in man. *Acta Physiol Scand* 1963; 59(Suppl 209):1–110.
3. Robin ED, Whaley RD, Crump CH, et al. Alveolar gas tensions, pulmo-

nary ventilation, and blood pH during physiologic sleep in normal subjects. *J Clin Invest* 1958; 37:981–989.
4. Block AJ, Boysen PG, Wynne JW, et al. Sleep apnea, hypopnea, and oxygen desaturation in normal subjects. *N Engl J Med* 1979; 300:513–517.
5. Webb P. Periodic breathing during sleep. *J Appl Physiol* 1974; 37:899.
6. Mellins R, Balfour H, Turino G, et al. Failure of autonomic control of ventilation (Ondine's curse). *Medicine* 1970; 49:487–504.
7. Tassinari C, Dalla Bernardina B, Cirignatta F, et al. Apnoeic periods and the respiratory related arousal patterns during sleep in the Pickwickian syndrome. *Bull Physiopathol Respir* 1972; 8:1087–1102.
8. Zwillich C, Sutton F, Pierson D, et al. Decreased hypoxic drive in the obesity hypoventilation syndrome. *Am J Med* 1975; 59:343–348.
9. Phillipson EA, Bowes G, Townsend ER, et al. Role of metabolic CO_2 production in ventilatory response to steady state exercise. *J Clin Invest* 1981; 68:768–774.
10. Phillipson EA, Duffin J, Cooper JD. Critical dependence of respiratory rhythmicity on metabolic CO_2 load. *J Appl Physiol* 1981; 50:45–54.
11. Weil J, Byrne-Quinn E, Sodal I, et al. Hypoxic ventilatory drive in normal man. *J Clin Invest* 1970;49: 1061–1072.
12. Read DJC. A clinical method for assessing the ventilatory response to carbon dioxide. *Australas Ann Med* 1967; 16:20–32.
13. Wiegand L, Zwillich C, White DP. Sleep and the ventilatory response to resistive loading in normal man. *J Appl Physiol* 1988; 64:1186–1195.
14. Hornbein TF. The relationship between stimulus to chemoreceptors and their response. *In* TW Torrance (ed). Arterial Chemoreceptors. Oxford, UK, Blackwell, 1968, pp 65–78.
15. Whipp BJ, Wasserman K. Carotid bodies and ventilatory control dynamics in man. *Fed Proc* 1980; 39:2668–2673.
16. Loeschcke HH. Review lecture: Central chemosensitivity and the reaction therapy. *J Physiol (London)* 1982; 332:1–24.
17. Skatrud J, Dempsey J. Interaction of sleep state and chemical stimuli in sustaining rhythmic ventilation. *J Appl Physiol* 1983; 55:813–822.
18. Eldridge FL, Kiley JP, Millhorn DE. Respiratory effects of carbon dioxide-induced changes of medullary extracellular fluid pH in cats. *J Physiol (London)* 1984; 355:177–189.
19. Lugliani R, Whipp BJ, Seard C, et al. Effect of bilateral carotid-body resection on ventilatory control at rest and during exercise in man. *N Engl J Med* 1971; 285:1105–1111.
20. White DP, Weil JV, Zwillich CW. Metabolic rate and breathing during sleep. *J Appl Physiol* 1985; 59:384–391.
21. Coleridge HM, Coleridge JCG. Reflexes evoked from tracheobronchial tree and lungs. *In* AP Fishman (ed). Handbook of Physiology, The Respiratory System, Vol II, Control of Breathing, Part I. Baltimore, American Physiology Society, 1986, pp 395–429.
22. Hering E, Breuer J. Die Selbststeuerung der Athmung durch den Nervus vagus. *Sitzungsber Akad Wiss Wien* 1868; 57:672–677.
23. Mills JE, Sellick H, Widdicombe JG. Activity of lung irritant receptors in pulmonary microembolism, anaphylaxis and drug-induced bronchoconstriction. *J Physiol (London)* 1969; 203:337–357.

24. Widdicombe J. Receptors in the trachea and bronchi of the cat. *J Physiol (London)* 1954; 123:71–104.
25. Coleridge JCG, Coleridge HM. Afferent vagal C-fiber innervation of the lungs and airways and its functional significance. *Rev Physiol Biochem Pharmacol* 1984; 99:1–110.
26. Scuirba FC, Owens GR, Sanders MH, et al. Evidence of an altered pattern of breathing during exercise in recipients of heart-lung transplants. *N Engl J Med* 1988; 319:1186–1192.
27. Cunningham DJC, Robbins, PA, Wolff CB. Integration of respiratory responses to changes in alveolar partial pressures of CO_2 and O_2 and in arterial pH. *In* AP Fishman (ed). Handbook of Physiology, The Respiratory System, Vol II, Control of Breathing, Part 2. Baltimore, American Physiology Society, 1986, pp 475–528, 1977.
28. Sullivan CE, Kozar LF, Murphy E, et al. Primary role of respiratory afferents in sustaining breathing rhythm. *J Appl Physiol* 1978; 45:11–17.
29. Phillipson EA. Control of breathing during sleep. *Am Rev Respir Dis* 1978; 118:909–939.
30. Sears TA, Newson Davis J. The control of respiratory muscles during voluntary breathing. *Ann NY Acad Sci* 1968; 155:183.
31. Proctor DF. Breathing mechanics during phonation and singing. *In* B Wyke (ed). Ventilatory and Phonatory Control Systems. London, Oxford University Press, 1974, p 39.
32. Cohen MI, Hugelin A. Suprapontine reticular control of intrinsic respiratory mechanisms. *Arch Ital Biol* 1965; 103:317–334.
33. Hugelin A, Cohen MI. The reticular activating system and respiratory regulation in the cat. *Ann NY Acad Sci* 1963; 109:586–603.
34. Orem J, Lydic R, Norris P. Experimental control of diaphragm and laryngeal abductor muscles by brain stem arousal systems. *Respir Physiol* 1979; 38:203–221.
35. Fink BR. Influence of cerebral activity in wakefulness on regulation of breathing. *J Appl Physiol* 1961; 16:15.
36. Rechtschaffen A, Kales A. A manual of standardized terminology, techniques, and scoring system for sleep stages of human subjects. Bethesda, Maryland, National Institute of Neurol Dis Blind, 1968, NIH Publ. 204.
37. Aserinsky E, Kleitman N. Regularly occurring periods of eye motility, and concomitant phenomena, during sleep. *Science* 1953; 118:273–274.
38. Berthon-Jones M, Sullivan CE. Ventilatory and arousal responses to hypoxia in sleeping humans. *Am Rev Respir Dis* 1982; 125:632–639.
39. Douglas NJ, White DP, Weil JV, et al. Hypoxic ventilatory response decreases during sleep in normal men. *Am Rev Respir Dis* 1982; 125: 286–289.
40. Hedemark LL, Kronenberg RS. Ventilatory and heart rate responses to hypoxia and hypercapnia during sleep in adults. *J Appl Physiol* 1982; 53:307–312.
41. White DP, Douglas NJ, Pickett CK, et al. Hypoxic ventilatory response during sleep in normal women. *Am Rev Respir Dis* 1982; 126:530–533.
42. Reed DJ, Kellogg RH. Effect of sleep on hypoxic stimulation of breathing at sea level and at altitude. *J Appl Physiol* 1960; 15:1130–1134.

43. Goethe B, Goldman MD, Cherniack NS, et al. Effect of progressive hypoxia on breathing during sleep. *Am Rev Respir Dis* 1982; 126:97–102.
44. White DP, Douglas NJ, Pickett CK, et al. Sexual influence on the control of breathing. *J Appl Physiol* 1983; 54:874–879.
45. Santiago TV, Scardella AT, Edelman NH. Determinants of the ventilatory response to hypoxia during sleep. *Am Rev Respir Dis* 1984; 130: 179–182.
46. Hudgel DW, Martin RJ, Johnson B, et al. Mechanics of the respiratory system and breathing during sleep in normal humans. *J Appl Physiol* 1984; 56:133–137.
47. Skatrud JB, Dempsey JA. Airway resistance and respiratory muscle function in snorers during NREM sleep. *J Appl Physiol* 1985; 59:328–335.
48. Wiegand L, Zwillich CW, White DP. Collapsibility of the human upper airway during normal sleep. *J Appl Physiol* 1989; 66:1800–1808.
49. Iber C, Berssenbrugge A, Skatrud J, et al. Ventilatory adaptations to resistive loading during wakefulness and non-REM sleep. *J Appl Physiol* 1982; 52:607–614.
50. Wiegand L, Zwillich CW, White DP. Sleep and the ventilatory response to resistive loading in normal man. *J Appl Physiol* 1988; 64:1186–1195.
51. White DP. Occlusion pressure and ventilation during sleep in normal humans. *J Appl Physiol* 1986; 61:1279–1287.
52. Phillipson EA, Sullivan CE, Read DJC, et al. Ventilatory and waking responses to hypoxia in sleeping dogs. *J Appl Physiol* 1978; 44:512–520.
53. Douglas NJ, White DP, Weil, JV, et al. Hypercapnic ventilatory response in sleeping adults. *Am Rev Respir Dis* 1982; 126:758–762.
54. Goethe B, Altose MD, Gotham MD, et al. Effect of quiet sleep on resting and CO_2 stimulated breathing in humans. *J Appl Physiol* 1981; 50:724–730.
55. Berthon-Jones M, Sullivan CE. Ventilatory and arousal responses to hypercapnia in normal sleeping adults. *J Appl Physiol* 1984; 57:59–67.
56. Honda Y, Hayashi F, Yoshida A, et al. Overall "gain" of the respiratory control system in normoxic humans awake and asleep. *J Appl Physiol* 1983; 55:1530–1535.
57. Bellville JW, Howland WS, Seed JC, et al. The effect of sleep on the respiratory response to carbon dioxide. *Anesthesiology* 1959; 20:628–634.
58. Reed DJ, Kellog RH. Changes in respiratory response to CO_2 during natural sleep at sea level and at altitude. *J Appl Physiol* 1958; 17:325–330.
59. Fink BR, Hanks EC, Ngal EH, et al. Central regulation of respiration during anesthesia and wakefulness. *Ann NY Acad Sci* 1963; 109:892–899.
60. Bainton CR, Mitchell RA. Posthyperventilation apnea in awake man. *J Appl Physiol* 1966; 21:411–415.
61. Tawadrous F, Eldridge F. Posthyperventilation breathing patterns after active hyperventilation in man. *J Appl Physiol* 1974; 37:353–356.
62. White DP, Zwillich CW, Weil JV. Metabolic rate and breathing during sleep. *J Appl Physiol* 1985; 59:384–391.
63. Brebbia DR, Altshuler KZ. Oxygen consumption rate and electroencephalographic stage of sleep. *Science* 1965; 150:1621–1623.
64. Buskirk ER, Thompson RH, Moore R, et al. Human energy expenditure studies in the National Institute of Arthritis and Metabolic Diseases metabolic chamber. *Am J Clin Nutr* 1960; 8:602–613.

65. Jamal K, McMahon G, Edgell G, et al. Cough and arousal responses to inhaled citric acid in sleeping humans. *Am Rev Respir Dis* 1983; 127(Suppl):237.
66. Power JT, Stewart IC, Connaughton JJ, et al. Nocturnal cough in patients with chronic bronchitis and emphysema. *Am Rev Respir Dis* 1984; 130:999–1001.
67. Farber JP, Marlow TA. Pulmonary reflexes and breathing pattern during sleep in the opossum. *Respir Physiol* 1976; 27:73–86.
68. Sullivan, Kozar LF, Murphy E, et al. Arousal, ventilatory, and airway responses to bronchopulmonary stimulation in sleeping dogs. *J Appl Physiol* 1979; 47:17–25.
69. Sullivan CE, Murphy E, Kozar L, et al. Ventilatory responses to CO_2 and lung inflation in tonic versus phasic REM sleep. *J Appl Physiol* 1979; 47:1304–1310.
70. Phillipson EA. Regulation of breathing during sleep. *Am Rev Respir Dis* 1977; 115(Suppl):217–224.
71. Remmers JE, Bartlett D, Putman MD. Changes in the respiratory cycle associated with sleep. *Respir Physiol* 1976; 28:227–238.
72. Baust W, Holzbach E, Zechlin O. Phasic changes in heart rate and respiration correlated with PGO-spike activity during REM sleep. *Pfluegers Arch* 1972; 331:113–123.
73. Sullivan CE, Kozar LF, Murphy E, et al. Primary role of respiratory afferents in sustaining breathing rhythm. *J Appl Physiol* 1978; 45:11–17.
74. Tabachnik E, Muller NL, Bryant AC, et al. Changes in ventilation and chest wall mechanics during sleep in normal adolescents. *J Appl Physiol* 1981; 51:557–564.
75. Gilbert R, Auchincloss JH, Brodsky J, et al. Changes in tidal volume, frequency and ventilation induced by their measurement. *J Appl Physiol* 1972; 33:252–254.
76. Bristow JD, Honour AJ, Pickering TG, et al. Cardiovascular and respiratory changes during sleep in normal and hypertensive subjects. *Cardiovasc Res* 1969; 3:476–485.
77. Krieger J, Turlot JC, Mangin P, et al. Breathing during sleep in normal young and elderly subjects: Hypopneas, apneas, and correlated factors. *Sleep* 1983; 6:108–120.
78. Lopes JM, Tabachnik E, Muller NL, et al. Total airway resistance and respiratory muscle activity during sleep. *J Appl Physiol* 1983; 54:773–777.
79. Millman RR, Knight H, Kline LR, et al. Changes in compartmental ventilation in association with eye movements during REM sleep. *J Appl Physiol* 1988; 65:1196–1202.
80. Kline LR, Hendricks JC, Davies RO, et al. Control of activity of the diaphragm in rapid eye-movement sleep. *J Appl Physiol* 1986; 61:1293–1300.
81. Gillam PMS. Patterns of respiration in human beings at rest and during sleep. *Bull Eur Physiopathol Respir* 1972; 8:1059–1070.
82. Mahan PJ, Kline LR, Grippi MA, et al. Changes in respiratory muscle activity during REM sleep in man. *Am Rev Respir Dis* 1987;135(Suppl): A47.
83. Read JC, Freedman S, Kafer ER. Pressures developed by loaded inspira-

tory muscles in conscious and anesthetized man. *J Appl Physiol* 1974; 37:207–218.
84. Lugaresi E, Coccagna G, Cirignotta F. Snoring and its clinical implications. *In* C Guilleminault, WC Dement (eds). Sleep Apnea Syndromes. New York, Alan R. Liss, 1978, pp 13–21.
85. Remmers JE, DeGrott WJ, Sauerland EK, et al. Pathogenesis of upper airway occlusion during sleep. *J Appl Physiol* 1978; 44:931–938.
86. Gould GA, Whyte KF, Rhind GB, et al. The sleep hypopnea syndrome. *Am Rev Respir Dis* 1988; 137:895–898.
87. Connolly CK. Diurinal rhythms in airway obstruction. *Br J Dis Chest* 1979; 73:357–366.
88. Ballard RD, Kelly PL, Martin RJ. Estimates of ventilation from inductance plethysmography in sleeping asthmatic patients. *Chest* 1988; 93: 128–133.
89. Ballard RD, Kelly PL, Tan WC, et al. Effects of sleep, before and after sleep deprivation, on ventilatory and arousal responses to induced bronchoconstriction. *Am Rev Respir Dis* 1988; 137(Suppl):A54.
90. Morgan AD, Rhind GB, Connaughton JJ, et al. Breathing patterns, ventilatin and hypoxaemic episodes during sleep in adult asthmatic patients. *Clin Sci* 1983; 65:39 pp.
91. Montplaisir J, Walsh J, Malo JL. Nocturnal asthma: Features of attacks, sleep and breathing patterns. *Am Rev Respir Dis* 1982; 125:18–22.
92. Neagley SR, White, DP, Zwillich CW. Does disordered breathing during sleep occur in stable asthmatics: The influence of inhaled bronchodilators. *Chest* 1986; 90:334–337.
93. Dougklas NJ, Calverley PMA, Leggett RJE, et al. Transient hypoxaemia during sleep in chronic bronchitis and emphysema. *Lancet* 1979; 1:1–4.
94. Wynne JW, Block AJ, Hemingway J, et al. Disordered breathing and oxygen desaturation during sleep in patients with chronic obstructive lung disease (COLD). *Am J Med* 1979; 56:573–579.
95. Catterall JR, Calverley PMA, MacNee W, et al. The mechanism of transient nocturnal hypoxemia in hypoxic chronic bronchitis and emphysema. *J Appl Physiol* 1985; 59:1698–1703.
96. Fletcher EC, Levin DC. Cardiopulmonary hemodynamics during sleep in subjects with chronic obstructive pulmonary disease. The effect of short and long term oxygen. *Chest* 1984; 85:6–14.
97. Fletcher EC, Gray BA, Levin DC. Nonapneic mechanisms of arterial oxygen desaturation during rapid eye movement sleep. *J Appl Physiol* 1983; 54:632–639.
98. Hudgel DW, Devadatta P. Decreases in functional residual capacity during sleep in normal humans. *J Appl Physiol* 1984; 57:1319–1322.
99. Catterall JR, Douglas NJ, Calverley PMA, et al. Transient hypoxemia during sleep in chronic obstructive pulmonary disease is not a sleep apnea syndrome. *Am Rev Respir Dis* 1983; 128:24–29.
100. Muller NL, Francis PW, Gurwitz D, et al. Mechanisms of hemoglobin desaturation during rapid-eye-movement sleep in normal subjects and in patients with cystic fibrosis. *Am Rev Respir Dis* 1980; 121:463–469.
101. Tusiewicz K, Moldofsky H, Bryan A, et al. Mechanisms of the rib cage and diaphragm during sleep. *J Appl Physiol* 1977; 43:600–602.

102. Mezon BL, West P, Israels J, et al. Sleep breathing abnormalities in kyphoscoliosis. *Am Rev Respir Dis* 1980; 122:617–621.
103. Bye P, Issa F, Berthon-Jones M, et al. Studies of oxygenation during sleep in patients with interstitial lung disease. *Am Rev Respir Dis* 1984; 129:27–32.
104. Perez-Padilla R, West P, Lertzman M, et al. Breathing during sleep in patients with interstitial lung disease. *Am Rev Respir Dis* 1985; 132:224–229.
105. McNicholas WT, Coffey M, Fitzgerald MY. Ventilation and gas exchange during sleep in patients with interstitial lung disease. *Thorax* 1986; 41:777–782.
106. Smith PEM, Calverley PMA, Edwards RHT, et al. Practical problems in the respiratory care of patients with muscular dystrophy. *N Engl J Med* 1987; 316:1197–1205.
107. Shatrud J, Iber C, McHugh W, et al. Determinants of hypoventilation during wakefulness and sleep in diaphragmatic paralysis. *Am Rev Respir Dis* 1980; 121:587–593.
108. Coccagna G, Mantovani M, Parchi C, et al. Alveolar hypoventilation and hypersomnia in myotonic dystrophy. *J Neurol Neurosurg Psychiatry* 1975; 38:977–984.
109. Cummiskey J, Lynne Davies P, Guilleminault C. Sleep study and respiratory muscle function in myotonic dystrophy. *In* C Guillerminault, WC Dement (eds). Sleep Apnea Syndromes. New York, Alan R. Liss, 1978, pp 295–308.
110. Veale D, Cooper BG, Gilmartin JJ, et al. Breathing during sleep in patients with myotonic dystrophy and non-myotonic respiratory muscle weakness. Thorax 1986; 41:710 (abstract).
111. Hirshman C, McCullough R, Weil J. Normal value for hypoxic and hypercapnic ventilatory drives in man. *J Appl Physiol* 1975; 38:1095–1098.
112. Rochester DF, Enson Y. Current concepts in the pathogenesis of the obesity–hypoventilation syndrome. *Am J Med* 1974; 57:402–420.
113. White DP, Lombard RM, Cadieux J, et al. Pharyngeal resistance in normal humans: Influence of gender, age, and obesity. *J Appl Physiol* 1985; 58:365–371.
114. Rapaport DM, Sorkin B, Garay SM, et al. Reversal of the "Pickwickian syndrome" by long-term use of nocturnal nasal airway pressure. *N Engl J Med* 1982; 307:931–933.
115. Weil JV, Byrne-Quinn E, Sodal IE, et al. Acquired attenuation of chemoreceptor function in chronically hypoxic man at altitude. *J Clin Invest* 1971; 50:186–194.
116. Guilleminault C, Van den Hoed J, Mitler M. Clinical overview of the sleep apnea syndromes. *In* C Guilleminault, WC Dement (eds). Sleep Apnea Syndromes. New York, Alan R. Liss, 1978, pp 1–11.
117. Roehrs T, Conway W, Wittig R, et al. Sleep–wake complaints in patients with sleep related respiratory disturbances. *Am Rev Respir Dis* 1985; 132:520–523.
118. Bixler E, Kales A, Soldatos C, et al. Sleep apneic activity in a normal population. *Res Commun Chem Pathol Pharmacol* 1982; 36:141–152.

119. Carskadon M, Dement W. Respiration during sleep in the aged human. *J Gerontol* 1981; 36:420–425.
120. Lugaresi E, Coccagna G, Cirignotta F, et al. Breathing during sleep in normal and pathological conditions. *Adv Exp Med Biol* 1978; 99:35–45.
121. Schroeder J, Motta J, Guilleminault C. Hemodynamic studies in sleep apnea. *In* C Guilleminault, WC Dement (eds). Sleep Apnea Syndromes. New York, Alan R. Liss, 1978, pp 177–196.
122. Podszus T, Bauer W, Mayer J, et al. Sleep apnea and pulmonary hypertension. *Klin Wochenschr* 1986; 64:131–134.
123. Bradley TD, Rutherford R, Grossman RE, et al. Role of daytime hypoxemia in the pathogenesis of right heart failure in the obstructive sleep apnea syndrome. *Am Rev Respir Dis* 1985; 131:835–839.
124. Fletcher EC, DeBehnke RD, Lovoi MS, et al. Undiagnosed sleep apnea in patients with essential hypertension. *Ann Intern Med* 1985; 103:190–195.
125. Roth T, Roehrs T, Conway W. Behavioral morbidity of apnea. Semin Respir Med 1988; 9:554–559.
126. Onal E, Lopata M, O'Connor T. Pathogenesis of apnea in hypersomnia-sleep apnea syndrome. *Am Rev Respir Dis* 1982; 125:167–174.
127. Weil J, Kryger M, Scoggin C. Sleep and breathing at high altitude. *In* C Guilleminault, WC Dement (eds). Sleep Apnea Syndromes. New York, Alan R. Liss, 1978, pp 119–136.
128. Lahiri S, Maret K, Sherpa MG. Dependence of high-altitude sleep apnea on ventilatory sensitivity to hypoxia. *Respir Physiol* 1983; 52:281–301.
129. White DP, Gleeson K, Pickett CK, et al. Altitude acclimatization: Influence on periodic breathing and chemoresponses during sleep. *J Appl Physiol* 1987; 63:401–412.
130. Bradley TD, McNicholas WT, Rutherford R, et al. Clinical and physiologic heterogeneity of the central sleep apnea syndrome. *Am Rev Respir Dis* 1986; 134:217–221.
131. Cherniack N. Sleep apnea and its causes *J Clin Invest* 1984; 73:1501–1506.
132. Oren J. Medullary respiratory neuron activity: Relationship to tonic and phasic REM sleep. *J Appl Physiol* 1980; 48:54–65.
133. McNicholas W, Tarlo S, Cole P, et al. Obstructive apneas during sleep in patients with seasonal allergic rhinitis. *Am Rev Respir Dis* 1982; 126: 625–628.
134. Zwillich C, Pickett C, Hanson F, et al. Disturbed sleep and prolonged apnea during nasal obstruction in normal man. *Am Rev Respir Dis* 1981; 124:158–160.
135. Suratt P, Turner B, Wilhoit S. Effect of intranasal obstruction on breathing during sleep. *Chest* 1986; 90:324–329.
136. White DP, Cadieux RJ, Lombard RM, et al. The effects of nasal anesthesia on breathing during sleep. *Am Rev Respir Dis* 1985; 132:972–975.
137. Gleeson K, Zwillich CW, Bendrick TW, et al. The effect of inspiratory nasal loading on pharyngeal patency. *J Appl Physiol* 1986; 60:1882–1886.
138. Issa F, Sullivan C. Reversal of central sleep apnea using nasal CPAP. *Chest* 1986; 90:165–171.
139. Davies AM, Koenig JS, Thach BT. Upper airway chemoreflex responses to saline and water in preterm infants. *J Appl Physiol* 1988; 64:1412–1420.

140. Alex C, Onal E, Lopata M. Upper airway occlusion during sleep in patients with Cheyne-Stokes respiration. *Am Rev Respir Dis* 1986; 133: 42–45.
141. Findley LJ, Zwillich CW, Ancoli-Israel S, et al. Cheyne-Stokes breathing during sleep in patients with left ventricular heart failure. *South Med J* 1985; 78:11–15.
142. Lange R, Hecht H. The mechanism of Cheyne-Stokes respiration. *J Clin Invest* 1962; 41:42–52.
143. Guyton A, Crowell J, Moore J. Basic oscillating mechanism of Cheyne-Stokes breathing. *Am J Physiol* 1979; 187:185–200.
144. Guilleminault C, Briskin J, Greenfield M, et al. The impact of autonomic nervous system dysfunction on breathing during sleep. *Sleep* 1981; 4: 263–278.
145. McNicholas WT, Rutherford R, Grossman R, et al. Abnormal respiratory pattern generation during sleep in patients with autonomic dysfunction. *Am Rev Respir Dis* 1983; 128:429–433.
146. Krieger A, Rosomoff H. Sleep induced apnea: A respiratory and autonomic dysfunction syndrome following bilateral percutaneous cervical cordatomy. *J Neurosurg* 1974; 39:168–180.
147. White D, Miller F, Erickson R. Sleep apnea and nocturnal hypoventilation following western equine encephalitis. *Am Rev Respir Dis* 1983; 127:132–133.
148. Levin B, Margolis G. Acute failure of autonomic respirations secondary to unilateral brainstem infarct. *Ann Neurol* 1977; 1:583–586.

4

The Sleep Apnea Syndrome: Obstructive and Mixed Apneas

Robert D. Ballard, M.D.

The clinical syndrome of sleep apnea has been described in medical literature dating to antiquity.[1] Only during the last three decades have we begun to fully recognize the widespread impact of this disorder. Sleep apnea currently affects 1%–5% of the adult population, frequently resulting in neuropsychological and behavioral consequences such as excessive daytime sleepiness, mood disorders, and cognitive impairment. Other clinical manifestations include pulmonary and systemic hypertension, cor pulmonale, and erythrocytosis. Evidence suggesting that untreated sleep apnea may result in reduced life expectancy has recently begun to accumulate.

The obvious clinical significance of this disorder has triggered increasing efforts to understand its pathophysiology. We now realize that in the sleep apnea syndrome both sleep and respiration are disturbed. The respiratory disturbances consist of sleep-related apneas that can be classified as central, obstructive, or mixed in origin, as determined by the presence or absence of respiratory effort. Obstructive apneas are the predominant respiratory disturbances in a majority of affected patients. In this chapter we will therefore discuss the factors contributing to obstructive and mixed apneas, including the respiratory function, control, and mechanics of the upper airway in both normal subjects and patients with obstructive sleep apnea. We

Martin RJ: Cardiorespiratory Disorders During Sleep, 2nd Edition. Futura Publishing Company, Inc., Mount Kisco, NY, © 1990.

will subsequently discuss various clinical manifestations of the sleep apnea syndrome.

Respiratory Function of the Upper Airway

The upper airway muscles are multifunctional, participating in many essential activities that include swallowing, airway protection, speaking, coughing, and respiration. The respiratory function of the upper airway is influenced by as many as 24 pairs of muscles, acting individually and in concert. The coordination of these muscles is complex in that the mechanical action of an individual muscle at a given moment can be determined by the simultaneous activities of other upper airway muscles. In general these muscles demonstrate phasic respiratory activity, typically with bursts of activity beginning prior to or at the beginning of mechanical inspiration. The net results of this pattern of activity are phasic changes in upper airway dimension such that the airway dilates during inspiration but constricts during expiration. Although we do not yet understand all of the specific sequelae resulting from the individual and coordinated activities of these muscles, we have some knowledge of their contribution to the respiratory function of the upper airway, as outlined in Table 1.

Table 1.
Upper Airway Respiratory Muscle Function

Muscle	*Time of major activity*	*Respiratory function*
Nasal alae	Inspiration	Nasal dilation
Genioglossus	Inspiration, some tonic expiration	Tongue protrusion
Geniohyoid	Inspiration	Ventral retraction of tongue, epiglottis
Tensor palatine	Inspiration, some tonic	Elevation soft palate
Stylopharygeus/ styloglossus	Inspiration	Ventral retraction of mandible
Pharyngeal constrictors	Expiration (? inspiration)	Pharyngeal constriction (? braking)
Posterior cricocarytenoid	Inspiration, decrescendo expiration	Glottic dilation
Thyroarytenoid	Expiration (when active)	Glottic constriction (? braking)

Nasal Dilation

The nasal alae demonstrate inspiratory bursts of activity, resulting in nasal flaring.[2] The resultant decrease in nasal and total airway resistance is substantial[2] and suggests that the nasal alae have a role in the regulation of inspiratory airflow. The potential significance of this function becomes more apparent after considering the magnitude of the contribution of nasal resistance to total airflow resistance.[3]

Pharyngeal Dilation

Several other upper airway muscles demonstrate inspiratory bursts of activity. These include the genioglossus, geniohyoid, tensor palatine, stylopharyngeus, styloglossus, and medial pterygoid.[4–6] The inspiratory activity of these muscles presumably maintains or increases pharyngeal patency in opposition to the negative pharyngeal pressure that accompanies inspiratory airflow and tends to collapse the upper airway.[7]

Pharyngeal Constriction

The superior, middle, and inferior pharyngeal constrictors constitute a thin band of muscle that forms the posterior and lateral walls of the pharynx. Multiple evaluations of the constrictors have suggested bursts of activity during both inspiration and expiration, although this remains uncertain.[8] One potential role for the expiratory activation of these muscles could be the production of pharyngeal "braking" of expiratory airflow.[9]

Laryngeal Abduction

The posterior cricoarytenoid muscle also demonstrates phasic respiratory activity. The inspiratory activity of this muscle results in widening of the glottic aperture and a subsequent reduction in upper airway resistance.[10,11] During expiration there occurs a rapid decrease in posterior cricoarytenoid activity, as shown in Figure 1. This results in a progressive narrowing of the glottic aperture and an increase in

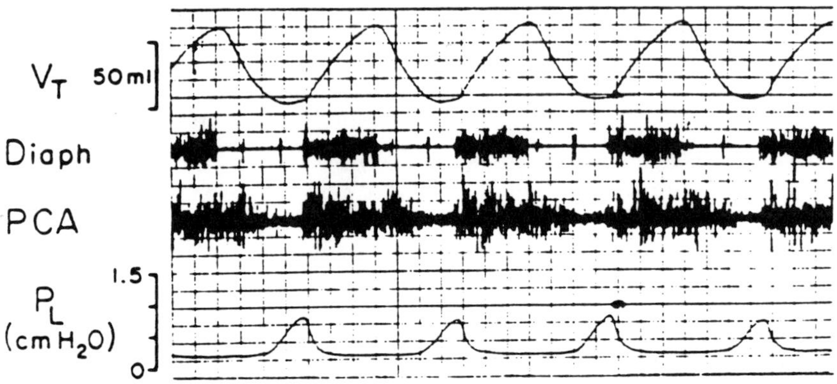

Figure 1. Tracings of tidal volume (V_t), diaphragm EMG (Diaph), posterior cricoarytenoid EMG (PCA) and transpulmonary pressure (P_L) taken during hypercapnic, spontaneous breathing in a cat. (From: reference 10, with permission.)

laryngeal resistance that contributes to expiratory braking and the determination of end-expiratory lung volume.[12,13]

Laryngeal Adduction

The thyroarytenoid muscle is phasically active on expiration during spontaneous breathing in awake humans, as shown in Figure 2.[14] This promotes the expiratory adduction of the vocal cords and contributes to an active laryngeal braking mechanism during expiration. Along with pharyngeal constriction, posterior cricoarytenoid relaxation, and tonic diaphragmatic and thoracic inspiratory muscle activity, this serves to retard expiratory airflow and to actively determine lung volume.[12]

Control of Upper Airway Muscle Activity

Like other respiratory muscles, the upper airway muscles rely upon impulses from the medullary respiratory control center to sustain rhythmic activity. During inspiration, augmenting inspiratory neurons undergo progressive depolarization with subsequent increases in firing rates.[15,16] Impulses from these neurons are transmitted via spinal neurons to inspiratory muscles, including upper airway muscles such as the genioglossus and nasal alae, which then contract to maintain or increase upper airway inspiratory patency. During the

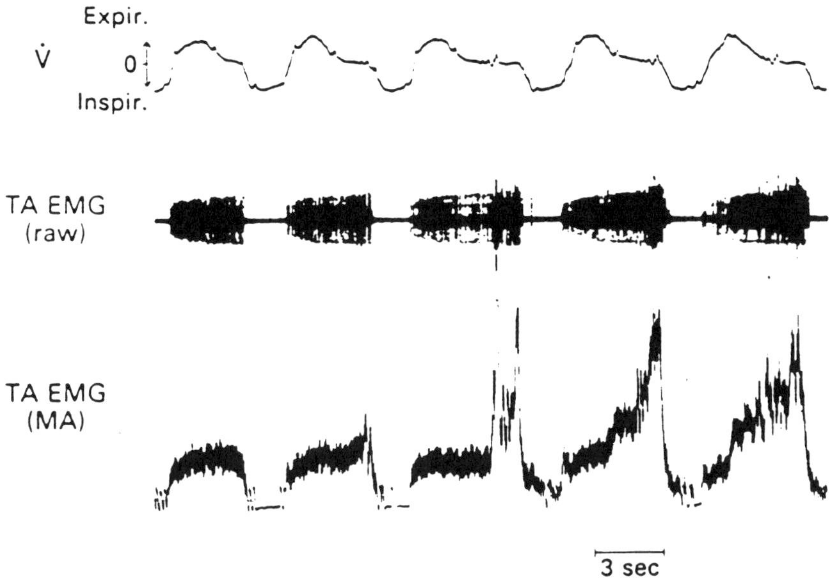

Figure 2. Thyroarytenoid (TA) raw and moving average (MA) EMG patterns during quiet breathing in an awake human. (From: reference 14, with permission.)

early postinspiratory phase, another group of respiratory neurons are immediately active, then fire in a rapidly decrescendo pattern. This occurs in conjunction with progressive decrements in thoracic inspiratory muscle activity and posterior cricoarytenoid activity (Fig. 1). This coordinated progressive decrease in thoracic and laryngeal respiratory muscle activity results in the braking of expiratory airflow.[11,12] During the early postinspiratory phase a third group of respiratory neurons are immediately disfacilitated. Approximately midway through mechanical expiration these neurons begin to progressively depolarize, generating impulses that are presumably transmitted to muscles with predominantly expiratory function, such as internal intercostals and abdominal expiratory muscles.

The muscles of the upper airway are similar to the other respiratory muscles in that their activity is modified in response to various stimuli including hypoxia, hypercapnia, chest wall and intrathoracic mechanical status, and a variety of mechanical stimuli originating from the upper airway itself. Other factors, such as level of consciousness, sedation, respiratory stimulants, hormones, and even body position, have also been shown to significantly alter upper airway muscle activity. To completely understand the pathophysiology of obstructive sleep apnea, it is useful to review the mechanisms responsible for upper airway muscle control, particularly as related to breathing.

Chemostimuli

Hypoxia and hypercapnia have both been observed in awake humans to stimulate electromyographic activity of the genioglossus muscle in a manner qualitatively similar to the response of the diaphragm.[4,17] Similar responses to chemostimuli have been observed from the posterior cricoarytenoid and nasal alae muscles (Fig. 3).[18] Fiberoptic visualization has demonstrated concurrent augmentation of respiratory motion of the glottis in response to both hypoxia and hypercapnia.[19] However, as we will discuss later, there is evi-

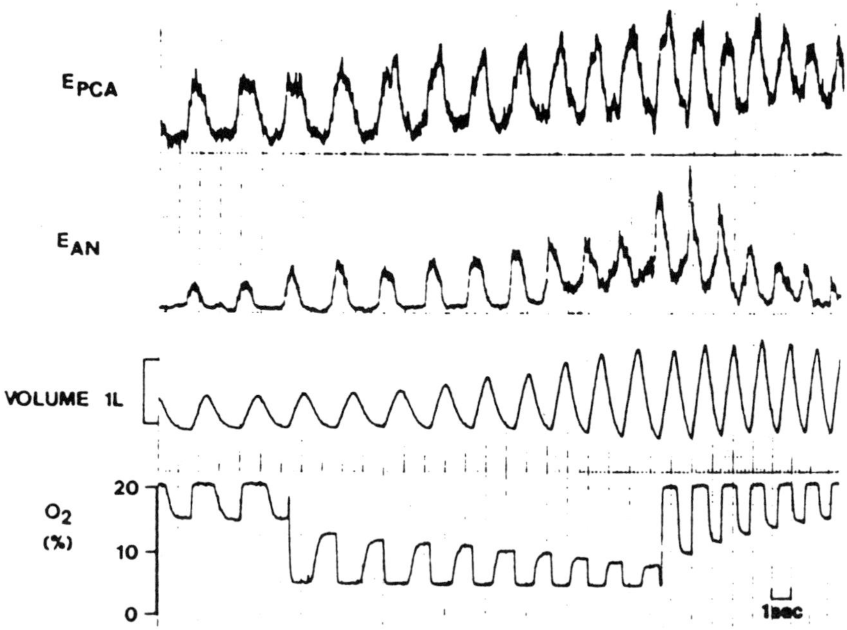

Figure 3. Integrated EMG activity of the posterior cricoarytenoid (E_{PCA}) and nasal alae (E_{AN}) muscles, tidal volume, and O_2 saturation during progressive isocapnic hypoxia in an awake human. (From: reference 18, with permission.)

dence that general anesthesia[20] and sleep[21,22] may disassociate the chemoregulatory response of the diaphragm and upper airway.

Pulmonary Proprioception

The upper airway muscles also respond to the inspiratory inhibiting and expiratory facilitating activities of pulmonary stretch receptors.[23,24] As shown in Figure 4, phasic inspiratory activity of the genioglossus is inhibited by lung inflation, an effect that is abolished after vagotomy. Airway occlusion produces augmentation of genioglossus activity on the first occluded inspiration, also an effect that is abolished after vagotomy (Fig. 5).[24] Furthermore, laryngeal motoneurons also receive proprioceptive feedback from intercostal muscle afferents, evidently inhibiting posterior cricoarytenoid inspiratory activity while augmenting thyroarytenoid expiratory activity.[25]

Upper Airway Stimuli

Recent investigations have established the presence of mechanoreceptors in the mucosa of the nasal cavity, pharynx, and larynx that respond to a variety of stimuli, including changes in intraluminal pressure, airflow, temperature, and upper airway muscle tone itself.[26–29] There is substantial evidence that sensory input from these receptors alters upper airway muscle activity in a reflex fashion. For example, negative upper airway pressure has been shown to increase genioglossus muscle activity in a rabbit model, an effect that can be blocked by topical anesthesia or section of the superior laryngeal nerve.[30,31] In the same model, diversion of respiratory airflow from the upper airway via a tracheostomy resulted in pharyngeal occlusion.[32] Phasic intrapharyngeal pressure changes subsequently restored patency to the upper airway, but this effect could also be abolished by topical pharyngeal anesthesia. Finally, studies of conscious and sleeping dogs have also demonstrated that upper airway pressure-sensitive receptors can reflexly augment genioglossus muscle activity.[33,34]

Studies of humans have produced more variable findings regarding the upper airway's sensory input into its own respiratory function. Topical nasal and oropharyngeal anesthesia have been shown to compromise patency of the upper airway in sleeping[35–37] and awake[37] humans. Laryngeal anesthesia also apparently interferes with the dilatory function of human upper airway muscles,[38] an effect that in anesthetized dogs was associated with reductions in superior laryngeal nerve activity.

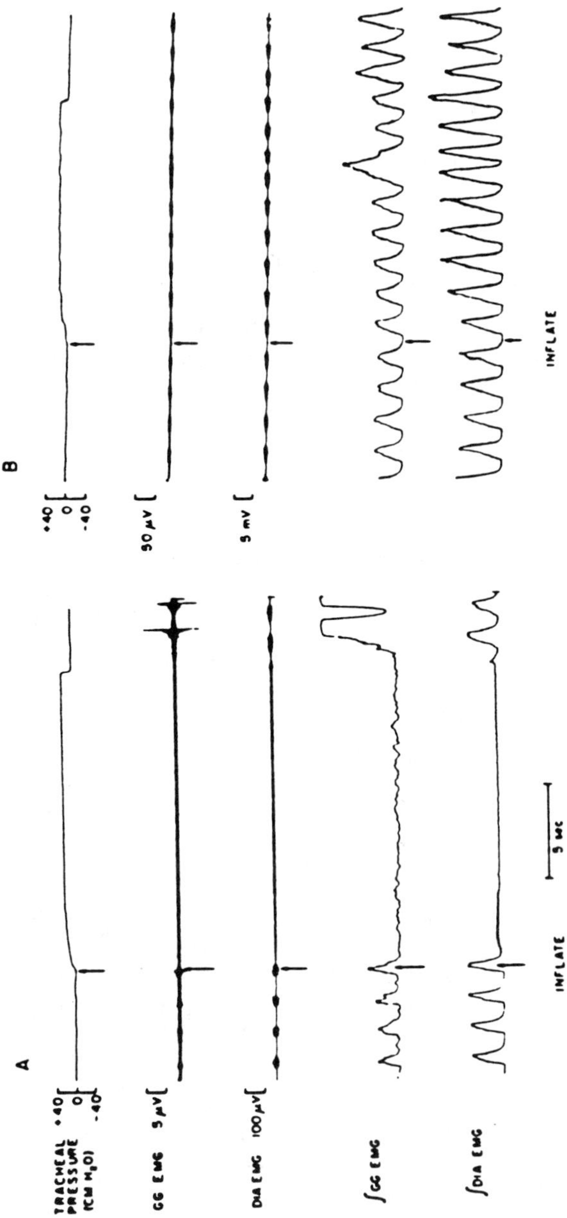

Figure 4. Effect of lung inflation on genioglossus (GG) and diaphragm (DIA) raw and integrated EMG activity before (A) and after (B) vagotomy in a rabbit. (From: reference 24, with permission.)

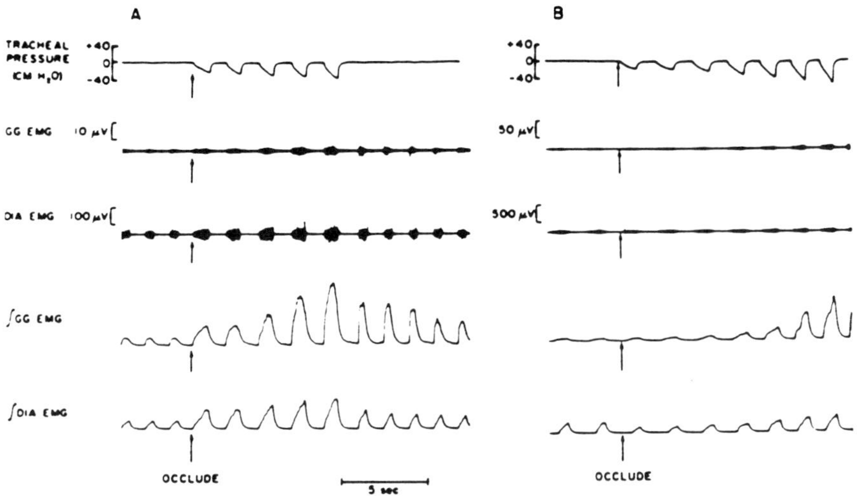

Figure 5. Effect of airway occlusion on genioglossus (GG) and diaphragm (DIA) raw and integrated EMG activity before (A) and after (B) vagotomy in a rabbit. (From: reference 24, with permission.).

On the other hand, studies of laryngectomized human subjects[39,40] and subjects with topically anesthetized upper airways[39] have revealed only minor contributions from upper airway sensory receptors to the ventilatory responses of either upper airway or thoracic respiratory muscles to hypercapnia and resistive inspiratory loading. These studies did, however, reemphasize the important contributions already discussed of chemostimuli and pulmonary proprioceptive feedback to the control of upper airway muscle activity.

Upper Airway Mechanics

Upper airway resistance typically constitutes about half the total airflow resistance in humans.[41] The major portion of upper airway resistance is contributed by the nasal cavity and remains relatively constant,[3] while the contributions of the pharynx and larynx are usually smaller. However, pharyngeal and laryngeal resistances are more variable for reasons primarily related to the respiratory function of the upper airway muscles, as already discussed. Phasic changes in upper airway muscle activity typically reduce inspiratory pharyngeal and laryngeal resistances that subsequently increase during expiration

This phasic pattern of activity can be modified in response to various stimuli, as already discussed, and is particularly affected by level of consciousness as we will discuss.

Other factors also influence upper airway resistance. For example, moving from the upright to the supine position significantly increases upper airway resistance[42] and decreases pharyngeal cross-sectional area.[43,44] This effect may be partly mediated by position dependent decrements in lung volume that can also be associated with increases in upper airway resistance[45] and decreased pharyngeal cross-sectional area.[46] However, other evidence suggests that the effect of position change is independent of associated changes in lung volume. Fouke and Strohl[44] used a continuous negative pressure cuirass to restore end-expiratory lung volume in the supine position to that previously measured in the upright position. This did not alter the supine reduction in cross-sectional area at any point along the upper airway.

Head position is another important determinant of upper airway patency. In the supine position flexion of the neck clearly increased upper airway resistance in conscious humans[47] and often completely occluded the pharynx in anesthetized humans.[48] Full extension of the neck significantly improved upper airway patency over the flexed and neutral positions. Additional findings suggested that body weight was an important factor in the flexion–extension determination of upper airway patency, as 95% of subjects with normal body weight but only 33% of obese subjects had a patent upper airway with the neck fully extended.[48] Finally, radiographic evaluation of the upper airway in supine anesthetized subjects by Safar et al. demonstrated a major role of the relapsing tongue in causing pharyngeal occlusion.[48]

Although nasal resistance is typically less variable than pharyngeal and laryngeal resistances, it can also be modified by position change. Anch et al.[42] found that the increase in upper airway resistance observed when changing from the upright to the supine position can be partially prevented by administration of nasal decongestants. This suggests that vascular congestion of the nasal mucosa may occur in the supine position and may contribute substantially to position-dependent changes in upper airway resistance. There is further evidence that other causes of increased nasal congestion, such as seasonal allergic rhinitis,[49] nasal polyps, and septal deviation[77] can either transiently or more chronically increase nasal and therefore total upper airway resistance.

Function of the Upper Airway during Sleep

It has been suggested that during wakefulness breathing is under the influence of a tonic excitatory input commonly referred to as the "wakefulness stimulus" or waking neural drive to ventilation.[50] With onset of sleep and loss of this tonic excitatory input, a reduction in chemical control and loss of voluntary control of breathing, there occurs a reduction in the spontaneous activity of respiratory muscles. The upper airway muscles clearly participate in this sleep-associated global reduction in respiratory activity. The sleep-associated reduction in genioglossus muscle activity allows pharyngeal narrowing and even occlusion in susceptible patients (Fig. 6).[7,51] Other studies revealed a sleep-associated decrease in inspiratory and expiratory posterior cricoarytenoid activity with a subsequent increase in upper air-

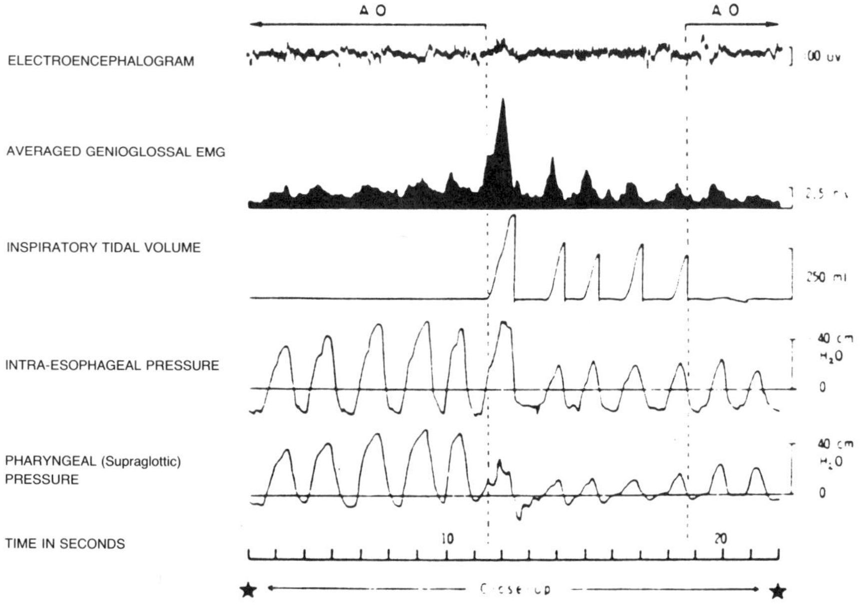

Figure 6. Tracings of EEG, genioglossal EMG, tidal volume, intraesophageal and pharyngeal pressures taken from an intermittently sleeping obstructive sleep apnea patient. Note that in the absence of alpha activity (i.e., with sleep onset) genioglossal activity decreases, allowing airway occlusion (AO) (From: reference 7, with permission.)

way resistance.[52–54] The respiratory activity of the thyroarytenoid muscle also has been observed to decrease with onset of sleep,[14] an effect that may counterbalance the increased expiratory laryngeal resistance anticipated with the decrease in posterior cricoarytenoid activity.

It is apparent from these studies and from our knowledge of the respiratory function of the upper airway muscles that their sleep-associated global reduction in respiratory activity compromises their ability to maintain upper airway patency. One recent study has clearly demonstrated in a dog model that the combined forces responsible for dilating the upper airway during wakefulness are reduced during slow-wave and REM sleep.[55] This probably accounts for the detection of sleep-associated increments in upper airway resistance.[7,41,52,53,56,57]

It is also apparent that the reduction in upper airway muscle activity is most significant during REM sleep. During REM sleep there appears to be ongoing activity of central respiratory neurons, but there occurs a reduction in afferent input[58] and apparent postsynaptic inhibition[59] that inhibits or even eliminates upper airway muscle activity. Although this additional reduction in respiratory activity does not necessarily further increase upper airway resistance to airflow,[41] it may have pronounced effects on pharyngeal compliance and the ability to maintain a patent pharynx in the presence of intraluminal negative pressure.

Upper Airway Responses to Stimuli during Sleep

Although ventilatory responses to hypoxia and hypercapnia clearly persist during sleep, they are substantially decreased when compared to wakefulness.[60,61] Upper airway muscle responses to chemostimuli also persist during sleep, although they may differ from those of the diaphragm. Parisi et al.[22] detected in unanesthetized goats a hypercapnic threshold for inspiratory activation of the genioglossus by CO_2 that was unaffected by sleep state except during REM sleep when genioglossus activity was markedly inhibited. This resulted in reduced genioglossus activity relative to the diaphragm during eupnea and mild hypercapnia. In a subsequent study,[62] the same authors demonstrated a hypoxic threshold for the activation of the genioglossus that was again unaffected by sleep state except during

REM sleep when goats aroused (at very low oxygen saturations) prior to genioglossus activation.

As previously described, Onal and associates[4,17] found a linear relationship between the electrical phasic activities of the genioglossus and diaphragm in response to hypoxia and hypercapnia in awake humans. Hudgel et al.[21] have more recently demonstrated a nonlinear relationship between upper airway and chest wall inspiratory muscle electrical activity during periodic breathing in sleep. Of interest, this nonlinear relationship between the activity levels of the two muscle groups was associated with fluctuations in upper airway resistance, such that resistance increased when the ratio between upper airway and chest wall EMG activity decreased below a critical level (Fig. 7).

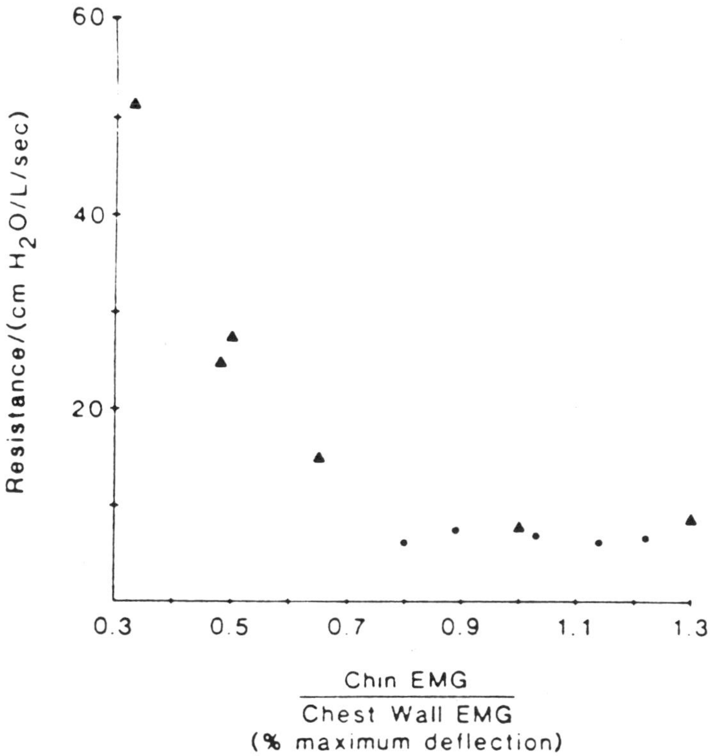

Figure 7. The effect on upper airway resistance from reductions in the ratio of chin EMG activity to chest wall EMG activity. Data obtained from sleeping periodically breathing humans. (From: reference 21, with permission.)

These findings are consistent with previous observations from anesthetized and naturally sleeping animals[22,62,63] and, as discussed later, may have important implications for the pathogenesis of sleep apnea.

The responses of respiratory muscles to resistive loading and even occlusion are also diminished in the presence of sleep.[34,64–66] This includes the responses of upper airway muscles[64] such as the genioglossus muscle.[34,67] Studies in a dog model comparing the genioglossus responses to both nasal and tracheal airway occlusions suggest that the previously mentioned upper airway mechanoreceptors may contribute more to the remaining upper airway muscle response to occlusion during sleep than lung/chest wall proprioception.[34] Such a preferential response to upper airway as opposed to lung/chest wall mechanoreceptors differs from previous observations of awake humans.[39,40] This suggests either a difference between animal and human responses or a specific effect of sleep on responses to lung/chest wall proprioception.

Upper Airway Mechanics during Sleep

After considering the substantial impact of sleep on upper airway muscle resting function and responses to various stimuli, one would expect sleep to also significantly affect upper airway mechanics. It has subsequently been demonstrated that with onset of sleep and concurrent with the sleep-associated reduction in upper airway respiratory activity, there occurs a significant increase in upper airway resistance.[41,68] As this increase in resistance was detected above the larynx and no sleep-associated increase in total nasal resistance was observed,[3] the site of increased resistance is localized primarily to the pharynx. Such an increase in pharyngeal resistance likely signifies a reduction in pharyngeal luminal size due to the inability of less active upper airway muscles to maintain pharyngeal patency during sleep.[7,55] This concept is lent support by the observations of Wiegand et al. that extrinsic inspiratory resistive loading may increase upper airway resistance more during non-REM sleep than during wakefulness, suggesting an increase in upper airway collapsibility during sleep.[68] In a similar study, Schwartz et al. were able to totally collapse the upper airways of normal subjects during non-REM sleep via the application of subatmospheric nasal pressure.[69] These findings underscore the significant implications of such sleep-associated reductions in upper airway dilator muscle activity.

Obstructive Sleep Apnea

In a significant portion of the population onset of sleep is associated with occlusion of the upper airway, resulting in the cessation of airflow despite ongoing ventilatory efforts. Cessations of airflow lasting at least 10 seconds in the presence of continuous ventilatory effort are usually referred to as obstructive apneas.[70] Each apnea results in progressive asphyxiation until an arousal from sleep occurs with a subsequent restoration of upper airway patency and airflow. A patient will then usually return to sleep quickly, resulting in another occlusion of the upper airway. In the more severe cases, this cycle may repeat itself hundreds of times each night, resulting in severely disturbed sleep, prolonged hypoxia and hypercapnia, and a variety of behavioral sequelae and clinical manifestations, as we will later discuss.

Pathogenesis of Obstructive and Mixed Apneas

As the majority of people maintain a patent upper airway during sleep and affected individuals clearly maintain airway patency while awake, much attention has been focused on differences between the upper airways of normals and obstructive sleep apnea patients. As already discussed, there is also increasing interest in the effect of sleep on upper airway function. From observations made in these areas have arisen several hypotheses about the pathogenesis of obstructive sleep apnea.

One increasingly plausible theory is demonstrated in Figure 8. With onset of sleep there occurs a reduction in the spontaneous activity of upper airway respiratory muscles[7,14,51–54], as already described. While in most subjects this is associated with only a small increase in upper airway resistance,[41,68] in affected individuals total occlusion of the upper airway occurs. Airway collapse therefore likely occurs as a result of the reduced ability of less active upper airway dilator muscles to oppose the collapsing tendency associated with negative intraluminal inspiratory pressures.

What factors predispose the airways of obstructive sleep apnea patients to collapse remains a focus of investigation. We have long recognized that a minority of affected patients have obvious anatomic abnormalities of the upper airway such as adenotonsillar hypertrophy,[71,72] micrognathia and retrognathia,[73,74] macroglossia,[75,76] and nasal septal deviation.[77] Presumably such pathologic abnormalities

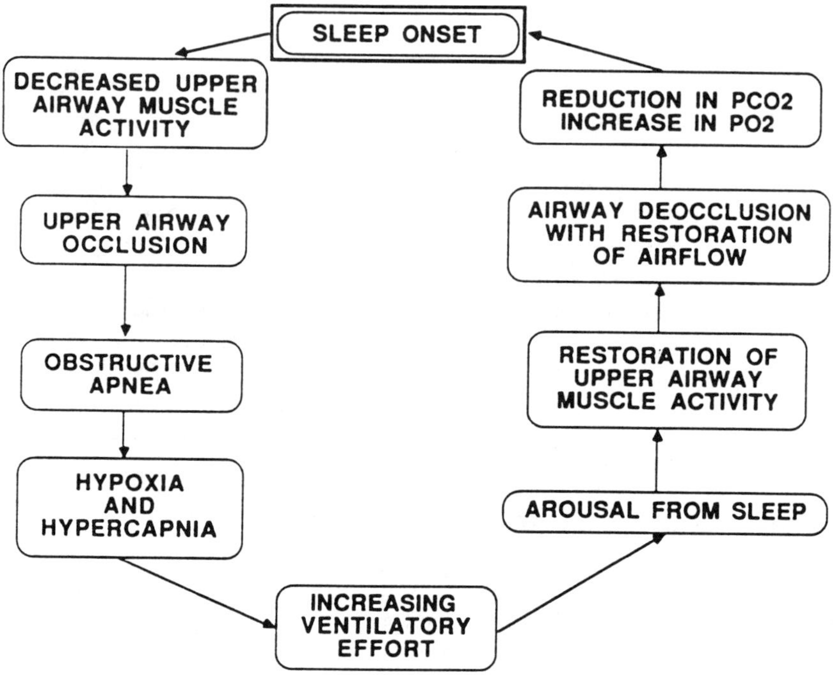

Figure 8. Proposed mechanism for the cyclic recurrence of obstructive apneas during sleep.

result in a narrowing of the upper airway that may promote occlusion of the involved segment (Bernoulli effect). Alternatively, to achieve airflow, such narrowing necessitates increasingly negative inspiratory pressures that may result in the collapse of upstream segments of the upper airway.

However, the majority of patients with obstructive sleep apnea on clinical examination do not have such obvious anatomic abnormalities. Using multiple different techniques, evaluations of such patients have often demonstrated more subtle narrowing of the oropharyngeal lumen. CT scanning of the upper airway revealed reduced pharyngeal cross-sectional area in obstructive sleep apnea patients when compared to unmatched controls,[78,79] and the reduction in pharyngeal size correlated with the severity of obstructive sleep apnea. When Stauffer et al. compared CT scans from the upper airways of affected patients with age- and weight-matched controls, they were unable to find differences in pharyngeal cross-sectional area between patients and controls.[80] They did observe that pharyngeal airflow resistance was significantly higher in the patients and that this measure correlated with the apnea–hypopnea index.[80] Acoustic reflectance measurements of pharyngeal area also demonstrated reduced pharyngeal cross-sectional area in obstructive sleep apnea patients when compared to matched controls,[46,81] a measurement that again correlated with the apnea–hypopnea index.

The cause of the reduced upper airway lumen in affected patients is not often apparent. Although many patients with obstructive sleep apnea are obese,[82] several studies have been unable to demonstrate via CT scanning excessive fatty infiltration of the pharyngeal walls.[78,79,83] However, external compression of the upper airway by an obese neck seems to be a reasonable alternative mechanism. Koenig and Thach recently demonstrated in a rabbit model that extrinsic mass loading of the upper airway caused changes in airway configuration and function similar to those seen in obstructive sleep apnea.[84] Finally, there are some reports that pharyngeal cross-sectional area decreases with reductions in lung volume,[46,85] suggesting that obesity reduces upper airway patency through associated reductions in functional residual capacity (FRC), especially in the supine position. However, as already noted, Fouke and Strohl found that changes in FRC had no effect on pharyngeal cross-sectional area in supine normals.[44] The exact relationship between obesity and upper airway patency therefore remains uncertain.

Other studies have evaluated craniofacial structure for contributions to upper airway narrowing. Cephalometric roentgenography has frequently revealed a small mandible that may have a slight posterior placement[86,87] and a displacement of the hyoid bone to a lower position than normal.[87] These changes may constitute a structural basis for airway narrowing in that they are associated with a reduction in the width of the posterior airway space and are a significant predictor of the severity of obstructive sleep apnea.[88]

Not only do obstructive sleep apnea patients have narrowing of the pharynx, but they also have an increase in pharyngeal compliance. Brown et al. demonstrated that the application of positive intrapharyngeal pressure results in a greater increase in pharyngeal area in obstructive sleep apnea patients than in control subjects.[43] In a similar fashion, Suratt et al. found that the application of subatmospheric pressure could completely collapse the pharyngeal airway in a majority of obstructive sleep apnea patients but could only partially collapse the airway in only a few control subjects.[89] These observations suggest that the pharyngeal walls of affected patients may be excessively "floppy" and therefore more easily collapsible than in normals.

Patients with obstructive sleep apnea are thus likely to have smaller, more compliant, and therefore more collapsible upper airways. To maintain adequate upper airway patency in such patients even while awake could require increased upper airway dilator muscle activity.[90,91] With the onset of sleep and its associated decrement in respiratory muscle activity, a reduction in pharyngeal patency or even complete upper airway occlusion may result in predisposed individuals. Recent evidence suggests that such sleep-associated airway occlusions most frequently occur in the region posterior to the palate or in the hypopharynx,[79,92] sites at which normal subjects also demonstrate substantial sleep-associated inspiratory narrowing.[93]

Returning to Figure 8, the subsequent obstructive apnea results in progressive and sometimes profound hypoxia and hypercapnia. The severity of hypoxemia developing during obstructive sleep apnea can vary significantly from one patient to another, apparently as determined by such factors as duration and frequency of apneas, awake Po_2, and lung volume.[94,95] These apnea-associated changes in Po_2 and Pco_2 stimulate ventilation, resulting in increasing inspiratory efforts (Fig. 9). Eventually the progressive hypoxemia and hypercapnia[60,61] and/or the associated increase in inspiratory effort[96] result in arousal of the patient (Fig. 9). With this usually transient arousal occurs augmentation of upper airway dilator muscle activity to an extent proportionately greater than the simultaneous augmentation of diaphragm activity.[7,97] This leads to deocclusion of the pharynx and restoration of airflow. During the subsequent brief period of ventilation, Po_2 rises and Pco_2 falls. However, the rapid resumption of sleep results in reocclusion of the upper airway. This cycle of events may therefore recur hundreds of times each night, triggering recurrent arousals that may contribute to many of the clinical features of obstructive sleep apnea, as we shall discuss.

It has been alternatively proposed that recurrent apneas of either the obstructive or central type could be caused either by sleep-associated instabilities in the feedback control of ventilation or by spontaneous oscillations in the ventilatory control system.[98,99] Onal et al. observed parallel, periodic fluctuations in genioglossus and diaphragm activities in sleeping obstructive sleep apnea patients.[97] They noted that obstructive apneas occurred at the nadir of these cyclic changes along with mixed apneas (cessation of ventilatory effort followed by resumption of ventilatory effort against an obstructed upper

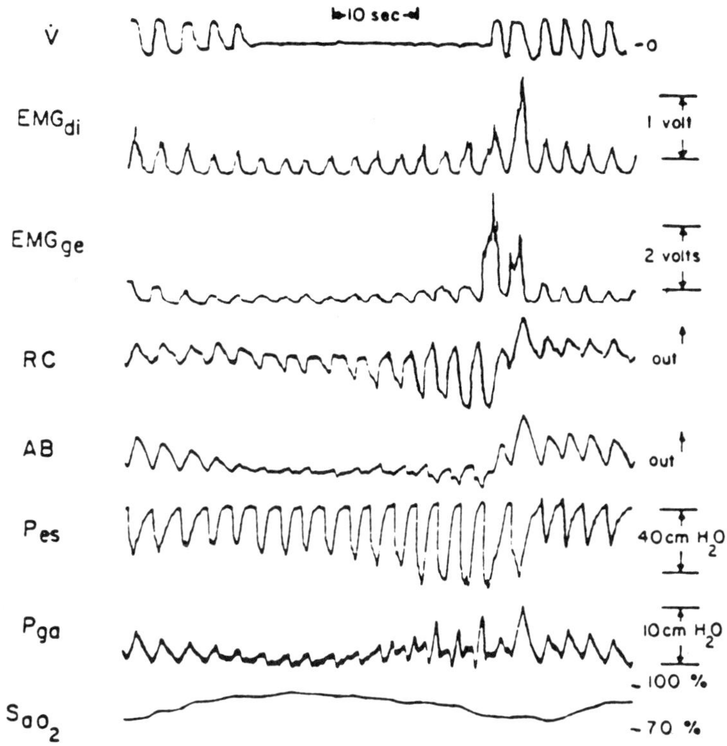

Figure 9. Increasing diaphragmatic (EMG_{di}) and genioglossus (EMG_{ge}) respiratory activity in the presense of progressive O_2 desaturation (SaO_2) during an obstructive apnea. Note that after the termination of the apnea as SaO_2 rises, EMG_{di} and EMG_{ge} decrease. (From: reference 97, with permission.)

airway), which they proposed to represent an extreme of this periodicity. More recently, Chapman et al. have observed spontaneous ventilatory oscillations in sleeping normals, noting that such oscillations could be converted to periodic breathing via augmentation of control system gain by artificially increasing the effect of ventilation on Sao_2.[100] Hypoxia-induced periodic breathing in normal subjects[101] and in snorers[102] has been observed to cause obstructive apneas and hypopneas at the nadirs of inspiratory muscle activity. These upper airway obstructions are presumably due to an excessive reduction in upper airway muscle activity relative to chest wall/diaphragm activity at the nadir of ventilatory effort.[7,21,24] Such evidence suggests that instabilities of ventilatory control may result in upper airway occlusion, especially in subjects with narrowing or increased compliance of the upper airway. This theory does not exclude our previous hypothesis (Fig. 8), and it seems likely that both mechanisms may play important roles in the pathogenesis of obstructive apneas.

As already noted, mixed apneas are also cessations of airflow lasting at least 10 seconds.[70] Mixed apneas are most typically central (no ventilatory effort) initially, followed by an obstructive component (resumption of ventilatory effort against an occluded upper airway). Mixed apneas were most often observed by Onal et al. at the nadirs of respiratory muscle activity in sleeping, periodically breathing, obstructive sleep apnea patients.[97] To better understand the potential mechanism of this association, we should consider the observations of Weiner et al.,[63] who observed in anesthetized dogs that the response of upper airway respiratory muscles to chemical stimuli had a different time course than the response of the diaphragm. That is, during passive hyperventilation, hypoglossal nerve activity ceased prior to the cessation of phrenic nerve activity and then did not return following the posthyperventilation apnea until after phrenic nerve activity had resumed. An analogous sequence of events has been demonstrated in sleeping, periodically breathing humans.[21] Thus, the resumption of diaphragm inspiratory activity at the conclusion of a "central" apnea may cause a reduction in intraluminal pressure that could collapse the upper airway until adequate upper airway dilator muscle activity returns, resulting in a mixed apnea. It therefore seems likely that sleep-associated instability of ventilatory control in conjunction with mismatching of upper airway muscle and diaphragm activity may result in mixed as well as obstructive apneas.

Clinical Manifestations of Obstructive Sleep Apnea

Although exact estimates of the prevalence of obstructive sleep apnea remain unavailable, current knowledge suggests it to be a common clinical problem, occurring in 1%–5% of the adult population.[103,104] It predominates in the male gender, with a male-to-female ratio of between 3:1 and 20:1.[82,105,106]

The role of gender remains uncertain, although it may relate to the observations that normal men have higher pharyngeal resistance than women and that only in men does pharyngeal resistance increase with age and obesity[107] while pharyngeal cross-sectional area decreases.[108] Alternatively, it has been observed that the prevalence of sleep-disordered breathing approaches that of males in postmenopausal women.[109] This suggests that hormones present in premenopausal women (such as progesterone) might be protective against sleep apnea. Progesterone therapy has been found to have utility in only the male patients with associated hypoventilation and hypercapnia.[110] However, a more recent study reported notable success in treating affected postmenopausal women with a combination of progesterone and estrogen,[111] reinforcing the concept that gender differences may be hormonally determined. Additional support for the potential role of sex hormones is derived from the observations that testosterone administration to hypogonadal males may result in substantial worsening of sleep apnea.[112]

Obstructive sleep apnea becomes more prevalent with age, peaking in the fifth and sixth decades. This would be anticipated in females, as we have already noted that sleep-disordered breathing increases after menopause.[109] In males the increasing prevalence with age may be related to the associated increases in pharyngeal resistance[107] and decreases in pharyngeal cross-sectional area.[108] As elderly subjects typically have reduced hypoxic/hypercapnic ventilatory responses that suggest a reduction in respiratory control system gain, it seems unlikely that sleep-associated instabilities in the feedback control of ventilation could account for the prevalence of obstructive sleep apnea in the elderly.[98]

Obstructive sleep apnea is therefore a disease predominantly, although not exclusively, of overweight, middle-aged to elderly males. Affected patients usually exhibit a preponderance of obstructive and mixed apneas.[82] As these apneas become more frequent and of longer duration, patients will be more likely to have clinically obvious manifestations of the disease.[113] In Table 2 we have listed, in

Table 2.
Signs and Symptoms of Obstructive Sleep Apnea

Signs	*Symptoms*
Obesity	Altered sleep behavior (snoring, agitation)
Male sex	Excessive daytime sleepiness
Hypertension	Intellectual deterioration
Cardiac arrhythmias	Personality, mood changes
Pulmonary hypertension	Morning headaches
Cor pulmonale	Sexual impotence
Erythrocytosis	Symptoms of heart failure (exertional dyspnea, decreased exercise tolerance

order of prevalence, the major symptoms and signs of adult patients presenting with obstructive sleep apnea.[99] To discuss these manifestations, we will divide them into cardiorespiratory and neuropsychological consequences.

Cardiorespiratory Consequences of Obstructive Sleep Apnea

Progressive asphyxia occurs during obstructive apneas, leading to at times profound hypoxia and hypercapnia. Pulmonary vasoconstriction with elevation of pulmonary artery pressure in response to apnea-associated hypoxia has been well-documented.[114,115] Such transient responses have been implicated in the development of sustained pulmonary hypertension and right ventricular failure,[114,116] presumably via chronic vascular remodeling. This occurs in 10%–15% of all sleep apnea patients. More recent evidence has suggested that the development of sustained pulmonary hypertension in obstructive sleep apnea patients also requires sustained daytime hypoxemia and is therefore more likely to be seen in affected patients with additional pulmonary disease such as diffuse obstructive airways disease.[117,118] Erythrocytosis evidently also requires the presence of persistent daytime hypoxemia before developing in obstructive apnea patients.[119]

Systemic artery pressure has also been observed to rise during obstructive apneas,[114,120] typically normalizing upon resolution of the apnea. However, persistent systemic hypertension may subsequently develop in some patients independent of their daytime gas exchange, ventilatory status, or obesity.[114,120] In fact, several recent studies have demonstrated a high incidence of sleep apnea in male hypertension patients.[121,122] These studies and other reports[120,123] have suggested that systemic hypertension often improves after effective therapy of the sleep apnea. Therefore, persistent systemic hypertension appears to be a documented sequela of obstructive sleep apnea, although the mechanisms underlying this association remain unknown.

Obstructive apneas have also been observed to influence cardiac rate and rhythm. Vagally mediated slowing of the heart has been commonly observed,[114,123,124] an effect apparently triggered by the apnea-associated hypoxemia.[125] Although periods of sinus arrest and atrioventricular block lasting more than 10 seconds have been reported, such extremes are uncommon and of uncertain pathologic significance. Although ventricular ectopy, including ventricular tachycardia, has also been observed in association with obstructive apneas,[124] premature ventricular contractions are most commonly encountered.[126] The cause of such ventricular ectopy has not been clearly established, although it may be related to the severity of arterial desaturation[126] and may also be more common in patients with co-existing coronary artery disease.[119] Despite its association with cardiac arrhythmias, the prevalence of serious arrhythmias in obstructive sleep apnea patients is apparently less than originally thought,[127,128] placing relatively few patients at risk.

However, evidence has recently begun to accumulate that untreated obstructive sleep apnea is associated with increased mortality. Partinen et al. observed a 5-year vascular mortality that was increased in untreated compared to tracheostomized obstructive sleep apnea patients.[129] Another retrospective study suggested that sleep apnea patients with apnea indices greater than 20 had a higher mortality than patients with apnea indices less than 20.[130] Although a third retrospective study was unable to show survival differences between obstructive sleep apnea patients and controls,[131] this study may have been flawed by inadequate population size. Pending the validation of these findings through a prospective study, we suspect that mortality is increased in untreated obstructive sleep apnea, although a relationship of disease severity to mortality remains uncertain.

Neurophysiological Consequences of Obstructive Sleep Apnea

Snoring is currently the most common cause of referral for sleep evaluation.[132] Snoring occurs as a result of reductions in upper airway patency in affected patients and is therefore not actually a consequence but rather a symptom of obstructive sleep apnea. The most typical pattern is that of recurrent periods of silence (apnea) alternating with explosive snoring during resumption of ventilation. In one survey of 200 consecutive obstructive sleep apnea patients, 100% reported nocturnal snoring.[132] The same survey determined that snoring had been present in 68% of the patients by their early twenties, noting that the symptomatology of obstructive sleep apnea increased in parallel with the intensity of snoring. Another preliminary study has demonstrated that the loudness of snoring can exceed 65 dB, above the noise levels considered safe in the workplace by OSHA.[132] It is therefore not surprising that obstructive sleep apnea patients often present for initial evaluation only after the strong encouragement of their spouse or other family members.

In addition to loud snoring during sleep, affected patients often demonstrate nocturnal restlessness and abnormal motor activity.[133] These bursts of activity are typically associated with the frequent arousals triggered by the recurrent apneas. They therefore most likely represent a waking response to the prior apnea-associated asphyxia. Such abnormal sleep behavior also frequently leads to a spouse's strong encouragement that the affected patient seek medical evaluation.

The recurrent, postapnea arousals result in the fragmentation of sleep and a reduction or loss of slow-wave and REM sleep. The majority of obstructive sleep apnea patients are unaware of the severity of their sleep disruption, but the frequent result is excessive daytime sleepiness.[99,132,133] Daytime sleepiness may be mild and manifest only by falling asleep while reading or watching television. Alternatively, affected patients may become pathologically hypersomnolent and therefore unable to perform daily activities such as working or driving automobiles.[134] Although clearly there is a relationship between the degree of sleep disruption and the severity of daytime sleepiness,[133,135,136] some studies have revealed substantial variability in the severity of daytime symptoms in patients with similar nocturnal respiratory and sleep patterns.[137,138] This suggests that we do not yet fully comprehend all factors that may contribute to the hypersomnolence of sleep apnea. Other factors that could potentially modify daytime symptomatology include the severity of apnea-associated hypoxia and hypercapnia and their effect on cerebral function. However, recent studies determined that the acute and chronic administration of nocturnal oxygen to obstructive sleep apnea patients did not improve daytime hypersomnolence.[139,140]

It seems likely that sleep disruption and daytime sleepiness account for other daytime symptoms of sleep apnea such as intellectual deterioration, personality changes, hallucinations, and automatic behavior,[103,105,132] although there is some evidence that recurrent episodes of apnea-associated hypoxia may also contribute to these symptoms.[141] Obstructive sleep apnea patients also frequently demonstrate somatic–neurotic personality traits that may contribute to cognitive dysfunction and memory deficits.[142] It is therefore apparent that the neuropsychological sequelae of obstructive sleep apnea may lead to substantial psychosocial problems and interfere with the affected patient's ability to achieve a normal lifestyle.[142]

Summary

Obstructive sleep apnea therefore most likely represents the interaction of sleep-associated changes in respiratory function with a predisposed, anatomically narrowed upper airway. This sets in motion a recurring cycle of sleep-associated upper airway occlusions followed by transient arousals with airway deocclusion. The cardiorespiratory and neuropsychological sequelae of such recurrent obstructive and/or mixed apneas may be attributable to the apnea-associated asphyxiation and sleep disruption, although the relative contributions of each and, perhaps, other factors remain unknown. Obstructive sleep apnea is therefore an important contributor to cardiovascular morbidity, neuropsychological dysfunction, and even mortality in the affected populations. Despite the obvious clinical significance of sleep apnea and a recent explosion of investigation into its mechanisms and consequences, our understanding of this disorder remains relatively primitive. A more complete understanding of the pathophysiology of sleep-associated respiratory disorders is necessary for the development of new, more effective strategies for therapeutic intervention.

References

1. Kryger MH. Sleep apnea, from the needles of Dionysius to continuous positive airway pressure. *Arch Intern Med* 1983; 143:2301–2303.
2. Strohl KP, O'Cain CF, Slutsky AS. Alae nasi activation and nasal resistance in healthy subjects. *J Appl Physiol* 1982; 52:1432–1437.
3. Hudgel DW, Robertson DW. Nasal resistance during wakefulness and sleep in normal man. *Acta Otolaryngol* 1984; 98:130–135.
4. Onal E, Lopata M, O'Connor TD. Diaphragmatic and genioglossal electromyogram responses to CO_2 rebreathing in humans. *J Appl Physiol* 1981; 50:1052–1055.
5. Rodenstein DO, Stanescu DC. The soft palate and breathing. *Am Rev Respir Dis* 1986; 134:311–325.
6. Sauerland EK, Mitchell SP. Electromyographic activity of intrinsic and extrinsic muscles of the human tongue. *Tex Rep Biol Med* 1975; 33:445–455.
7. Remmers JE, deGroot WJ, Sauerland EK, et al. Pathogenesis of upper airway occlusion during sleep. *J Appl Physiol* 1978; 44:931–938.
8. Hairston LE, Sauerland EK. Electromyography of the human pharynx: Discharge patterns of the superior pharyngeal constrictor during respiration. *Electromyogr Clin Neurophysiol* 1981; 21:299–306.
9. England SJ, Bartlett D, Daubenspeck JA. Influence of human vocal cord

movements on airflow and resistance during eupnea. *J Appl Physiol* 1982; 52:773–779.
10. Bartlett D, Remmers JE, Gautier H. Laryngeal regulation of respiratory airflow. *Respir Physiol* 1973; 18:194–204.
11. Brancatisano TP, Dodd DS, Engel LA. Respiratory activity of posterior cricoarytenoid muscle and vocal cords in humans. *J Appl Physiol* 1984; 57:1143–1149.
12. Remmers JE, Bartlett D. Reflex control of expiratory airflow and duration. *J Appl Physiol* 1977; 42:80–87.
13. Collett PW, Brancatisano TP, Engel LA. Upper airway dimensions and movements in bronchial asthma. *Am Rev Respir Dis* 1986; 133:1143–1149.
14. Kuna ST, Insalaco G, Woodson GE. Thyroarytenoid muscle activity during wakefulness and sleep in normal adults. *J Appl Physiol* 1988; 65: 1332–1339.
15. Richter DW. Generation and maintenance of the respiratory rhythm. *J Exp Biol* 1982; 100:93–107.
16. Berger AJ, Mitchell RA, Severinghaus JW. Regulation of respiration. *N Engl J Med* 1977; 297:92–97, 138–143, 194–201.
17. Onal E, Lopata M, O'Connor TD. Diaphragmatic and genioglossal electromyographic responses to isocapnic hypoxia in humans. *Am Rev Respir Dis* 1981; 127:215–217.
18. Brancatisano TP, Dodd DS, Engel LA. Responses of the posterior cricoarytenoid and alae nasi muscles to increased chemical drive in man. *Respir Physiol* 1986; 64:177–189.
19. England SJ, Bartlett D. Changes in respiratory movements of human vocal cords during hyperpnea. *J Appl Physiol* 1982; 52:780–785.
20. Bruce EN, Mitra J, Cherniack NS. Central and peripheral chemoreceptor inputs to phrenic and hypoglossal motoneurons. *J Appl Physiol* 1982; 53:1504–1511.
21. Hudgel DW, Chapman KR, Faulks C, et al. Changes in inspiratory muscle electrical activity and upper airway resistance during periodic breathing induced by hypoxia during sleep. *Am Rev Respir Dis* 1987; 135:899–906.
22. Parisi RA, Neubauer JA, Frank MM, et al. Correlation between genioglossal and diaphragmatic responses to hypercapnia during sleep. *Am Rev Respir Dis* 1987; 135:378–382.
23. Cohen MI. Phrenic and recurrent laryngeal discharge patterns and the Hering-Breuer reflex. *Am J Physiol* 1975; 228:1489–1496.
24. Brouillette RT, Thach BT. Control of genioglossus muscle inspiratory activity. *J Appl Physiol* 1980; 49:801–808.
25. Remmers JE. Extra-segmental reflexes derived from intercostal afferents: Phrenic and laryngeal responses. *J Physiol* 1973; 233:45–62.
26. Hwang JC, St. John WM, Bartlett D. Receptors responding to changes in upper airway pressure. *Respir Physiol* 1987; 55:355–366.
27. Mathew OP, Sant'Ambrogio G, Fisher JT, et al. Laryngeal pressure receptors. *Respir Physiol* 1984; 57:113–122.
28. Sant'Ambrogio G, Mathew OP, Fisher JT, et al. Laryngeal receptors responding to transmural pressure, airflow and local muscle activity. *Respir Physiol* 1983; 54:317–330.

29. Sant'Ambrogio G, Mathew OP, Sant'Ambrogio FB, et al. Laryngeal cold receptors. *Respir Physiol* 1985; 59:35–44.
30. Mathew OP, Abu-Osba YK, Thach BT. Influence of upper airway pressure changes on genioglossus muscle respiratory activity. *J Appl Physiol* 1982; 52:438–444.
31. Mathew OP, Abu-Osba YK, Thach BT. Genioglossus muscle responses to upper airway pressure changes. *J Appl Physiol* 1982; 52:445–450.
32. Abu-Osba YK, Mathew UP, Thach BT. An animal model for airway sensory deprivation producing obstructive apnea with postmortem findings of sudden infant death syndrome. *Pediatrics* 1981; 68:796–801.
33. McNamara SG, Issa FG, Szeto E, et al. Influence of negative pressure applied to the upper airway on the breathing pattern in unanesthetized awake dogs. *Respir Physiol* 1986; 65:315–329.
34. Issa FQ, Edwards P, Szeto E, et al. Genioglossus and breathing responses to airway occlusion: Effect of sleep and route of occlusion. *J Appl Physiol* 1988; 64:543–549.
35. White DP, Cadieux RJ, Lombard RM, et al. The effects of nasal anesthesia on breathing during sleep. *Am Rev Respir Dis* 1985; 132:972–975.
36. McNicholas WT, Coffey M, McDonnell T, et al. Upper airway obstruction during sleep in normal subjects after selective topical oropharyngeal anesthesia. Am Rev Respir Dis 1987; 135:1316–1319.
37. DeWeese EL, Sullivan TY. Effects of upper airway anesthesia on pharyngeal patency during sleep. *J Appl Physiol* 1988; 64:1346–1353.
38. Kuna ST, Woodson GE, Sant'Ambrogio G. Effect of laryngeal anesthesia on pulmonary function testing in normal subjects. *Am Rev Respir Dis* 1988; 137:656–661.
39. Redline S, Strohl KP. Influence of upper airway sensory receptors on respiratory muscle activation in humans. *J Appl Physiol* 1987; 63:368–374.
40. O'Donnell DE, Sanii R, Younes M. External mechanical loading in conscious humans: Role of upper airway mechanoreceptors. *J Appl Physiol* 1988; 65:541–548.
41. Hudgel DW, Martin RJ, Johnson B, et al. Mechanics of the respiratory system and breathing pattern during sleep in normal humans. *J Appl Physiol* 1984; 56:133–137.
42. Anch AM, Remmers JE, Bunce H. Supraglottic airway resistance in normal subjects and patients with occlusive sleep apnea. *J Appl Physiol* 1982; 53:1158–1163.
43. Brown IB, McClean PA, Boucher R, et al. Changes in pharyngeal cross-sectional area with posture and application of continuous positive airway pressure in patients with obstructive sleep apnea. *Am Rev Respir Dis* 1987; 136:628–632.
44. Fouke JM, Strohl KP. Effect of position and lung volume on upper airway geometry. *J Appl Physiol* 1987; 63:375–380.
45. Van de Graaff WB. Thoracic influence on upper airway patency. *J Appl Physiol* 1988; 65:2124–2131.
46. Hoffstein V, Zamel N, Phillipson EA. Lung volume dependence of pharyngeal cross-sectional area in patients with obstructive sleep apnea. *Am Rev Respir Dis* 1984; 130:175–178.

47. Spann RW, Hyatt RE. Factors affecting upper airway resistance in conscious man. *J Appl Physiol* 1971; 31:708–712.
48. Safar P, Escarraga LS, Chang F. Upper airway obstruction in the unconscious patient. *J Appl Physiol* 1959; 14:760–764.
49. McNicholas WT, Tarlo S, Cole P, et al. Obstructive apneas during sleep in patients with seasonal allergic rhinitis. *Am Rev Respir Dis* 1982; 126: 625–628.
50. Bulow K. Respiration and wakefulness in man. *Acta Physiol Scand Suppl* 1963; 209:1–110.
51. Sauerland EK, Harper RM. The human tongue during sleep: Electromyographic activity of the genioglossus muscle. *Exp Neurol* 1976; 51:160–170.
52. Orem J, Netick A, Dement WC. Increased upper airway resistance to breathing during sleep in the cat. *Electroencephalogr Clin Neurophysiol* 1977; 43:14–22.
53. Orem J, Lydic R. Upper airway function during sleep and wakefulness: Experimental studies on normal and anesthetized cats. *Sleep* 1978; 1: 49–68.
54. Sherrey JH, Megirian D. Respiratory EMG activity of the posterior cricoarytenoid, cricothyroid and diaphragm muscles during sleep. *Respir Physiol* 1980; 39:355–365.
55. Goh AS, Issa FG, Sullivan CE. Upper airway dilating forces during wakefulness and sleep in dogs. *J Appl Physiol* 1986; 61:2148–2155.
56. Lopes JM, Tabachnik E, Muller NL, et al. Total airway resistance and respiratory muscle activity during sleep. *J Appl Physiol* 1983; 54:773–777.
57. Skatrud JB, Dempsey JA. Airway resistance and respiratory muscle function in snorers during NREM sleep. *J Appl Physiol* 1985; 59:328–335.
58. Foutz AS, Netick A, Dement WC. Sleep state effects on breathing after spinal cord transection and vagotomy in the cat. *Respir Physiol* 1979; 37:89–100.
59. Orem J. Neuronal mechanisms of respiration in REM sleep. *Sleep* 1980; 3:251–267.
60. Douglas NJ, White DP, Weil JV, et al. Hypoxic ventilatory response decreases during sleep in normal man. *Am Rev Respir Dis* 1982; 125: 286–289.
61. Douglas NJ, White DP, Weil JV, et al. Hypercapnic ventilatory response in sleeping adults. *Am Rev Respir Dis* 1982; 126:758–762.
62. Parisi RA, Santiago TV, Edelman NH. Genioglossal and diaphramatic EMG responses to hypoxia during sleep. *Am Rev Respir Dis* 1988; 138: 610–616.
63. Weiner D, Mitra J, Salamone J, et al. Effect of chemical stimuli on nerves supplying upper airway muscles. *J Appl Physiol* 1982; 52:530–536.
64. Hudgel DW, Mulholland M, Hendricks C. Neuromuscular and mechanical responses to inspiratory resistive loading during sleep. *J Appl Physiol* 1987; 63:603–608.
65. Iber C, Bersenbrugge A, Skatrud JB, et al. Ventilatory adaptations to resistive loading during wakefulness and non-REM sleep. *J Appl Physiol* 1982; 52:604–617.
66. Wiegand L, Zwillich CW, White DP. Sleep and the ventilatory response to resistive loading in normal man. *J Appl Physiol* 1988; 64:1186–1195.

67. Kuna ST, Smickley J. Response of genioglossus muscle activity to nasal airway occlusion in normal sleeping adults. *J Appl Physiol* 1988; 64:347–353.
68. Wiegand L, Zwillich CW, White DP. Collapsibility of the human upper airway during normal sleep. *J Appl Physiol* 1989; 66:1800–1809.
69. Schwartz AR, Smith PL, Wise RA, et al. Induction of upper airway occlusion in sleeping individuals with subatmospheric nasal pressure. *J Appl Physiol* 1988; 64:535–542.
70. American Thoracic Society. Indications and standards for cardiopulmonary sleep studies. *Am Rev Respir Dis* 1989; 139:559–568.
71. Mangat E, Orr WC, Smith RO. Sleep apnea, hypersomnolence and upper airway obstruction secondary to adenotonsillar enlargement. *Arch Otolarygol* 1977; 103:383–386.
72. Orr WC, Martin RJ. Obstructive sleep apnea associated with tonsillar hypertrophy in adults. *Arch Intern Med* 1981; 141:990–992.
73. Bear SE, Priest JH. Sleep apnea syndrome: Correction with surgical advancement of the mandible. *J Oral Maxillofac Surg* 1980; 38:543–549.
74. Imes NK, Orr WC, Smith RO, et al. Retrognathia and sleep apnea: A life-threatening condition masquerading as narcolepsy. *JAMA* 1977; 237: 1596–1597.
75. Mezon BJ, West P, MacLean JP, et al. Sleep apnea in acromegaly. *Am J Med* 1980; 69:615–618.
76. Orr WC, Males JL, Imes NK. Myxedema and obstructive sleep apnea. *Am J Med* 1981; 70:1061–1066.
77. Luke M, Mehrizi A, Folger G, et al. Chronic nasopharyngngeal obstruction as a cause of cardiomegaly, cor pulmonale, and pulmonary edema. *Pediatrics* 1966; 37:762–768.
78. Haponik EF, Smith PL, Bohlman ME, Computerized tomography in obstructive sleep apnea. *Am Rev Respir Dis* 1983; 127:221–226.
79. Suratt PM, Dee P, Atkinson RL, et al. Fluoroscopic and computed tomographic features of the pharyngeal airway in obstructive sleep apnea. *Am Rev Respir Dis* 1983; 127:487–492.
80. Stauffer JL, Zwillich CW, Cadieux RJ, et al. Pharyngeal size and resistance in obstructive sleep apnea. *Am Rev Respir Dis* 1987; 136:623–627.
81. Rivlin J, Hoffstein V, Kalbfleish J, et al. Upper airway morphology in patients with obstructive sleep apnea. *Am Rev Respir Dis* 1984; 129:355–360.
82. Guilleminault C, Tilkian A, Dement WC. The sleep apnea syndromes. *Annu Rev Med* 1976; 27:465–484.
83. Bohlman ME, Haponik EF, Smith PL, et al. CT demonstration of pharyngeal narrowing in adult obstructive sleep apnea. *AJR* 1983; 140:543–548.
84. Koenig JS, Thach BT. Effects of mass loading on the upper airway. *J Appl Physiol* 1988; 64:2294–2299.
85. Series F, Cormier Y, Lampron N, et al. Increasing the functional residual capacity may reverse obstructive sleep apnea. *Sleep* 1988; 11:349–353.
86. Guilleminault C, Riley R, Powell N. Obstructive sleep apnea and abnormal cephalometric measurements. *Chest* 1984; 86:793–794.

87. Jameison A, Guilleminault C, Partinen M, et al. Obstructive sleep apneic patients have craniomandibular abnormalities. *Sleep* 1986; 9:469–477.
88. Partinen M, Guilleminault C, Quera-Salva M, et al. Obstructive sleep apnea and cephalometric roentgenograms. *Chest* 1988; 93:1199–1205.
89. Suratt PM, Wilhoit SC, Cooper K. Induction of airway collapse with subatmospheric pressure in awake patients with sleep apnea. *J Appl Physiol* 1984; 57:140–146.
90. Suratt PM, McTier RF, Wilhoit SC. Upper airway muscle activation is augmented in patients with obstructive sleep apnea compared with that in normal subjects. *Am Rev Respir Dis* 1988; 137:889–894.
91. White DP. Genioglossal responses to respiratory stimuli in apnea patients versus controls. *Am Rev Respir Dis* 1989; 139:A446.
92. Hudgel DW. Variable site of airway narrowing among obstructive sleep apnea patients. *J Appl Physiol* 1986; 61:1403–1409.
93. Hudgel DW, Hendricks C. Palate and hypopharynx—sites of inspiratory narrowing of the upper airway during sleep. *Am Rev Respir Dis* 1988; 138:1542–1547.
94. Bradley TD, Martinez D, Rutherford R, et al. Physiological determinants of nocturnal arterial oxygenation in patients with obstructive sleep apnea. *J Appl Physiol* 1985; 59:1364–1368.
95. Findley LJ, Ries AL, Tisi GM, et al. Hypoxemia during apnea in normal subjects: mechanisms and impact of lung volume. *J Appl Physiol* 1983; 55:1777–1783.
96. Gleeson K, Zwillich CW, White DP. Arousal from sleep in response to ventilatory stimuli occurs at a similar degree of ventilatory effort irrespective of the stimulus. *Am Rev Respir Dis* 1989; 139:A82.
97. Onal E, Lopata M, O'Connor T. Pathogenesis of apneas in hypersomnia-sleep apnea syndrome. *Am Rev Respir Dis* 1982; 125:167–174.
98. NHLBI Workshop Summary. Respiratory disorders of sleep: Pathophysiology, clinical implications, and therapeutic approaches. *Am Rev Respir Dis* 1987; 136:755–761.
99. Strohl KP, Cherniack NS, Gothe B. State of art: Physiologic basis of therapy for sleep apnea. *Am Rev Respir Dis* 1986; 134:791–802.
100. Chapman KR, Bruce EN, Gothe B, et al. Possible mechanisms of periodic breathing during sleep. *J Appl Physiol* 1988; 64:1000–1008.
101. Onal E, Burrows DL, Hart RH, et al. Induction of periodic breathing during sleep causes upper airway obstruction in humans. *J Appl Physiol* 1986; 61:1438–1443.
102. Warner G, Skatrud JB, Dempsey JA. Effect of hypoxia-induced periodic breathing on upper airway obstruction during sleep. *J Appl Physiol* 1987; 62:2201–2211.
103. Lavie, P. Sleep disturbances in industry workers. *Sleep Res* 1980; 9:209–211.
104. Lavie P. Incidence of sleep apnea in a presumably healthy working population: A significant relationship with excessive daytime sleepiness. *Sleep* 1983; 6:312–318.
105. Guilleminault C, Vanden Hoad J, Mitler M. Clinical overview of the sleep apnea syndromes. *In* C Guilleminault, WC Dement (eds). Sleep Apnea Syndromes. New York, Alan R. Liss, 1978, pp 1–12.

106. Kales A, Cadieux RJ, Bixler EO, et al. Severe obstructive sleep apnea I: Onset, clinical course, and characteristics. *J Chron Dis* 1985; 38:419–425.
107. White DP, Lombard RM, Cadieux RJ, et al. Pharyngeal resistance in normal humans: Influence of gender, age, and obesity. *J Appl Physiol* 1985; 58:365–371.
108. Brown IG, Zamel N, Hoffstein V. Pharyngeal cross-sectional area in normal men and women. *J Appl Physiol* 1986; 61:890–895.
109. Block AJ, Wynne JW, Boysen PG. Sleep disordered breathing and nocturnal oxygen saturation in postmenopausal women. *Am J Med* 1980; 69:75–79.
110. Sutton FD, Zwillich CW, Creagh CE, et al. Progesterone for outpatient treatment of Pickwickian Syndrome. *Ann Intern Med* 1975; 83:476–479.
111. Pickett CK, Regensteiner JG, Woodard WD, et al. Progestin and estrogen reduce sleep-disordered breathing in post menopausal women. *J Appl Physiol* 1989; 66:1656–1661.
112. Schneider BK, Pickett CK, Zwillich CW, et al. Influence of testosterone on breathing during sleep. *J Appl Physiol* 1986; 61:618–623.
113. Guilleminault C, Dement WC. Sleep apnea syndromes and related sleep disorders. *In* RL Williams, I Karacan, CA Moore (eds). Sleep Disorders: Diagnosis and Treatment. New York, John Wiley & Sons, 1988, pp 47–71.
114. Tilkian AG, Guilleminault C, Schroeder JS, et al. Hemodynamics in sleep-induced apnea. *Ann Intern Med* 1976; 85:714–719.
115. Buda AJ, Schroeder JS, Guilleminault C. Abnormalities of pulmonary artery wedge pressures in sleep-induced apneas. *Int J Cardiol* 1981; 1: 67–74.
116. Fletcher EC, Schaaf JW, Miller J, et al. Long-term cardiopulmonary sequelae in patients with sleep apnea and chronic lung disease. *Am Rev Respir Dis* 1987; 135:525–533.
117. Bradley TD, Rutherford R, Grossman RF, et al. Role of daytime hypoxemia in the pathogenesis of right heart failure in the obstructive sleep apnea syndrome. *Am Rev Respir Dis* 1985; 131:835–839.
118. Weitzenblum E, Kreiger J, April M, et al. Daytime pulmonary hypertension in patients with obstructive sleep apnea syndrome. *Am Rev Respir Dis* 1988; 138:345–349.
119. Bradley TD, Phillipson EA. Pathogenesis and pathophysiology of the obstrucive sleep apnea syndrome. *Med Clin North Am* 1985; 69:1169–1185.
120. Scharf SM. Influence of sleep state and breathing on cardiovascular function. *In* NA Saunders, CE Sullivan (eds). Sleep and Breathing, Lung Biology in Health and Disease, Vol 21. New York, Marcel Dekker, 1984, pp 221–239.
121. Fletcher EC, DeBehnke R, Lovoi M, et al. Undiagnosed sleep apnea in patients with essential hypertension. *Ann Intern Med* 1985; 103:190–195.
122. Kales A, Bixler EO, Cadieux RJ, et al. Sleep apnea in a hypertensive population. *Lancet* 1984; 2:1005–1008.
123. Motta J, Guilleminault C, Schroeder JS, et al. Tracheostomy and hemodynamic changes in sleep-induced apnea. *Ann Intern Med* 1978; 89:454–458.

124. Tilkian AG, Guilleminault C, Schroeder JS, et al. Sleep-induced apnea syndrome: Prevalence of cardiac arrhythmias and their reversal after tracheostomy. *Am J Med* 1977; 63:348–358.
125. Zwillich CW, Devlin J, White DP, et al. Bradycardia during sleep apnea: Its characteristics and mechanisms. *J Clin Invest* 1982; 69:1286–1292.
126. Shepard JW, Garrison MW, Grither DA, et al. Relationship of ventricular ectopy to oxygemoglobin desaturation in patients with obstructive sleep apnea. *Chest* 1985; 88:335–340.
127. Guilleminault C, Connolly SJ, Winkle RA. Cardiac arrhythmia and conduction disturbances during sleep in 400 patients with sleep apnea syndrome. *Am J Cardiol* 1983; 52:490–494.
128. Miller WP. Cardiac arrhythmias and conduction disturbances in the sleep apnea syndrome. *Am J Med* 1982; 73:317–321.
129. Partinen M, Jamieson A, Guilleminault C. Long-term outcome for obstructive sleep apnea syndrome patients: Mortality. *Chest* 1988; 94:1200–1204.
130. He J, Kryger MH, Zorick FJ, et al. Mortality and apnea index in obstructive sleep apnea: Experience in 385 male patients. *Chest* 1988; 94:9–14.
131. Gonzalez-Rothi RJ, Foresman GA, Block AJ. Do patients with sleep apnea die in their sleep? *Chest* 1988; 94:531–538.
132. Guilleminault C. Clinical features and evaluation of obstructive sleep apnea. *In* MH Kryer, T Roth, WC Dement (eds). Principles and practice of sleep medicine. New York, W.B. Saunders, 1989, pp 552–558.
133. Roehrs T, Conway W, Wittig R, et al. Sleep-wake complaints in patients with sleep-related respiratory disturbances. *Am Rev Respir Dis* 1985; 132: 520–523.
134. Findley LJ, Unverzagt ME, Suratt PM. Automobile accidents involving patients with obstructive sleep apnea. *Am Rev Respir Dis* 1988; 138:337–340.
135. Roth T, Hartse KM, Zorick F, et al. Multiple naps and the evaluation of daytime sleepiness in patients with upper airway sleep apnea. *Sleep* 1980; 3:425–439.
136. Guilleminault C, Partinen M, Quera-Salva M, et al. Determinants of daytime sleepiness in obstructive sleep apnea. *Chest* 1988; 94:32–37.
137. Orr WC, Martin RJ, Imes NK, et al. Hypersomnolent and nonhypersomnolent patients with upper airway obstruction during sleep. *Chest* 1979; 75:418–422.
138. Sink J, Bliwise D, Dement WC. Self-reported excessive daytime somnolence and impaired respiration in sleep. *Chest* 1986; 90:177–180.
139. Smith PL. Haponik EF, Bleeker ER. The effects of oxygen in patients with sleep apnea. *Am Rev Respir Dis* 1984; 130:958–963.
140. Gold AR, Schwartz AR, Bleeker ER, et al. The effect of chronic nocturnal oxygen administration upon sleep apnea. *Am Rev Respir Dis* 1986; 134: 925–929.
141. Gibson GE, Pulsinelli W, Blass JP, et al. Brain dysfunction in mild to moderate hypoxia. Am J Med 1981; 70:1247–1254.
142. Kales A, Caldwell AB, Cadieux RJ, et al. Severe obstructive sleep apnea II: Associated psychopathology and psychosocial consequences. J Chron Dis 1985; 38:427–443.

5

The Management of Sleep-Disordered Breathing

Mark H. Sanders, M.D.

As our understanding of sleep-disordered breathing has increased over the last several decades, so have the therapeutic options available to clinicians managing these patients. Initially, there was only tracheotomy for the treatment of obstructive sleep apnea but now there are diverse approaches from which the physician can and must choose in treating individuals with breathing abnormalities during sleep. The heterogeneity of treatment options probably reflects current uncertainty regarding the pathogenesis of sleep-disordered breathing. In addition, the observation that all the available modalities are successful in treating some but not all patients probably reflects the heterogeneity of pathophysiologic mechanisms leading to the final common pathway of sleep-disordered breathing. In this chapter the currently employed therapies for sleep-disordered breathing will be discussed and critically evaluated in order that the reader may decide the appropriate place for each modality in the management of each patient. While I will try to channel the chapter in terms of increasing order of therapeutic aggressiveness, or invasiveness, it should be understood that the discussion is not meant to describe a treatment algorithm or protocol. It is essential that therapy match the

Supported by Merit Review funding from the Veterans Administration and the Competitive Medical Research Fund of Presbyterian-University Hospital, Pittsburgh, PA.
Martin RJ: Cardiorespiratory Disorders During Sleep, 2nd Edition. Futura Publishing Company, Inc., Mount Kisco, NY, © 1990.

requirements of the patient. Unfortunately, identifying these requirements is not always an easy task.

The initial, and hidden, decision in the management of sleep-disordered breathing is determining which patient requires treatment at all. In essence, this issue asks the physician to distinguish between sleep-disordered breathing as just an abnormality and as a disease entity. An abnormality may be defined as "different from the average; unusual; irregular,"[1] while a disease is a condition of ill-health[1] or a process that adversely effects the quality or quantity of life. There is a large body of literature indicating that sleep apnea is prevalent in the general population, particularly in the elderly, many of whom are asymptomatic and otherwise healthy.[2–11] The magnitude of the negative impact of this sleep-disordered breathing on both the quantity and quality of life is controversial, however. Some authors have reported that sleep apnea may not necessarily be associated with cardiovascular or cognitive dysfunction or subjective decrease in daytime alertness,[3,5,7,11] while others have detected abnormalities of daytime alertness and sleep quality on specific questioning or testing of individuals with sleep-disordered breathing who had not spontaneously sought medical attention.[3,9,10] It is clear that we do not currently know the critical level and duration of nocturnal hypoxia that is ultimately harmful to an individual's well-being, nor do we as yet recognize the cutoff frequency of sleep-disordered breathing events at which a breathing abnormality becomes a breathing disease.[12–14] The natural history of untreated, truly asymptomatic sleep-disordered breathing is uncertain and long-term multicenter studies are needed, in this regard.[15] It is generally agreed, however, that treatment is indicated in cases where sleep-disordered breathing causes or contributes to physiologic and/or psychophysiologic morbidity.[15] It is on this patient population that the remainder of this chapter will center.

Management of Sleep-Disordered Breathing Associated with Upper Airway Dysfunction

Reduction or Elimination of Risk Factors for Upper Airway Obstruction

In the following section agents, conditions, and circumstances that precipitate or augment upper airway dysfunction during sleep will be discussed. A reasonable first step in the management of patients with sleep-disordered breathing is the identification and subsequent elimination, or avoidance, of these elements. In selected individuals, further, more aggressive intervention may not be needed.

Alcohol

The destabilizing impact of alcohol on the upper airway may represent a window on the pathogenesis of obstructive sleep-disordered breathing. Alcohol ingestion has been shown in animals to selectively reduce the output of the hypoglossal nerve.[16] Since this cranial nerve is responsible for innervating the upper airway dilator muscles, the activity of these muscles is diminished after alcohol consumption. The result is an alteration of the balance between those forces that tend to promote upper airway collapse and those that maintain upper airway patency, favoring collapse.[17–21] That alcohol similarly reduces the activity of upper airway dilator muscles in man and thus increases upper airway collapsibility was demonstrated by Krol et al.[22] and Issa and Sullivan.[23] In the clinical setting, these data translate into an increased frequency of obstructive sleep-disordered breathing events following alcohol ingestion. Taasan and coworkers[24] observed that only 2 cc/kg of 100 proof vodka at bedtime increased the frequency of sleep-disordered breathing events, including episodes of oxyhemoglobin desaturation, in a group of healthy men, some of whom had no sleep-disordered breathing in the absence of alcohol ingestion. In contrast, Scrima et al.[25] noted that while 3 ounces of alcohol prior to bedtime increased the frequency of sleep-disordered breathing events in patients with preexisting obstructive sleep apnea, 0.8 g/kg of alcohol had no provocative effect in this regard on subjects without preexisting sleep apnea. Issa and Sullivan[26] reported that alcohol increased the frequency of sleep-disordered breathing events in patients with obstructive sleep disordered breathing, and it precipitated apnea in individuals who otherwise had only chronic snoring. These authors, as well as Guilleminault and Rosekind,[27] documented an increase in apnea duration as well as an increase in apnea frequency, after alcohol consumption. The prolongation of apnea following the ingestion of alcohol is probably due to its depressant effects on the arousal response to hypoxia and hypercapnia.[28,29]

In summary, the adverse effects of alcohol on upper airway stability during sleep and the arousal response to chemical stimuli mandate that patients with sleep-disordered breathing be instructed to abstain from alcohol. Most clinicians will readily recognize the impact of alcohol on sleep-disordered breathing from their interviews with patients and their bed-partners, who usually relate augmentation of snoring, apneic periods, and daytime fatigue following alcohol consumption. This only reinforces the importance of educating patients regarding the properties of alcohol that are particularly detrimental to their health.

Obesity

Although not invariably associated with obstructive sleep-disordered breathing, obesity is usually present in this patient population.[30–32] The mechanism responsible for this association is unclear. Studies employing computerized tomography have indicated that the pharyngeal airway is abnormally narrow in sleep apnea patients and it has been postulated that obesity, in some fashion, plays a pathogenetic role in this regard.[33–35] This link, however, does not appear to be deposition of adipose tissue along the inner pharyngeal wall, although "marbling" of the tissues cannot be excluded. Recent studies employing the acoustic reflection technique have shown that during wakefulness there is a direct relationship between lung volume and pharyngeal cross-sectional area and that the dependency of pharyngeal cross-sectional area on lung volume is greater in patients with sleep apnea.[36] It has therefore been postulated that obesity, by virtue of a reduction in lung volumes,[37,38] results in pharyngeal narrowing thus predisposing to occlusion during sleep. Interpretation of the results obtained by the acoustic reflection technique is confounded by the fact that the data were collected in awake individuals. Extrapolation to sleeping subjects and patients remains to be validated. In addition, other studies have found no relationship between functional residual capacity and the severity of obstructive sleep-disordered breathing.[39] Finally, a recent, thought-provoking paper reported that mass loading of the anterior cervical neck in animals resulted in concentric narrowing of the pharynx and increased pharyngeal airway resistance.[40] This raises the possibility, which remains to be investigated, that the mass of cervical soft tissue is the operative mechanism responsible for the association between obesity and sleep-disordered breathing. These and other data suggest that while there is no direct relationship between the magnitude of obesity and the severity of sleep-disordered breathing,[41] weight loss in obese sleep apnea patients is almost always of value. Weight reduction resulting in substantial amelioration of sleep-disordered breathing may be achieved on a medical regimen and need only be moderate in degree in certain patients.[39,41–43] Alternatively, surgical weight reduction may also result in marked improvement in upper airway function and oxygenation during sleep.[44–47] Indeed, it is possible that, in part, improved baseline oxygenation in patients following weight reduction may, independently, have a beneficial effect on breathing pattern during sleep. This will be discussed below.

The important message is that weight reduction may result in significant improvement in sleep-disordered breathing, nocturnal oxygenation, and sleep quality[43,48] and may obviate the need for further therapeutic intervention. Unfortunately, as most clinicians realize, it is very difficult to obtain meaningful and lasting weight loss in patients. Efforts in this regard represent a major, life-long therapeutic challenge, best approached by utilizing the multidisciplinary resources of the physician, nutritionist, psychologist and a peer support system.

Influence of Sleep Position on Obstructive Sleep-Disordered Breathing

The relationship between sleep in the supine position and augmentation of snoring and sleep apnea in some patients is apparent both during interviews with the bed-partner and polysomnography. Several investigations have documented a decreased incidence of sleep-disordered breathing events during sleep in the lateral decubitus position.[49–55] It has been hypothesized that the effects of gravity in promoting posterior movement of the tongue with apposition against the posterior pharyngeal wall are magnified in the supine position. The possibility that any consequences of increased soft tissue in the anterior neck relative to reducing pharyngeal circumference[40] is also intriguing as a mechanism for position-dependence of sleep-disordered breathing. In this context, recent data by Cartwright et al.[50] and George et al.[56] suggests that position-dependence may be less prevalent in extremely obese individuals, who appear to have comparable degrees of sleep-disordered breathing in both the supine and lateral decubitus postures. Conceivably, the effects of cervical mass loading reach a threshold where there is sufficient weight on the pharyngeal structures in all positions to promote upper airway instability during sleep. This hypothesis, however, remains to be tested.

Manipulation of sleep position has been suggested as a therapy for patients with documented position-dependence of sleep-disordered breathing.[50] Data in a recent report by George and coworkers,[56] however, indicate that sleep in the lateral decubitis position results in substantial reduction of apnea plus hypopnea frequency only during non-rapid eye movement sleep, while there is no position-dependence of sleep-disordered breathing during rapid eye movement (REM) sleep. Apnea duration was unchanged by altering sleep position in this study. These data suggest that sleep posture may influence upper airway stability primarily during non-REM sleep, which is not associated with as great a suppression of upper airway dilator muscle tone as is REM sleep. It has no influence on the arousal response regardless of sleep stage, however. Thus, the effectiveness of sleep-position therapy may be modified by the interaction between sleep stage and sleep position in a given patient on a given night.

Based upon our current knowledge, it seems reasonable to investigate the possibility of position-dependence of sleep-disordered breathing in individual patients. This should be done during the interview with the patient and his or her bed partner and as part of the polysomnographic evaluation. Having identified a patient with supine position-dependent apnea, especially one in whom the severity of sleep-disordered breathing is acceptably low during REM sleep, the "sleep-ball" technique may be employed to assist the patient in maintaining the lateral decubitus position during sleep. The "sleep-ball" technique consists of creating a pocket in the back of the patient's sleeping garment. A tennis ball, or similar object, is placed in this pocket so that if the patient rolls into the supine position, he or she will be promptly stimulated to resume sleeping in the lateral decubitus posture. A gravity-sensitive sleep position monitor and alarm has been designed to accomplish the same goal: to train the patient over time to sleep exclusively on his or her side.[50] A recent paper by McEvoy et al.[54] suggested that vertical manipulation of the sleep position, such that the patient sleeps upright, at a 60-degree angle, is also effective in reducing the frequency of sleep-disordered breathing events and improving nocturnal oxygenation. There was no comparison of the effects of sleeping in the lateral decubitus position and sleeping semiupright in that study, however. Of interest, in contrast to the inverse relationship reported between the magnitude of obesity and the effectiveness of sleeping in the lateral decubitus position,[49] McEvoy and coworkers observed that those individuals who improved most in the semiupright posture were the more obese, hypoxic, and hypercapnic patients.[54]

In conclusion, although manipulation of the sleeping position is not an effective therapy for the majority of patients with sleep-disordered breathing, it may be all that is needed in selected individuals. The presence of position-dependence of sleep-disordered breathing should therefore be sought in all patients undergoing evaluation. Along similar lines, the effect of sleep position on breathing during sleep should be kept in mind when comparing pre- and postintervention polysomnogram data (i.e., before and after surgery, nasal continuous positive airway pressure, oral appliance therapy, etc.) in order to avoid attributing therapeutic success to the intervention when it may have been due, at least in part, to sleeping in a more "favorable" posture.

Hypothyroidism

Over the last decade anecdotal reports have been published suggesting an association between obstructive sleep-disordered breathing and hypothyroidism.[57] More recently, Rajagopal et al.[58] confirmed this association. These investigators studied 11 consecutive hypothyroid patients and noted obstructive sleep apnea in nine of them, with apnea indices (number of apneas per hour of sleep) ranging from 17 to 176. This is particularly important from a therapeutic perspective because initiation of thyroid replacement medication has been shown to reverse sleep-disordered breathing, independent of changes in weight.[57,58]

The mechanism responsible for the association between sleep-disordered breathing and hypothyroidism is not clear. Certainly, to the extent that these individuals have macroglossia, this anatomic factor may play a pathogenetic role in predisposing the upper airway to obstruction during sleep.

Since hypothyroidism may not always be readily apparent to the clinician, all patients with sleep-disordered breathing should undergo laboratory assessment of thyroid function as a routine part of the work-up.

Drug-Related Risk Factors

Certain pharmacologic agents may precipitate obstructive sleep-disordered breathing in individuals who otherwise do not have abnormal breathing or worsen it in those who do have preexisting sleep-disordered breathing (Table 1). One such agent is the benzodiazepine flurazepam, which has been associated with an abnormal frequency of sleep-disordered breathing events.[59,60] It has been postulated that the "hangover" experienced after flurazepam use is related to this association. There has been recent information that may provide insight regarding the mechanism by which benzodiazepines can elicit or augment upper airway dysfunction during sleep. Diazepam, another benzodiazepine, has been found to selectively reduce the output of the hypoglossal nerve.[61,62] This results in a selective loss of upper airway dilator muscle tone and creation of an imbalance between those forces that tend to promote upper airway closure and those that maintain airway patency during sleep. The influence of benzodiazepines on ventilatory chemosensitivity and its relationship to the association between these agents and sleep-disordered breathing is arguable. Some investigators have observed a depression of hypercapnic ventilatory responsiveness during wakefulness following flurazepam, while others have found no change in hypoxic and hypercapnic responsiveness during sleep after flurazepam administration.[63–65] Similarly, sleep-disordered breathing events may be prolonged by a depressant effect of benzodiazepines on the arousal response to chemical stimuli, although not all investigators have been able to confirm such an effect.[64,65] Currently available information thus suggests that benzodiazepines are quite likely to have an adverse impact on breathing during sleep in people who have an underlying predisposition to or already have sleep-disordered breathing. Thus, these agents should be avoided in this patient population.

Barbiturates, in the usual clinical dosages, have mild ventilatory depressant properties. These agents, however, may reduce upper airway dilator muscle tone and thereby predispose patients to airway instability during sleep.[19] In light of this information, these drugs are to be avoided in patients with sleep-disordered breathing.

Table 1

Drugs that Worsen Breathing during Sleep

Alcohol
Benzodiazepines
Barbiturates
Narcotics (especially parenteral)
Testosterone (?)

Narcotics, when administered parenterally, and in sufficient oral dosages, have been demonstrated to reduce minute ventilation, depress hypoxic and hypercapnic ventilatory chemosensitivity, and raise arterial carbon dioxide tension. A recent study has suggested that usual clinical doses of hydromorphine hydrochloride, administered to individuals without sleep apnea syndrome, do not evoke clinically significant sleep-disordered breathing.[66] The authors are careful to caution, however, that this may be a dose-related observation and that narcotic administration is not to be recommended in patients with sleep-disordered breathing. Importantly, in this regard, life-threatening upper airway obstruction has been anecdotally reported following narcotic administration to patients with sleep apnea syndrome.[67] Concern about the safety of narcotic administration in sleep apnea patients is particularly relevant should these patients require surgery for any reason. Indeed, the postoperative period may be particularly risky for these patients since general anesthetic agents may selectively depress the activity of the upper airway dilator muscles[68] and increase the likelihood of upper airway instability during the postoperative recovery period. Therefore, patients with sleep-disordered breathing should be carefully monitored in the pre- and postoperative period when the administration of agents with potentially destabilizing upper airway properties and/or depressant effects on ventilatory or arousal responses cannot be avoided.

Finally, the observation that sleep-disordered breathing is more prevalent in males and postmenopausal females has suggested that androgenic hormones may confer a particular risk for this disorder or, conversely, that progesterone, or similar hormones, may provide a protective effect.[5,69] Along these lines, several papers published over the last decade have reported worsening of sleep-disordered breathing following androgenic hormone administration.[70–72] The mechanism responsible for this association has not been conclusively defined, and the number of subjects in the published studies is small. It is possible that testosterone elicits anatomic changes that predispose to upper airway closure during sleep,[71] although one investigation failed to document changes in upper airway dimensions and resistance in hypogonadal individuals who experienced increased sleep-disordered breathing during testosterone therapy.[72] Given the limited data currently available, it is prudent to consider the possibility that sleep-disordered breathing is a potential complication of therapy with androgenic drugs.

Treatment with Pharmacologic Agents

Protriptyline

Overnight apnea time may be reduced and overnight oxygenation may be improved in some patients by the administration of protriptyline. This agent is a nonsedating, tricyclic antidepressant that has REM sleep suppressant properties. Data reported by Brownell and coworkers[73] indicated that improvement in nocturnal breathing with this agent was due to the reduction of time spent in REM sleep, which is particularly associated with more prolonged and frequent apneas as well as the more severe episodes of oxyhemoglobin desaturation. Thus, standardizing the apnea time for sleep stage by separately determining apnea time during non-REM sleep and REM sleep revealed no significant difference before and during protriptyline therapy. Although the overnight apnea time was reduced in their patients, Brownell et al. did not observe a significant reduction in the apnea frequency, taken across the night of study, nor did they document a reduction in the arousal frequency (one measure of sleep fragmentation). Conway et al.[74] did, however, observe a reduction in overnight apnea frequency in four of nine patients given 5–20 mg of protriptyline at bedtime; patients with more severe apnea did not respond as well as those with milder disorders. Smith et al.[75] treated 12 patients with protriptyline at bedtime and found that during non-REM sleep there was no change in the frequency of all sleep-disordered breathing events. There was, however, a shift in the pattern of these events, with a reduction in the apnea frequency and an increase in the hypopnea frequency. Thus apnea time during non-REM sleep decreased. There was no change in apnea frequency, duration, or time, nor was there a shift in the pattern of sleep-disordered breathing events during REM sleep although there was a reduction in the amount of time spent in REM sleep, thus reducing the number of more severe sleep-disordered breathing events. Nocturnal oxygenation was improved during protrityline therapy.

Thus, it appears that there are two mechanisms responsible for the beneficial effects of this drug on sleep-disordered breathing: (1) the dominant mechanism is probably related to the suppressant effects on REM sleep, and (2) a shift from apnea to hypopneas, which are generally associated with less severe oxyhemoglobin desaturation. This alteration in the pattern of abnormal events may be related to selective activation of the upper airway dilator muscles.[61] Unfortunately, most studies report incomplete amelioration of sleep-disordered breathing by protriptyline, particularly in those patients with more than mild disease.[73–77] Nonetheless, many patients report a decrease in daytime sleepiness and/or fatigue while receiving protriptyline.[73–77] Clearly, this effect cannot be solely attributed to improved sleep quality or reduced sleep-disordered breathing event frequency. It has therefore been postulated that this agent has specific "alerting" properties, over and above any influence on breathing and sleep architecture.[73–77] The clinical implication of this observation is that one cannot rely on the patient's subjective report of improvement to reflect a favorable physiologic response to protriptyline. A repeat polysomnogram is needed to document the effectiveness of therapy in this regard.

Unfortunately, protriptyline is not without side effects. These are primarily due to its anticholinergic properties in a population that is largely comprised of middle-aged males. Thus, a substantial number of patients are forced to withdraw from this drug due to urinary hesitancy or retention, dry mouth, constipation, confusion, ataxia, impotence, and/or loss of libido.[74–76] Hair loss has also been reported.[76] Tachyarrhythmias have not been a clinically significant problem during protriptyline therapy.

In summary, protriptyline may be useful in treating patients with relatively mild sleep-disordered breathing. Its utility may be limited, however, by it side effects, and the clinician cannot depend upon the patient's subjective response to mirror the physiologic response to therapy. Follow-up polysomnography is therefore mandatory.

Supplemental Oxygen

In recent years, several investigations have indicated that supplemental oxygen therapy has beneficial effects in at least some patients with sleep-disordered breathing.[78,79] In eucapnic sleep apnea patients, Martin et al.[78] noted that, after 30 minutes of sleep while receiving supplemental oxygen, there was a significant reduction in apnea time due to a lower apnea frequency and no change in apnea duration. Concomitantly, oxyhemoglobin saturation was improved and apnea-related alterations in heart rate were minimized. A subsequent report by Smith and coworkers[79] confirmed the beneficial impact of oxygen supplementation on sleep-disordered breathing.

Martin et al. further demonstrated that improvement in sleep-disordered breathing during acute oxygen administration is sustained during chronic home oxygen therapy.[78]

Any or all of several mechanisms may be responsible for the favorable influence of supplemental oxygen on sleep-disordered breathing.[78] The maintenance of normal or supernormal oxyhemoglobin saturation may prevent hypoxic ventilatory depression.[80,81] Oxygen may augment ventilation by reducing cerebral blood flow with a consequent increase in cerebral carbon dioxide tension. Alternatively, oxygen therapy may interrupt a pathophysiologic vicious cycle by preventing central nervous system (CNS) dysfunction on the basis of apnea-related hypoxia. Since it is recognized that hypoxia may induce CNS respiratory center instability, which in turn may predispose to upper airway occlusion, supplemental oxygen may prevent excessive respiratory control system oscillation, periodic breathing, and sleep apnea.[82–84]

Supplemental oxygen should not be casually administered to patients with sleep-disordered breathing, however. During the initial several minutes of oxygen administration, Martin et al.[78] noted substantial apnea prolongation, although after 30 minutes of therapy apnea duration had shortened back to approximately baseline values. Others similarly have observed marked prolongation of apnea and respiratory acidosis during the first 5 minutes of oxygen therapy in sleep apnea patients without and with concomitant chronic obstructive pulmonary disease.[85,86] It is therefore advisable to monitor the patient polysomnographically during the initial trial of oxygen therapy. This will document the safety of this therapeutic modality, confirm its beneficial effects (and justify its use), and establish the liter flow necessary to achieve therapeutic benefit in the individual patient.

Progestational Agents

The known ventilatory-stimulating properties of medroxyprogesterone acetate (MPA) theoretically make it an attractive therapeutic alternative for patients with sleep-disordered breathing.[87,88] Several studies, each involving small numbers of patients, concluded that certain individuals might obtain clinically significant reductions in sleep-disordered breathing on MPA therapy, even though for the group of patients as a whole there was no significant change with administration of this agent.[89–91] In a more recent, controlled study of eucapnic sleep apnea patients, however, Rajagopal et al.[92] noted that there was no improvement in sleep-disordered breathing during MPA administration despite significant augmentation of hypercapnic ventilatory responsiveness during wakefulness. The failure of MPA to exert a beneficial effect was documented for apnea frequency, duration, and oxyhemoglobin saturation. The absence of a beneficial effect on sleep-disordered breathing despite an increase in ventilatory drive should not, perhaps, be surprising in view of the failure of the potent respiratory stimulant doxepram to have a favorable impact on this disorder.[93,94]

It appears, therefore, that at best, MPA is not uniformly successful in treating eucapnic sleep apnea patients. The effectiveness of this agent in the treatment of those sleep apnea patients who are hypercapnic during wakefulness remains to be reported. MPA treatment may be an alternative in patients with "central" sleep apnea and primary alveolar hypoventilation.[95,96] This will be discussed below.

Other Pharmacologic Agents

Tryptophan

Investigations suggesting that ventilation can be modified by central neural serotininergic systems, have led to the hypothesis that L-tryptophan may be useful in the treatment of sleep-disordered breathing. Limited studies have been conducted in this regard.[97,98] Administration of 2.5–3 g of L-tryptophan, either as a single dose or in divided doses, reduced apnea and hypopnea frequency in 15 patients. There was no change in apnea duration, however. In addition, L-tryptophan was less effective in those individuals with more severe obstructive sleep-disordered breathing and was ineffective in reducing the frequency of "central" apnea. There are no data regarding the effect of L-tryptophan on nocturnal oxygenation. Thus, currently available information is incomplete regarding the utility of this agent, and more study is required to better define its therapeutic role in the management of patients with sleep-disordered breathing.

Theophylline

Theoretically, theophylline is an attractive therapeutic prospect for the management of sleep-disordered breathing. It has long been known to increase ventilatory chemoresponsiveness,[99,100] and it has been shown to minimize Cheyne-Stokes breathing, a form of periodic breathing, in humans.[100,101] In this regard, periodic breathing has been postulated to be important in the pathogenesis of obstructive sleep-disordered breathing.[82,84] Theophylline has also been reported to decrease apnea attacks associated with the apnea of prematurity; however, there was no distinction between obstructive and central events.[102] Better definition of the role of theophylline in treating adults with sleep apnea has recently become available.[103] Espinoza and coworkers[103] observed that aminophylline infusion had no effect on the frequency or duration of obstructive apneas or on nocturnal oxygenation. There was, however, a significant decrease in the frequency of central apneas and central components of mixed apneas. With respect to sleep architecture and quality, aminophylline administration (compared with a saline control) was associated with significantly reduced sleep efficiency and greater sleep fragmentation. It must be concluded, therefore, on the basis of currently available although still somewhat limited information, that theophylline (or at least aminophylline) is not therapeutically useful in the treatment of obstructive sleep-disordered breathing. A possible place in the management of central apnea will require further study.

Nicotine

A recent and thought-provoking paper has identified nicotine as an agent that may have a beneficial effect on upper airway function during sleep. Gothe et al.[104] observed a significant reduction in obstructive and mixed apnea frequency one hour following the administration of 14 mg of nicotine (nicotine-containing chewing gum). Two hours after the nicotine administration, the frequency of mixed apneas was not significantly different from baseline, predrug values, but the obstructive apnea frequency was significantly lower than baseline. Neither central apnea frequency nor the average duration of all apneas was affected by the nicotine. There was no mention of adverse consequences. The beneficial effect of nicotine on obstructive and mixed apnea frequency may be attributed, at least in part, to its enhancement of upper airway dilator muscle activity and consequent reduction in upper airway resistance.[105–107] There is only one study published thus far that addresses the therapeutic use of nicotine for sleep apnea, and therefore the number of patients evaluated is much too small to allow any firm conclusions to be drawn. In addition, the apparent benefits are only transient, and this problem will need to be addressed as well, before serious consideration can be given to the clinical use of this agent.

Acetazolamide

Attempts have been made utilizing this agent to treat sleep-disordered breathing based on the knowledge that metabolic acidosis normally evokes ventilatory augmentation. Studies in this regard, however, have included only small numbers of subjects. Nonetheless, the results do not appear encouraging. Sharp et al.[108] noted that the creation of a metabolic acidosis with acetazolamide had no effect on obstructive apneas and converted central apneas into events with an obstructive pattern. More recently, Whyte and coworkers[109] observed that acetazolamide decreased the apnea + hypopnea index in 4 of 10 obstructive sleep apnea patients, with no effect on apnea duration. Perplexingly, there was no symptomatic improvement in any of the patients receiving this therapy. In addition, the majority of patients complained of parasthesias on acetazolamide, precluding long-term use in all but one of the patients in whom it was prescribed for chronic therapy. The other problematic side effect was dry mouth, although apparently this was not as severe as the parasthesias. The authors concluded that acetoazolamide has a limited role in the treatment of mild to moderate sleep apnea.

Agents without Benefit

The hypothesis that endogenous opioids are operative in the pathogenesis of sleep-disordered breathing has led to the investigation of the utility of naloxone, an opiate antagonist, in the treatment of sleep apnea. Unfortunately, there does not appear to be a beneficial effect in this regard.[110] Similarly, there is no apparent role for bromocriptine,[110] baclofen,[111] atropine,[112] or almitrine.[113] Finally, agents including chlorimiprimine, prochlorperizine, and strychnine[114–116] should not be used because there is too little information available regarding their effectiveness and safety.

Devices that Maintain Upper Airway Patency

Nasal Continuous Positive Airway Pressure (CPAP)

Nasal CPAP has been increasingly recognized as an important therapeutic modality in the treatment of sleep-disordered breathing.[117] As first described by Sullivan et al. in 1981,[118] CPAP was applied through nasal prongs sealed within the nares using silicon rubber, to five patients with obstructive sleep apnea. There was a dramatic relief of apnea and oxyhemoglobin desaturation in these patients at CPAP levels ranging from 4.5 to 10 cm H_2O. Subsequently, Sanders et al.[119,120] and Rapoport and coworkers[121] employed self-sealing masks to apply nasal CPAP with great success in treating obstructive sleep apnea patients. Since these reports, a variety of different systems have been developed to deliver nasal CPAP (Figure 1). While commercially available off-the-shelf nasal mask units are the most widely used in current clinical practice, other devices, including nasal prongs and custom-molded nasal masks, have been used with success.[122,123] At the present time the selection of a particular nasal CPAP delivery system remains one of personal choice.

In addition to being therapeutically effective in obstructive sleep apnea, Sanders[120] has reported that nasal CPAP effectively reduces or eliminates mixed apneas, including both the "central" and obstructive components. In that study, there appeared to be a tendency for nasal CPAP to also reduce the frequency of central apneas, an observation that was subsequently confirmed by Issa and Sullivan.[124] This therapeutic modality has also been shown to result in significant improvement in cor pulmonale in hypercapnic obstructive sleep apnea patients,[121,125] with improved cardiac function as well as better awake oxygenation and reduced hypercapnia after a relatively short period of therapy. In addition to providing rapid physiologic improvement, clinicians have recognized that in most patients there is almost immediate improvement in daytime alertness, relief of morning headaches and, in general, a remission from the symptoms of sleep apnea after the institution of nasal CPAP therapy. In this context, Rajagopal and associates[126] reported improvement in a subjective sleepiness index following one night of nasal CPAP.

In order for a therapeutic modality to be considered successful, it

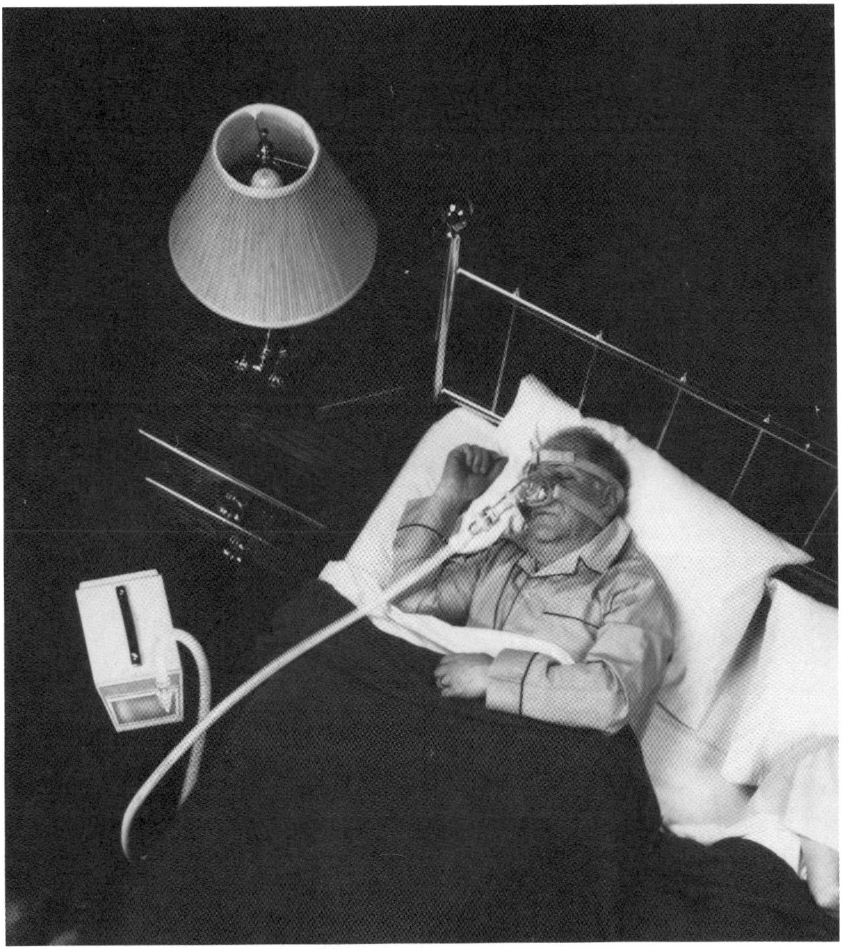

Figure 1. This sleep apnea patient is using nasal CPAP during sleep.

must be acceptable to patients as well as effective in reversing the disease process. Many studies have documented a high level of patient compliance with nasal CPAP therapy.[127–131] It has been estimated that 75–85% of patients will be compliant during long-term, home therapy. In order to facilitate good patient compliance, it is essential that the physician and/or the sleep laboratory act as an educational resource for the patient as well as being available to answer questions or address problems that may arise. In addition, I have found that an organization of the patients themselves provides much needed peer support and relief from the sense of isolation experienced by a large number of these patients who have for years been accused of malingering, when in fact their lassitude resulted from sleep-disordered breathing (Figure 2).

Given that considerable levels of pressure have been applied via nasal CPAP, the side effects are surprisingly few and mild. To our knowledge, there are no reports of pneumomediastinum and/or pneumothorax associated with nasal CPAP application. Nor are there reported cases of clinically important hypotension. There is, however, one report of hypoxemia associated with nasal CPAP.[132] These considerations mandate that the initial application of nasal CPAP to sleep

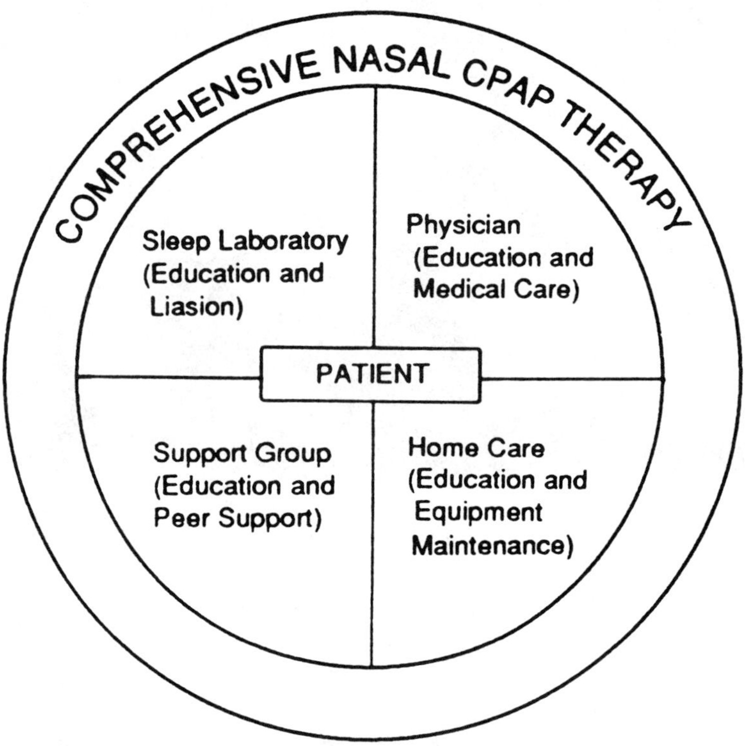

Figure 2. Unless all groups take part in the nasal CPAP therapy, the patient will not derive the maximal benefit and failure could ensue.

apnea patients be conducted in a sleep laboratory. Not only will this define the required pressure, it will, as best as possible, ensure the safety of this pressure as well as the patient's ability to tolerate it. These issues notwithstanding, however, the majority of complaints regarding nasal CPAP include nasal congestion, rhinorrhea, conjunctivitis, dry mouth, and nose, and discomfort and inconvenience from the nasal mask (Table 2). An occasional patient will complain of daytime chest discomfort or generalized heaviness following nights using nasal CPAP. In these cases, evaluation for cardiac and/or pulmonary causes is usually negative and the discomfort is attributed to a musculoskeletal source.

While there are several possible mechanisms by which nasal CPAP maintains upper airway patency during sleep in patients with sleep-disordered breathing, many investigators believe that the positive intrapharyngeal pressure acts as a pneumatic splint, stabilizing the airway (Figure 3).[20,21,118,133] Alternatively, the data obtained in awake individuals suggesting that pharyngeal cross-sectional area varies with lung volume[36] has led to the hypothesis that nasal CPAP promotes airway patency perhaps reflexly, by raising functional residual capacity (FRC). Indeed, there are isolated reports of apparent improvement in sleep apnea in association with increases in FRC.[134] Against this theory, are the data of Rapoport et al.[135] and Strohl and Redline[136] indicating that the application of nasal CPAP may, in fact, be associated with a reduction in upper airway dilator muscle electromyogram activity. This is inconsistent with a reflex mechanism. In addition, recent animal studies by Fouke and Strohl suggest that passive increases in FRC do not alter upper airway geometry.[137] This is in line with studies in my laboratory indicating that the application of up to -15 cm H_2O of continuous negative end-expiratory pressure (NEEP) to the chest wall does not reduce the frequency of obstructive apnea (unpublished studies). Finally, it has been suggested that nasal CPAP relieves nocturnal oxyhemoglobin desaturation and thereby

Table 2
Potential Side Effects of Nasal CPAP

Nasal congestion
Rhinorrhea
Nasal/throat dryness
Conjunctivitis
Mask discomfort
Chest discomfort (usually of musculoskeletal etiology)

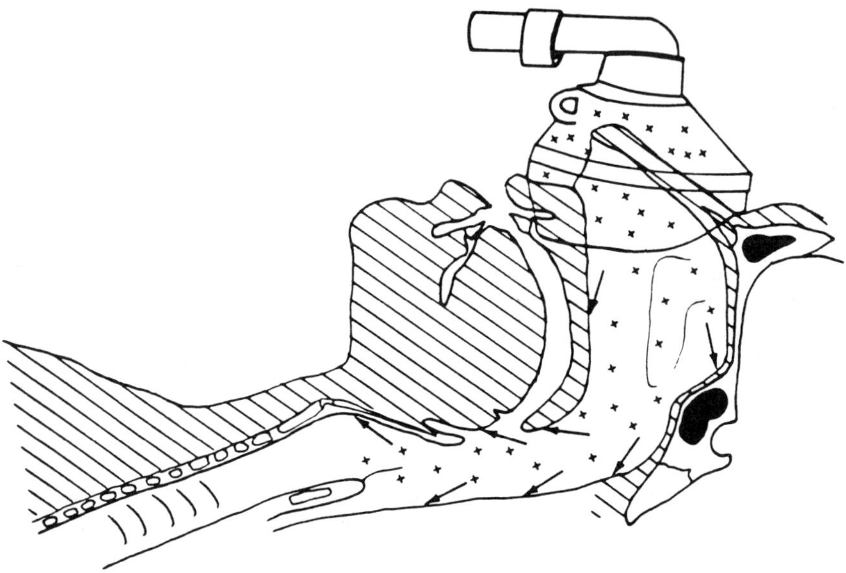

Figure 3. Nasal CPAP works by providing positive intrapharyngeal pressure, thus producing a pneumatic splint.

relieves hypoxia-induced ventilatory depression and/or ventilatory controller instability, thus reducing the apnea.[138–140] All of these authors conclude that relief of nocturnal hypoxia by nasal CPAP may eliminate a potentiating factor in the pathophysiology of sleep-disordered breathing. However, since the apnea/hypopnea must first be (and is) eliminated by this modality in order to improve nocturnal oxygenation, the improvement in oxyhemoglobin saturation cannot be the primary mechanism of action of nasal CPAP.

There have been several variations on the theme of nasal CPAP that deserve brief mention. Several years ago Mahadevia et al.[140] reported the successful amelioration of obstructive sleep apnea by the application of nasal expiratory positive airway pressure (EPAP). The authors concluded that the beneficial effect was probably mediated by improved nocturnal oxygenation, increased FRC, stimulation of the upper airways, or a combination of these. Since these data were published, Sanders and associates[141,142] reported that expiratory as well as inspiratory airway resistance were elevated in conjunction with the onset of obstructive apnea and that the airway may actually become occluded during expiration. Even more recent information supports this concept, since it has been shown that in sleep apnea patients, intraluminal pharyngeal pressures need not be negative, relative to atmospheric pressure, in order for the upper airway to collapse.[20] Thus the mechanism explaining the benefit of EPAP in obstructive sleep-disordered breathing may still be a splinting action, specifically during the expiratory phase of the ventilatory cycle. In any case, EPAP therapy for sleep apnea has not become a widely used modality, perhaps because of poor patient acceptance.

Occasionally, one hears of the application of CPAP via full-face mask in the treatment of obstructive sleep-disordered breathing. I and others have not had consistent success in alleviating upper airway obstruction using this technique (unpublished data).[21] In addition, there is the potential problem of an increased possibility of nocturnal aspiration. Finally, the fact that both the oral and the nasal breathing routes are covered by a mask during sleep mandates the incorporation of an alarm and fail-safe mechanism to preserve a way for the patient to breathe in the event of machine malfunction.

In addition to the treatment of sleep-disordered breathing, nasal CPAP may be a valuable diagnostic tool. Clinicians occasionally encounter a patient whose symptoms seem disproportionately severe relative to the degree of sleep-disordered breathing recorded during polysomnography. Nasal CPAP can be used as a noninvasive means to abolish the sleep-disordered breathing events and to determine if this results in improvement in the patient's symptoms. Such an improvement will establish a cause-and-effect relationship between the objective findings on the sleep study and the patient's subjective reports. The formulation of further therapeutic plans will be facilitated by this information. Conversely, patients who claim to be completely asymptomatic despite severe sleep-disordered breathing may likewise be given a therapeutic trial of nasal CPAP to determine if reversal of the abnormal breathing during sleep impacts favorably on the way the patient feels. Occasionally patients do not realize how poorly they felt until the sleep-disordered breathing is relieved.

Nasal CPAP has become an important tool in the care of patients with sleep-disordered breathing. It is an available therapy that is highly successful and well-accepted by patients.

Tongue-Retaining Device

There has been increasing interest in the use of an oral appliance in the treatment of obstructive sleep-disordered breathing. The hypothesis is that such a device will advance the tongue and/or mandible, thereby promoting pharyngeal patency. A tongue-retaining device (TRD) was described in 1982 by Cartwright and Samelson.[143] During a one-half night trial, these authors noted a reduction in apnea frequency in eight of 12 patients. Although reduced, two of the eight individuals continued to experience a substantially high apnea frequency, however. Ten patients subsequently were studied after home use of the TRD for a period ranging from 4 to 6 months. Again, half-night studies were conducted, and it was observed that on the two half-nights, five and six of the patients demonstrated clinical relief of apnea (less than seven apneas per hour of sleep). Thus, these data suggested that the TRD would be successful in 50%–60% of patients. In addition, the authors determined patient compliance with TRD therapy utilizing questionnaires. Sixty-one percent of the patients used the device "regularly," although this term was not defined. The effect of the TRD on nocturnal oxygenation was not assessed in this study. Subsequently, Cartwright reported that position-dependence of obstructive sleep-disordered breathing was a predictor of success with the TRD.[144] Those patients in whom sleep-disordered breathing was more severe in the supine position appeared to respond better to the device. Since, as previously noted, patients who tend to be less obese also tend to be more position-dependent, it is understandable how these investigators observed that lesser degrees of obesity also seemed to predict a better result from TRD therapy. This information suggests that a particular upper airway configuration (one that tends to collapse during sleep in the supine position) is more amenable to the TRD. The favorable predictive feature of supine-position dependence and lower body weight as well as the approximate 60% long-term compliance were subsequently demonstrated again.[145] Several other reports have been published indicating that there are some patients who can obtain some degree of relief from nocturnal upper airway obstruction using an oral appliance.[146,147] Unfortunately, all the studies reported to date have involved very limited numbers of patients, incomplete data regarding nocturnal oxygenation, poor control of other potentially confounding factors such as weight changes, and/or incomplete documentation of functional patient improvement. There are also no substantive data regarding the success of this device over a period of greater than one year. In addition, although there are relatively few studies, the available information indicates that patient compliance with an oral appliance may not be better than it is with other nonsurgical treatments, such as nasal CPAP. Clearly, long-term systematic studies are needed in larger numbers of patients before oral appliances can be considered for an established role in the management of patients with sleep-disordered breathing.

Nasopharyngeal Airway

In an attempt to stent the pharynx open during sleep, several investigators have inserted a nasopharyngeal airway (trumpet) in sleep apnea patients.[147,149] In my experience (unpublished) and those of others,[149] this technique is not useful in the long-term management of these patients. In some individuals the airway needs to be inserted so far down in order to prevent occlusion that the gag reflex is activated. Other patients simply cannot tolerate the device despite nightly alternation of the nares and the application of a topical anesthetic jelly. In summary, the nasopharyngeal airway does not appear to be a promising approach to the treatment of this patient population.

Surgical Management of Obstructive Sleep-Disordered Breathing

Surgery for obstructive sleep-disordered breathing is designed either to bypass the obstructing region of the upper airway or to modify the upper airway in such a fashion that it is less likely to lose patency. The obstruction may result either from a wide variety of structural aberrations, such as nasal deformity, nasal polyps, hypertrophic tonsils and/or adenoids, craniofacial disproportion, neoplasms in the oro- or hypophyarynx, macroglossia, or, as in most cases, no detectable anatomic abnormalities. Accordingly, a variety of surgical procedures has been applied to the management of these patients (Table 3). As much as possible, the specific abnormality should be identified, and using this information, the most appropriate operative procedure should be selected. As with nonsurgical therapy, this decision is often confounded by difficulty in defining the precise pathophysiologic pathway in a given individual that culminates in upper airway occlusion during sleep.

Table 3
Surgical Procedures for Sleep-Disordered Breathing

Location	*Procedure*	*Comments*
Neck	Tracheostomy	Assures a patient airway; potentially associated with high morbidity
Oro/hypopharynx	Tonsillectomy	Low success rate in absence of grossly hypertrophied tonsils
	Removal of vallecular cysts/tumors	Corrects a specific anatomic lesion
	Uvulopalatopharyngoplasty	Generally successful in 50% of patients
	Partial glossectomy	Little published data; no published trials
Maxillofacial	Maxillomandibular advancement: sagittal splitting osteotomy; vertical osteotomy	For maxillomandibular retrognathia, limited number of centers where performed; limited clinical trials

Uvulopalatopharyngolplasty (UPPP)

In 1964, Ikematsu described the relief from snoring after surgical excision of the mucosa of the tonsillar pillars and partial excision of the uvula.[150] Subsequently, Fujita et al. described a modification of this technique, called uvulopalatopharyngoplasty or UPPP, for the treatment of obstructive sleep-disordered breathing.[151] In this technique and most of its subsequent modifications,[152–155] the patient undergoes a bilateral tonsilectomy. Excess submucosal tissue is removed via an incision over the palate lateral to the glossopalatal arch, in a curvilinear fashion from the inferior pole of the tonsil (bilaterally) to the tip of the uvula. A variable portion of the posterior margin of the soft palate is also removed and the palatopharyngeus muscle may also be resected.

To date, there is no consensus regarding the criteria that should be applied in the assessment of surgical success.[13] Most studies addressing UPPP for sleep apnea have liberally defined a "response" as at least a 50% reduction in sleep-disordered breathing events. Using this definition, the response rate for UPPP ranges from 40% to 70%, with the usually quoted figure of 50%.[151,152,156–160] In the absence of weight gain or other confounding factors, the success has been shown to be sustained for at least one year postoperatively.[160] Given the physiologic improvement in breathing during sleep in only approximately half the individuals undergoing the procedure, it is of interest that over 80% report increased daytime alertness.[157,159] It should be noted when considering these data that many patients were lost to post-UPPP follow-up and were therefore not included in the results. A placebo effect also needs to be considered. The message here, however, is that the subjective reports of the patient, suggesting relief of daytime fatigue and/or sleepiness, cannot be assumed to reflect physiologic improvement in breathing during sleep. Thus, a repeat polysomnogram is necessary to assess the therapeutic outcome of surgery. Highlighting this dissociation between subjective and objective results of UPPP, 70% of nonresponders to UPPP may report reduced daytime sleepiness but have no reduction in sleepiness as assessed objectively by Multiple Sleep Latency Testing (MSLT). MSLT should be considered in the postoperative evaluation of UPPP patients, especially those in whom the significance of the physiologic improvement in breathing and sleep architecture is unclear.

UPPP surgery does entail some morbidity, although this is not unacceptably high in most patients. Postoperative pain is usually significant during the initial 2–3 days following surgery, gradually diminishing over two weeks. Nasal regurgitation may be present in at least 50% of patients in the immediate postoperative period but this is a persistent problem in only about 5%.[152] Although most surgeons have not reported a high incidence of voice alterations of an objectionable nature to the patient, such changes, including rhinolalia, may certainly occur. Patients should be counseled regarding these possible undesirable outcomes before undertaking surgery. Along similar lines, although not common, there have been reports of early post-UPPP deaths.[161,162] Because of concern regarding swelling and upper airway compromise in the postoperative period, several surgeons have recommended concomitant tracheostomy, especially in patients with severe obstructive sleep apnea.[163]

In order to better assess the acute effects of UPPP, we recently performed polysomnograms on patients on the second postoperative night.[164] For the group, there was no difference between the pre- and post-UPPP apnea, hypopnea, or apnea + hypopnea indices. Examining the data from individual patients, however, we found that there was a reciprocal relationship between the apnea and hypopnea indices, such that when one went up postoperatively, the other went down. The mean nadir of oxyhemoglobin desaturation was unchanged for the group in the pre- and postoperative periods; however, it is critical to note that several patients required supplemental oxygen during wakefulness postoperatively and thus received oxygen during their post-UPPP sleep study. In these patients, the awake arterial blood gases indicated a reduction in oxygen tension that mandated oxygen therapy (independent of consideration of sleep apnea). Thus, it is quite reasonable to assume that without oxygen administration, and with persistent sleep-disordered breathing, these individuals would have become substantially, if not dangerously, hypoxic during sleep following surgery. It is also important to note that all patients in this study were normocapnic in the awake, preoperative period and that these results may not be extrapolated to hypercapnic sleep apnea patients. It was concluded that, all other things being equal, in normocapnic sleep apnea patients, prophylactic tracheotomy was not necessary. Arterial blood gases should be obtained postoperatively, and these individuals should be placed in a monitored nursing unit until stability and adequate nocturnal oxygenation is assured. In selected patients considered at high risk, consideration should be given to early post-UPPP polysomnography.

With all these data in mind, it becomes clear that a major difficulty in applying UPPP to the treatment of sleep apnea is the inability to adequately predict who will respond in a meaningful way to the procedure. Fujita and coworkers[159] found that patients in whom the level of obstruction, as determined by laryngoscopy in the awake individual, is in the oropharynx do better than those in whom it is in the hypopharynx. This makes sense since the surgery addresses the former but not the latter. Conceivably, visualizing the upper airway via a fiberoptic laryngoscope, while the patient performs a Mueller maneuver, and localizing the level at which the airway tends to narrow will facilitate identification of the obstructing segment during sleep.[165] Along similar lines, somnofluoroscopy has been used to identify the obstructing segment.[166] Patients with apnea-related airway collapse only at the upper portion of the airway fared better than patients with collapse at lower levels or at both the upper and lower levels. It should be noted, however, that in this study 20% of the patients (albeit of only 15 patients) who exhibited obstruction only in the upper segment of the airway were, nonetheless, not surgical successes. Some authors have suggested that the patient's body weight has predictive value regarding the likelihood of successful UPPP. Fujita et al.[159] observed that no patients who were less than 125% of ideal body weight had a response to this surgery, while approximately 50% of those over 125% were considered responders. Other studies, however, are not consistent with these observations. Guilleminault et al.[167] and Gislason et al.[168] found that the response rate was actually lower in their more obese patients, while others have concluded that weight has no predictive value.[169,170] There are similarly conflicting data regarding the predictive value of the preoperative severity of sleep-disordered breathing. Caldarelli et al.[169] concluded that UPPP was more likely to be successful in patients with apnea indices greater than 70, while Gislason and coworkers concluded that those with mild to moderate sleep apnea are most likely to benefit.[168] Schoen and Anand,[170] on the other hand, found that apnea severity carried no predictive power.

It thus appears that UPPP is an imperfect treatment for obstructive sleep-disordered breathing. The uncertainties regarding the proper predictive parameters for surgical success greatly limit optimal patient selection. This problem is compounded by the invasive nature of the procedure and uncommon but potentially significant operative and postoperative complications. It deserves mention, however, that the UPPP procedure remains a good alternative for those individuals who have unacceptable snoring. UPPP successfully alleviates this problem in over 90% of cases. The decision as to whether snoring, in the absence of physiologically significant sleep-disordered breathing, is a problem of sufficient magnitude to warrant an operative procedure must be left up to the fully informed patient. Finally, in this regard, clinicians should recognize that even sleep apnea patients who are UPPP failures will probably have substantial reduction in snoring, despite persistent apnea. Thus, as is the case with subjective reports of decreased daytime sleepiness after UPPP, subjective reports of amelioration of snoring cannot be assumed to reflect physiologic improvement in breathing during sleep.

Maxillofacial Surgery

Patients with mandibular malposition, retrognathia, or micrognathia are predisposed to upper airway collapse during sleep. Increasing experience with cephalometric examination of sleep apnea patients has suggested that many have maxillofacial abnormalities that are too subtle to be consistently detected on routine clinical examination.[172] Accordingly, a variety of surgical procedures are being developed in order to normalize the bony relationships of the maxilla and mandible in order to minimize the likelihood of airway collapse during sleep.[173–175] Many of these procedures are preceded by UPPP and, if the results are unsatisfactory, a second stage involving mandibular advancement (variably consisting of inferior sagittal osteotomy, horizontal osteotomy, hyoid resuspension, to name a few techniques) is undertaken. Preliminary reports regarding the surgical results are very encouraging (Riley RW, Powell NB, Guilleminault C, personal communications); however, it is important to remember that the operations are complex in nature and require a great deal of specific surgical skill and experience. In addition, a great deal of expertise is necessary on the part of the anesthesia services in order to control the airway during the procedure as well as in the postoperative period. Following surgery, the participation of an experienced pulmonologist is also of great benefit in the management of the ventilatory and airway problems to which these individuals are very susceptible. Finally, it is noteworthy that even after the mandibular surgery itself is completed, the patient may be obligated to orthodontic manipulation to restore or create proper occlusion and subsequently to intermaxillary fixation for a prolonged period creating a nutritional and psychologic management challenge.

These considerations, the absence of established and proven patient selection criteria, and large, multicenter studies of the long-term effectiveness, morbidity, and mortality of these procedures indicate that these surgical techniques are not ready for inclusion in the routine treatment of sleep apnea patients. The area, however, seems to hold much promise and the needed data are eagerly awaited.

Nasal Surgery

Theoretically, nasal obstruction should promote upper airway instability during sleep by allowing the generation of excessively negative intrapharyngeal pressures that overcome the dilating forces of the upper airway musculature. Indeed, Olsen et al.[176] observed an increase in obstructive apneas and hypopneas during sleep after packing of the anterior nose. Similarly, Zwillich et al.[177] noted an increase in sleep-disordered breathing events after nasal packing in otherwise normal individuals. On the basis of these data, nasal surgery has been performed on sleep apnea patients with evidence of nasal obstruction in an effort to reduce the predisposition to collapse during sleep.

Heimer et al. found this to be effective in three patients.[178] Nonetheless, our clinical experience and that of others[179] suggests that nasal obstruction, per se, is likely to cause only mild sleep apnea and more commonly is associated with snoring alone. Along these lines, it is not surprising that Rubin et al.[180] found that only a small percentage (less than 30%) of sleep apnea patients with nasal obstruction derived clinically significant benefit from nasal surgery alone.

The fact that nasal surgery alone is, in general, a relatively low-yield procedure for sleep apnea should not deter the clinician from evaluating the possible pathophysiologic contribution of the nasal airway. Information regarding nasal patency may be useful in planning therapy relative to considering corrective nasal surgery in combination with other operative procedures in the hopes of improving the likelihood of surgical success, nasal surgery alone, or even simply to improve the olfactory sense and/or breathing of the individual during wakefulness.

Tonsillectomy/Adenoidectomy

Tonsillar and adenoidal enlargement are the most common cause of obstructive sleep-disordered breathing in children. In most children with tonsillar hypertrophy and obstructive sleep-disordered breathing, there is a satisfactory response to tonsillectomy and adenoidectomy.[181–185] The clinician can usually develop a high index of suspicion for adenotonsillar enlargement as the etiology of nocturnal upper airway obstruction in childhood from visual examination of the airway and, if necessary, lateral neck roentgenograms. It is relatively uncommon, however, for adenotonsillar enlargement to precipitate obstructive sleep-disordered breathing in adults, especially in the absence of neoplastic lymphoid involvement.[186] In selected adult cases, tonsillectomy may be beneficial but the yield is surprisingly low.[180] It is reasonable to undertake this procedure, without a concomitant UPPP in those sleep apnea patients with clearly enlarged tonsils that compromise the airway lumen even during wakefulness. Deciding which patients with lesser degrees of obstruction will respond to tonsillectomy alone, without a simultaneous UPPP, is a difficult clinical decision.

Tracheotomy

Historically, this has been the treatment for obstructive sleep apnea.[187,188] The advantages of this procedure include the immediate relief of sleep-associated upper airway obstruction, improvement in nocturnal oxygenation, and improved sleep quality.[189,190] The disadvantages are considerable, however. The surgical procedure itself may be difficult from the outset with many of these obese, short-necked patients presenting difficulty in tracheal intubation. Experienced anesthesiology personnel are necessary for safe and successful intubation of these patients. In fact, the presence of at least two qualified individuals in this regard is desirable in case of intubation failure and the need to ventilate manually with a resuscitation bag–valve–mask unit. This, of course, may be said of any operative procedure in these patients. The creation of the tracheotomy itself may be problematic due to the anterior adipose tissue and the posterior location of the trachea in these patients.[191,192] Following a tracheotomy, further difficulties may be encountered as a result of stomal bleeding, stricture, stomal and/or tracheal granulation tissue, or acute and chronic tracheitis. In large measure, some of these problems are avoided by the use of skin flaps.[191–193] Proper fit of the tracheotomy tube is also essential.[194] Lateral tomograms of the neck with the tube in place may be of assistance in assessing this, particularly in view of the posterior location of the trachea. In this regard, customized tubes may be of benefit. An additional problem associated with the tube size is the presence of an inadequate airway when the tube is plugged, as it is during the day. This results from a tube diameter that is too large relative to the diameter of the patient's trachea. In these cases a narrower or fenestrated tracheotomy tube may provide relief. Another, potentially serious problem after tracheotomy is aspiration of oral contents. Tracheotomy may alter the mechanical ability of the larynx to adequately close during swallowing. The relatively fixed tracheotomy tube can limit the rostrocaudal movement of the laryngotracheal apparatus, which limits sufficient elevation to achieve complete closure of the airway.[195] Finally, and perhaps of greatest functional significance, there is often substantial psychosocial morbidity associated with the cosmetic consequences of the procedure.[193] Not only does tracheotomy obligate the patient to a different lifestyle and wardrobe, patients have encountered employers who were reluctant to hire them. Depression, therefore, is a relatively common management problem in these individuals.

The utilization of tracheotomy for obstructive sleep-disordered breathing has lessened in recent years, primarily as a result of the development of other successful modalities, notably nasal continuous positive airway pressure. It has been suggested that tracheotomy be reserved for those individuals who frequently desaturate to levels below 50%, who have cyclic bradycardia to rates below 40–45 beats/min, excessive pharyngeal tissue, morbid obesity, and/or significant apnea-related cardiac arrhythmias.[194] It is the opinion of this author that tracheotomy be reserved for those patients who have physiologically or functionally significant sleep-disordered breathing who either have not responded to or are intolerant of other interventions that are less invasive, deforming, or adversely altering of lifestyle.

Therapy of Central Sleep Apnea

Patients presenting with predominantly central sleep apnea are relatively uncommon (approximately 10% of patients). There is a wide variety of therapies for central sleep apnea (Table 4) but, because the condition is uncommon, there have not been large clinical trials of any of them. In fact, many patients referred to our laboratory with a polysomnographic diagnosis of central sleep apnea are found to have a significant obstructive component when polysomnography is repeated using quantitative recording of esophageal pressure and airflow.

There is a variety of disorders associated with central sleep apnea. These include brain-stem lesions (either infectious or neoplastic), spinal surgery, cervical cordotomy, encephalitis, bulbar poliomyelitis, and spinal malformations.[196] Other conditions that predispose to periodic breathing are cardiac and/or cerebrovascular diseases. These entities are thought to introduce a phase-lag in the feedback mecha-

Table 4
Therapy of Central Sleep Apnea

Pharmacologic
Acetazolamide
Medroxyprogesterone acetate
Theophylline
Oxygen
Devices
Nasal CPAP
Diaphragm pacing
Nocturnal mechanical ventilation
Via tracheotomy
Via nasal mask

nisms within the central nervous system that govern ventilatory timing.[82] Alternatively, hypoxia, whether as a result of alteration in ventilatory chemoresponsiveness associated with sleep or altitude, can also induce periodic breathing.[196,197]

It is a clinical truism that the most appropriate way to treat a disorder is to address the underlying cause. Thus, in patients with central apnea and significant cardiac and/or cerebrovascular disease, all attempts should be made to optimize therapy in this regard. In selected patients oxygen therapy may be of benefit.[78,198]

Acetazolamide

In one report, the carbonic anhydrase inhibitor acetazolamide reduced central apnea in six patients.[199] Long-term follow-up was conducted in two of these patients, in one of whom acetazolamide lost its effectiveness. In using this agent to treat central sleep apnea, the report by Sharp et al.[108] should be kept in mind. These investigators found that administration of acetazolamide to patients with predominantly mixed apnea increased the frequency of obstructive apneas and worsened nocturnal oxygenation. The authors concluded that the increased ventilatory drive associated with the drug-induced metabolic acidosis resulted in greater augmentation of phrenic output than hypoglossal output, thereby favoring upper airway collapse. Subsequent data indicating that central apneas may be associated with increased upper airway collapsibility heighten concern in this regard.[142,200] The key message however, is that the studies of acetazolamide and central sleep apnea are too small and too few as well as lacking in long-term follow-up to provide any meaningful insight into the utility of this agent in patients.

Progestational Agents (Medroxyprogesterone Acetate, MPA)

As is the case with acetazolamide, there is inadequate information available regarding the use of MPA in central sleep apnea. Sutton et al.[201] and Lyons and Huang[202] have reported that progesterone augments alveolar ventilation in patients with awake hypercarbia. No formal sleep evaluations were performed on these patients, however. Thus, one should not have high expectations when treating a patient with central sleep apnea, especially in the absence of awake hypercarbia, with progestational agents.

Theophylline

This agent, a known ventilatory stimulant, has been reported to successfully reverse Cheyne-Stokes breathing in adults and central apnea in children.[101,203–205] Large studies have not been performed, however, to facilitate the usefulness of this agent in the treatment of central sleep apnea patients. The clinician must recall the relatively high risk–benefit ratio and the narrow therapeutic window of this agent if it is prescribed to patients.

Nasal Continuous Positive Airway Pressure (CPAP)

Sanders, in a study of the effect of nasal CPAP on the various apnea patterns, found that this modality eliminated the central as well as the obstructive components of mixed apnea.[120] In addition, the data suggested that some central apneas may be abolished by this therapy.[120] Subsequently, Issa and Sullivan[124] confirmed the beneficial effect of nasal CPAP on central apnea. These authors believed that this effect was consistent with other data suggesting that there is an obstructive component in central apnea.[142,200] They further speculated that nasal CPAP acted by stimulating sensory receptors in the mucosa of the upper airway. Alternatively, it is possible that the prolongation of the expiratory phase, which is what central apnea usually represents, is related to an altered volume history of the respiratory system, which, in turn, is due to expiratory upper airway obstruction. The altered volume history modifies the expiratory off-switch and delays the ensuing inspiratory effort. Nasal CPAP splints the upper airway open during expiration as well as during inspiration, and thus may normalize the expiratory volume history of the system and tend to normalize the ventilatory pattern.

Notwithstanding theoretical considerations and the observations that nasal CPAP may reduce central apnea in some individuals, a substantial proportion of these patients are not benefited by this modality. Thus, nasal CPAP is worth trying in this population of patients, but it should not be expected to be of universal benefit. All of these issues support the concept that central apnea is a pattern of breathing with a heterogeneous pathophysiology; some events represent an obstructive phenomenon, while others represent a true suspension of ventilatory cycling in the central nervous system.

Diaphragm Pacing

Diaphragmatic pacing has been employed in patients with abnormal ventilatory control or failure of neural transmission and alveolar hypoventilation.[206,207] Although requiring considerable technical skill and substantial bioengineering resources, this methodology can maintain awake alveolar ventilation at acceptable levels. Unfortunately, diaphragm pacing may precipitate upper airway occlusion during sleep due to dysynchrony between activation of the diaphragm and the upper airway and laryngeal dilators.[208,209] Thus, tracheotomy must be performed concomitantly with diaphragm pacing.[207,208] This, of course, complicates both the medical management and, importantly, the quality of life for these patients. These difficulties, in conjunction with the resource-intensive nature of the procedure and subsequent care have made this technique one that is infrequently employed in the clinical setting of central sleep apnea.

Nocturnal Mechanical Ventilation

Nighttime mechanical ventilation of patients with alveolar hypoventilation has been shown by Garay et al. to result in improvement in awake arterial blood gases in some individuals as well as providing an improved quality of life.[210] These investigators used a variety of mechanical ventilation modalities, including negative-pressure devices (chest cuirass, tank ventilators) as well as positive-pressure devices, in conjunction with tracheotomy. It should be noted however, that their patients were diagnosed as having alveolar hypoventilation and not solely central sleep apnea. In addition, the use of negative pressure ventilators has, like diaphragm pacing, been shown to predispose to upper airway occlusion during sleep.[211] Until recently, the only remaining alternative was positive pressure via tracheotomy. The use of nasal masks with small, positive-pressure ventilators has been reported to successfully support alveolar hypoventilating patients during sleep with improvement in oxygenation (especially during REM sleep), well-being, and sleep architecture.[212]

This technique can confer all the advantages of nocturnal ventilation without the disadvantages of tracheotomy and/or devices that are cumbersome (i.e., negative pressure wraps) or that require a very precise fit, such as the chest cuirass. Clearly, nasal positive-pressure ventilation is a promising new modality for the treatment of nocturnal hypoventilation and, although not yet specifically reported, possibly for patients with clinically and/or physiologically significant central sleep apnea.

Conclusions

It is evident that our biotechnical and pharmacologic skills have increased enormously over the last decade, such that most patients with sleep-disordered breathing can be treated by means other than tracheotomy. There are now treatments available with various gradations of invasiveness and risk–benefit ratios. Unfortunately, our understanding of the basic pathophysiology of sleep-disordered breathing has not increased to the point where each individual patient can be treated with the intervention that best reverses their particular pathophysiologic sequence. Under these circumstances it is difficult, although nonetheless critically important, to try to tailor the therapy to the specific needs of the patient. If, for example, a patient has clearly obstructing tonsils and is not an inordinate operative risk, it would seem inappropriate to administer protriptyline. Similarly, patients should be involved in the decision-making process regarding choice of therapy. The choice of treatment should be based upon the historical, physical, and polysomnographic data with the recommendation of a knowledgable, experienced, and compassionate physician as well as input from a well-informed patient. Except for the rare patient with an immediately life-threatening sleep-disordered breathing problem, surgery, particularly surgery that does not carry a high cure rate such as UPPP, should be considered after other, less invasive treatments, particularly nasal CPAP, have been tried. If successful, the patient will have a better appreciation of the potential benefits associated with relief of sleep-disordered breathing, and if unsuccessful, either because of poor physiologic response or poor patient acceptance, they are no longer in line as therapeutic options. Finally, having tried all appropriate, noninvasive therapies, the patient is in a better position to assess the potential risks and benefits of surgery. Thus, it is evident that an educated, informed patient, an understanding and experienced physician, and a competent, supportive staff in the sleep laboratory are all essential elements in the optimal management of sleep-disordered breathing.

References

1. Funk and Wagnalls Standard Encyclopedic Dictionary. Ramsey, NJ, Funk and Wagnalls. 1966.
2. Knight H, Millman RP, Gur RC, et al. Clinical significance of sleep apnea in the elderly. *Am Rev Respir Dis* 1987; 136:845–850.
3. Carskadon MA, Dement WC. Respiration during sleep in the aged human. *J Gerontol* 1981; 36:420–423.
4. Bixler EO, Kales A, Cadieux RJ, et al. Sleep apneic activity in older healthy adults. *J Appl Physiol* 1985; 58:1597–1601.
5. Block AJ, Boysen PG, Wynne JW, et al. Sleep apnea, hypopnea and oxygen desaturation in normal subjects: A strong male predominance. *N Engl J Med* 1979; 300:513–517.
6. Reynolds CF, Kupfer D, Taska LS, et al. Sleep of healthy seniors: A revisit. *Sleep* 1985; 8:20–29.
7. Berry DTR, Phillips BA, Cook YR, et al. Sleep-disordered breathing in healthy aged persons: possible daytime sequelae. *J Gerontol* 1987; 42: 620–626.
8. Bliwise DL, Carey E, Dement WC. Nightly variation in sleep-related respiratory disturbance in older adults. *Exp Aging Res* 1983; 9:77–81.
9. Lavie P. Incidence of sleep apnea in a presumably healthy working population: A significant relationship with excessive daytime sleepiness. *Sleep* 1983; 6:312–318.
10. Gislason T, Almqvist M, Eriksson G, et al. Prevalence of sleep apnea syndrome among Swedish men—an epidemiological study. *J Clin Epidemiol* 1988; 41:571–576.
11. Catterall JR, Calverley PMA, Shapiro CM, et al. Breathing and oxygenation during sleep are similar in normal men and women. *Am Rev Respir Dis* 1985; 132:86–88.
12. Berry DTR, Webb WB, Block AJ. Sleep apnea syndrome: A critical review of the apnea index as a diagnostic criterion. *Chest* 1984; 86:529–531.
13. Sanders MH, Rogers RM. Sleep apnea: When does better become benefit? *Chest* 1985; 88:320–321.
14. Littner M, McGinty D. Asymptomatic disordered breathing during sleep in older persons. Disease or not. *Arch Intern Med* 1985; 145:223–234.
15. Weil JV, Cherniack NS, Dempsey JA, et al. Respiratory disorders of sleep, NHLBI Workshop Summary, *Am Rev Respir Dis* 1987; 136:755–761.
16. Bonora M, Shields GI, Knuth SL, et al. Selective depression by ethanol of upper airway respiratory motor activity in cats. *Am Rev Respir Dis* 1984; 130:156–161.
17. Anch AM, Remmers JE, Bunce H. Supra-glottic airway resistance in

normal subjects and patients with occlusive apnea. *J Appl Physiol* 1982; 53:1158–1163.
18. Remmers JE, DeGroot WJ, Sauerland EK, et al. Pathogenesis of upper airway occlusion during sleep. *J Appl Physiol* 1978; 44:931–938.
19. Brouillette RT, Thach BT. A neuromuscular mechanism maintaining extrathorcic airway patency. *J Appl Physiol* 1979; 46:772–779.
20. Schwartz AR, Smith PL, Wise RA, et al. Induction of upper airway occlusion in sleeping individuals with subatmospheric nasal pressure. *J Appl Physiol* 1988; 64:535–542.
21. Smith PL, Wise RA, Gold AR, et al. Upper airway pressure-flow relationships in obstructive apnea. *J Appl Physiol* 1988; 64:789–795.
22. Krol RC, Knuth SL, Bartlett D Jr. Selective reduction of genioglossal muscle activity by alcohol in normal human subjects. *Am Rev Respir Dis* 1984; 129:247–250.
23. Issa FG, Sullivan CE. Upper airway closing pressures in snorers. *J Appl Physiol* 1984; 57:528–535.
24. Taasan VC, Block AJ, Boysen PG, et al. Alcohol increases sleep apnea and oxygen desaturation in asymptomatic men. *Am J Med* 1981; 71:240–245.
25. Scrima L, Broudy M, Nay KN, et al. Increased severity of obstructive sleep apnea after bedtime alcohol ingestion: Diagnostic potential and proposed mechanism of action. *Sleep* 1982; 5:318–328.
26. Issa FG, Sullivan CE. Alcohol, snoring and sleep apnea. *J Neurol Neurosurg Psychiatr* 1982; 45:353–359.
27. Guilleminault C, Rosekind M. The arousal threshold: Sleep deprivation, sleep fragmentation, and obstructive sleep apnea syndrome. *Bull Eur Physiopathol Respir* 1981; 17:341–349.
28. Anthonisen NR, Kryger M. Ventilatory and arousal responses to hypoxemia in sleep. *Am Rev Respir Dis* 1982; 126:1–2.
29. Remmers JE. Obstructive sleep apnea: a common disorder exacerbated by alcohol. *Am Rev Respir Dis* 1984; 130:153–155.
30. Remmers JE, Anch AM, DeGroot WJ. Respiratory disturbances during sleep. *Clin Chest Med* 1980; 1:57–71.
31. Block AJ. Sleep apnea and related disorders. *Disease-a-Month* 1985; 31: 1–56.
32. Guilleminault C, Tilkian A, Dement WC. The sleep apnea syndromes. *Annu Rev Med* 1976; 27:465–484.
33. Bohlman ME, Haponik EF, Smith PL, et al. CT demonstration of pharyngeal narrowing in adult sleep obstructive apnea. *Am J Roentgenol* 1983; 140:543–548.
34. Suratt PM, Dee P, Atkinson P, et al. Fluoroscopic and computed tomographic features of the pharyngeal airway in obstructive sleep apnea. *Am Rev Respir Dis* 1983; 127:487–492.
35. Haponik EF, Smith PL, Bohlman ME, et al. Computerized tomography in obstructive sleep apnea. 1983; 127:221–226.
36. Hoffstein V, Zamel N, Phillipson EA. Lung volume dependence of pharyngeal cross-sectional area in patients with obstructive sleep apnea. *Am Rev Respir Dis* 1984; 130:175–178.
37. Sugerman HJ. Pulmonary function in morbid obesity. *Gastroenterol Clin North Am* 1987; 16:225–237.

38. Ray CS, Sue DY, Bray G, et al. Effects of obesity on respiratory function. *Am Rev Respir Dis* 1983; 128:501–506.
39. Suratt PM, McTier RF, Findley LJ, et al. Changes in breathing and the pharynx after weight loss in obstructive sleep apnea. *Chest* 1987; 4:631–637.
40. Koenig JS, Thach BT. Effects of mass loading on the upper airway. *J Appl Physiol* 1988; 64:2294–2299.
41. Wittels EH. Obesity and hormonal factors in sleep and sleep apnea. *Med Clin North Am* 1985; 69:1265–1280.
42. Browman CP, Sampson MG, Yolles SF, et al. Obstructive sleep apnea and body weight. *Chest* 1984; 85:435–436.
43. Smith PL, Gold AR, Meyers DA, et al. Weight loss in mildly to moderately obese patients with obstructive sleep apnea. *Ann Intern Med* 1985; 103:850–855.
44. Harman EM, Wynne JW, Block AJ. The effect of weight loss on sleep-disordered breathing and oxygen desaturation in morbidly obese men. *Chest* 1982; 82:291–294.
45. Peiser J, Lavie P, Ovnat A, et al. Sleep apnea syndrome in the morbidly obese as an indication for weight reduction surgery. *Ann Surg* 1984; 199:112–115.
46. Sugarman HJ, Fairman RP, Baron PL, et al. Gastric surgery for respiratory insufficiency of obesity. *Chest* 1986; 90:81–86.
47. Sugarman HJ, Baron PL, Fairman RP, et al. Hemodynamic dysfunction in obesity hypoventilation syndrome and the effects of treatment with surgically induced weight loss. *Ann Surg* 1988; 207:604–613.
48. Charuzi I, Ovnat A, Peiser J, et al. The effect of surgical weight reduction on sleep quality in obesity-related sleep apnea syndrome. *Surgery* 1985; 97:535–538.
49. Cartwright RD. Effect of sleep position on sleep apnea activity. *Sleep* 1984; 7:110–114.
50. Cartwright RD, Lloyd S, Lilie J, et al. Sleep position training as treatment for sleep apnea syndrome: A preliminary study. *Sleep* 1985; 8:87–94.
51. Chaudhary BA, Chaudhary TK, Kolbeck RC, et al. Therapeutic effect of posture in sleep apnea. *South Med J* 1986; 79:1061–1063.
52. Kavey NB, Blitzer MA, Gidro-Frank S, et al. Sleeping position and sleep apnea syndrome. *Am J Otolaryngol* 1985; 6:373–377.
53. Phillips BA, Okeson J, Paesani D, et al. Effect of sleep position on sleep apnea and parafunctional activity. *Chest* 1986; 90:424–430.
54. McEvoy RD, Sharp DJ, Thornton AT. The effects of posture on obstructive sleep apnea. *Am Rev Respir Dis* 1986; 133:662–666.
55. Lerner SA, Cecil WT. The effect of posture on obstructive sleep apnea. *Chest* 1984; 26:327.
56. George CF, Millar TW, Kryger MH. Sleep apnea and body position during sleep. *Sleep* 1988; 11:90–99.
57. Skatrud J, Iber C, Ewart R, et al. Disordered breathing during sleep in hypothyroidism. *Am Rev Respir Dis* 1981; 124:325–329.
58. Rajagopal KR, Abbrecht PH, Derderian SS, et al. Obstructive sleep apnea in hypothyroidism. *Ann Intern Med* 1984; 101:491–494.

59. Mendelson WB, Garnett D, Gillin JC. Flurazepam-induced sleep apnea syndrome in a patient with insomnia and mild sleep-related respiratory changes. *J Nerv Ment Dis* 1981; 169:261–264.
60. Dolly FR, Block AJ. Effect of flurazepam on sleep-disordered breathing and nocturnal oxygen desaturation in asymptomatic subjects. *Am J Med* 1982; 73:239–243.
61. Bonora M, St. John WM, Bledsoe TA. Differential elevation by protriptyline and depression by diazepam of upper airway respiratory muscle activity. *Am Rev Respir Dis* 1985; 131:41–45.
62. Leiter JC, Knuth SL, Krol RC, et al. The effect of diazepam on genioglossal muscle activity in normal subjects. *Am Rev Respir Dis* 1985; 132: 216–219.
63. Geddes DM, Rudolf M, Saunders KB. Effect of nitrazepam and flurazepam on the ventilatory response to carbon dioxide. *Thorax* 1976; 31: 548–551.
64. Hedemark LL, Kronenberg RS. Flurazepam attenuates the arousal response to sleep in normal subjects. *Am Rev Respir Dis* 1983; 128:980–983.
65. Gothe B, Cherniack NS, Williams L. Effect of hypoxia on ventilatory and arousal response to CO_2 during n-REM sleep with and without flurazepam in young adults. *Sleep* 1986; 9:24–37.
66. Robinson RW, Zwillich CW, Bixler EO, et al. Effects of oral narcotics on sleep-disordered breathing in healthy adults. *Chest* 1987; 91:197–203.
67. Rafferty TD, Ruskis A, Sasaki C, et al. Perioperative considerations in the management of tracheostomy for the obstructive sleep apnea patient. *Br J Anaesth* 1980; 52:619–621.
68. Nishino T, Shirahata M, Yonezawa T, et al. Comparison of changes in the hypoglossal and phrenic nerve activity in response to increasing depth of anesthesia in cats. *Anesthesiology* 1984; 60:19–24.
69. Block AJ, Boysen PG, Wynne JW. Sleep-disordered breathing and nocturnal oxygen desaturation in post-menopausal women. *Am J Med* 1980; 69:75–79.
70. Sandblom RE, Matsumoto AM, Schoene RB, et al. Obstructive sleep apnea syndrome induced by testosterone administration. *N Engl J Med* 1983; 308:508–510.
71. Johnson MW, Anch AM, Remmers JE. Induction of the obstructive sleep apnea syndrome in a woman by exogenous androgen administration. *Am Rev Respir Dis* 1984; 129:1923–1925.
72. Schneider BK, Pickett CK, Zwillich CW, et al. Influence of testosterone on breathing during sleep. *J Appl Physiol* 1986; 61:618–623.
73. Brownell LG, West P, Sweatman P, et al. Protriptyline in obstructive sleep apnea. A double blind trial. *N Engl J Med* 1982; 307:1037–1042.
74. Conway WA, Zorick F, Piccione P, et al. Protriptyline in the treatment of sleep apnoea. *Thorax* 1982; 37:49–53.
75. Smith PL, Haponik EF, Allen RP, et al. The effects of protriptyline in sleep-disordered breathing. *Am Rev Respir Dis* 1983; 127:8–13.
76. Brownell LG, Perez-Padilla R, West P, et al. The role of protriptyline in obstructive sleep apnea. *Bull Eur Physiopathol Respir* 1983; 19:621–624.
77. Popkin J, Rutherford R, Grossman R, et al. One year randomized trial of

nasal CPAP versus protriptyline in the management of obstructive sleep apnea. *Am Rev Respir Dis* 1988; 137(part 2):311.
78. Martin RJ, Sanders MH, Gray BA, et al. Acute and long-term ventilatory effects of hyperoxia in the adult sleep apnea syndrome. *Am Rev Respir Dis* 1982; 125:175–180.
79. Smith PL, Haponik EF, Bleecker ER. The effects of oxygen in patients with sleep apnea. *Am Rev Respir Dis* 1984; 130:958–963.
80. Ou LC, Miller MJ, Tenney SM. Hypoxia and carbon dioxide as separate and interactive depressants of ventilation. *Respir Physiol* 1976; 28:347–358.
81. Morrill CG, Meyer JR, Weil JV. Hypoxic ventilatory depression in dogs. *J Appl Physiol* 1975; 38:143–146.
82. Longobardo GS, Gothe B, Goldman MD, et al. Sleep apnea considered as a control system instability. *Respir Physiol* 1982; 50:311–333.
83. Onal E, Burrows DL, Hart RH, et al. Induction of periodic breathing during sleep causes upper airway obstruction in humans. *J Appl Physiol* 1986; 61:1438–1443.
84. Onal E, Lopata M. Periodic breathing and the pathogenesis of occlusive sleep apneas. *Am Rev Respir Dis* 1982; 126:676–680.
85. Motta J, Guilleminault C. Effects of oxygen administration in sleep-induced apneas. *In* C Guilleminault, W Dement (eds). Sleep Apnea Syndromes: Kroc Foundation Series, Vol 2. New York, Alan R. Liss, 1978, pp 137–144.
86. Guilleminault C, Cummiskey J, Motta J. Chronic obstructive airflow disease and sleep studies. *Am Rev Respir Dis* 1980; 122:397–406.
87. Skatrud JB, Dempsey JA, Kaiser DG. Ventilatory response to medroxyprogesterone acetate in normal subjects: Time course and mechanisms. *J Appl Physiol* 1978; 44:939–944.
88. Skatrud JB, Dempsey JA, Bhansali P, et al. Determinants of carbon dioxide retention and its correction in humans. *J Clin Invest* 1980; 65:813–821.
89. Orr WC, Imes NK, Martin RJ. Progesterone therapy in obese patients with sleep apnea. *Arch Intern Med* 1979; 139:109–111.
90. Hensley MJ, Saunders NA, Strohl KP. Medroxyprogesterone treatment of obstructive sleep apnea. *Sleep* 1980; 3:441–446.
91. Strohl KP, Hensley MJ, Saunders NA, et al. Progesterone administration and progressive sleep apneas. *J Am Med Assoc* 1981; 245:1230–1232.
92. Rajagopal KR, Abbrecht PH, Jabbari B. Effects of medroxyprogesterone acetate in obstructive sleep apnea. *Chest* 1986; 90:815–821.
93. Suratt PM, Wilhoit SC, Brown ED, et al. Effect of doxepram on obstructive sleep apnea. *Bull Eur Physiopathol Respir* 1986; 22:127–131.
94. Suratt PM, Wilhoit SC, Brown ED, et al. Treatment of obstructive sleep apnea with a respiratory stimulant. *Sleep Res* 1985; 14:220.
95. Lyons HA, Huang CT. Therapeutic use of progesterone in alveolar hypoventilation associated with obesity. *Am J Med* 1968; 44:881–888.
96. Skatrud JB, Dempsey JA. Relative effectiveness of acetazolamide versus medroxyprogesterone in correction of carbon dioxide retention. *Am Rev Respir Dis* 1983; 127:405–412.

97. Schmidt HS. L-Tryptophan in the treatment of impaired respiration during sleep. *Bull Eur Physiopathol Respir* 1983; 19:625–629.
98. Schmidt HS. Combined L-tryptophan and protriptyline in the treatment of obstructive sleep apnea. *Sleep Res* 1985; 14:209.
99. Lakshminarayan S, Sahn SA, Weil JV. Effect of aminophylline on ventilatory responses in normal man. *Am Rev Respir Dis* 1978; 117:33–38.
100. Dowell AR, Heyman A, Sieker HO, et al. Effect of aminophylline on respiratory-center sensitivity and in pulmonary emphysema. *N Engl J Med* 1963; 273:1447–1453.
101. Marias OAS, McMichael J. Theophylline ethylenediamine in Cheyne-Stokes breathing. *Lancet* 1937; 2:437–430.
102. Dietrich J, Krauss AN, Reidenberg M, et al. Alterations in state in apneic pre-term infants receiving theophylline. *Clin Pharmacol Ther* 1978; 24: 474–478.
103. Espinoza H, Antic R, Thornton AT, et al. The effects of aminophylline on sleep and sleep-disordered breathing in patients with obstructive sleep apnea syndrome. Am Rev Respir Dis 1987; 136:80–84.
104. Gothe B, Strohl KP, Levin S, et al. Nicotine: A different approach to treatment of obstructive sleep apnea. *Chest* 1985; 87:11–17.
105. Haxhiu MA, van Lunteren E, Mitra J, et al. Responses to chemical stimulation of upper airway muscles and the diaphragm in awake cats. *J Appl Physiol* 1984; 54:397–493.
106. Haxhiu MA, Van de Graaf W, Mitra J, et al. The effect of pharmacologic stimulation on phrenic and hypoglossal nerve activity. *Clin Res* 1982; 30:784.
107. Strohl KP, Gottfried SB, Van de Graaf WB, et al. Physical and pharmacologic manipulation of upper airway resistance in anesthetized dogs. *Clin Res* 1982; 30:751.
108. Sharp JT, Druz WS, D'Souza V, et al. Effect of metabolic acidosis upon sleep apnea. *Chest* 1985; 87:619–624.
109. Whyte KF, Gould GA, Airlie AA, et al. Role of protriptyline and acetazolamide in the sleep apnea/hypopnea syndrome. *Sleep* 1988; 11:463–472.
110. Guilleminault C, Hayes B. Naloxone, theophylline, bromocriptine, and obstructive sleep apnea. *Bull Eur Physiopathol Respir* 1983; 19:632–634.
111. Guilleminault C, Flagg WH, Coburn SC, et al. Baclofen trial in myotonic dystrophy patients. *Acta Neurol Scand* 1978; 57:232–238.
112. Tilkian AG, Guilleminault C, Schroeder JS, et al. Sleep induced apnea syndrome: Prevalence of cardiac arrhythmias and their reversal after tracheostomy. *Am J Med* 1977; 63:348–358.
113. Krieger J, Mangin P, Kurtz D. Effects of almitrine in the treatment of sleep apnea syndromes. *Bull Eur Physiopathol Respir* 1983; 19:630.
114. Krieger J, Mangin P, Kurtz D. Sleep apnea syndrome: Effects of chlorimiprimine in subjects with stable body weight. *Rev Electroencephalogr Neurophysiol Clin* 1979; 9:250–257.
115. Olson LG, Hensley MJ, Saunders NA. Breathing during sleep: The responses to asphyxia and prochlorperizine in normal subjects and patients with obstructive sleep apnoea. *Aust NZ J Med* 1983; 13:613–620.

116. Remmers JE, Anch AM, deGroot WJ, et al. Oropharyngeal muscle tone in obstructive sleep apnea before and after strychnine. *Sleep* 1980; 3: 447–453.
117. Block AJ, Hughs RL. Factors influencing upper airway closure. *Chest* 1984; 86:114–122.
118. Sullivan CE, Issa FG, Berthon-Jones M, et al. Reversal of obstructive sleep apnoea by continuous positive airway pressure applied through the nares. *Lancet* 1981; 1:862–865.
119. Sanders MH, Moore SE, Eveslage J. CPAP via nasal mask: A treatment for occlusive sleep apnea. *Chest* 1983; 83:144–145.
120. Sanders MH. Nasal CPAP effect on patterns of sleep apnea. *Chest* 1984; 86:839–844.
121. Rapoport DM, Sorkin B, Garay SM, et al. Reversal of the "Pickwickian syndrome" by long term use of nocturnal airway pressure. *N Engl J Med* 1982; 307:931–933.
122. Wilhoit SC, Brown ED, Suratt PM. Treatment of obstructive sleep apnea with continuous nasal airflow delivered through nasal prongs. *Chest* 1984; 85:170–173.
123. Remmers JE, Sterling JA, Thorarinsson B, et al. Nasal airway positive pressure in patients with occlusive sleep apnea. Methods and feasibility. *Am Rev Respir Dis* 1984; 130:1152–1155.
124. Issa FG, Sullivan CE. Reversal of central sleep apnea using nasal CPAP. *Chest* 1986; 90:165–171.
125. Sullivan CE, Berthon-Jones M, Issa FG. Remission of severe obesity–hypoventilation syndrome after short-term treatment during sleep with nasal continuous positive airway pressure. *Am Rev Respir Dis* 1983; 128: 177–181.
126. Rajagopal KR, Bennett LL, Dillard TA, et al. Overnight nasal CPAP improves hypersomnolence in sleep apnea. *Chest* 1986; 90:172–176.
127. Sullivan CE, Berthon-Jones M, McCauley VB, et al. Home treatment of obstructive sleep apnoea with continuous positive airway pressure applied through a nose-mask. *Bull Eur Physiopathol Respir* 1984; 20:49–54.
128. Schmidt-Nowara WW. Continuous positive airway pressure for long-term treatment of sleep apnea. *Am J Dis Child* 1984; 138:82–84.
129. McEvoy RD, Thornton AT. Treatment of obstructive sleep apnea syndrome with nasal continuous positive airway pressure. *Sleep* 1984; 7: 313–325.
130. Frith RW. Severe obstructive sleep apnoea treated with long term nasal continuous positive airway pressure. *Thorax* 1985; 40:45–50.
131. Sanders MH, Gruendl CA, Rogers RM. Compliance of patients with nasal CPAP therapy for sleep apnea. *Chest* 1986; 90:330–333.
132. Krieger J, Weitenblum E, Monassier JP, et al. Dangerous hypoxaemia during continuous positive airway pressure treatment of obstructive sleep apnoea. *Lancet* 1983; 2:1429–1430.
133. Alex CG, Aronson RM, Onal E, et al. Effects of continuous positive upper airway pressure on upper airway and respiratory muscle activity. *J Appl Physiol* 1987; 62:2026–2030.
134. Series F, Cormier Y, Lampron N, et al. Increasing functional residual capacity may reverse obstructive sleep apnea. *Sleep* 1988; 11:349–353.

135. Rapoport DM, Garay SM, Goldring RM. Nasal CPAP in obstructive sleep apnea: Mechanisms of action. *Bull Eur Physiopathol Respir* 1983; 19:616–620.
136. Strohl KP, Redline S. Nasal CPAP therapy, upper airway muscle activation, and obstructive sleep apnea. *Am Rev Respir Dis* 1986; 134:555–558.
137. Fouke JM, Strohl KP. Effect of position and lung volume on upper airway geometry. *J Appl Physiol* 1987; 63:375–380.
138. Sullivan CE, Issa FG, Berthon-Jones M. Reduced severity of obstructive sleep apnoea following short-term treatment with continuous positive airway pressure applied through the nose. *Aust NZ J Med* 1982; 12:224.
139. Berthon-Jones M, Issa FG, Sullivan CE. Acute upward shift in ventilatory response to CO_2 after reversal of obstructive sleep apnoea by pneumatic splinting. *Aust NZ J Med* 1982; 12:224–225.
140. Mahadevia AK, Onal E, Lopata M. Effects of expiratory positive airway pressure on sleep-induced respiratory abnormalities in patients with hypersomnia-sleep apnea syndrome. *Am Rev Respir Dis* 1983; 128:708–711.
141. Sanders MH, Moore SE. Inspiratory and expiratory partitioning of airway resistance during sleep in patients with sleep apnea. *Am Rev Respir Dis* 1983; 127:554–558.
142. Sanders MH, Rogers RM, Pennock BE. Prolonged expiratory phase in sleep apnea. A unifying hypothesis. *Am Rev Respir Dis* 1985; 131:401–408.
143. Cartwright RD, Samelson CF. The effects of non-surgical treatment for obstructive sleep apnea: The tongue-retaining device. *J Am Med Assoc* 1982; 248:705–709.
144. Cartwright RD. Predicting response to the tongue-retaining device for sleep apnea syndrome. *Arch Otolaryngol* 1985; 111:385–388.
145. Cartwright RD, Stefoski D, Calderelli D, et al. Toward a treatment logic for sleep apnea: The place of the tongue-retaining device. *Behav Res Ther* 1988; 26:121–126.
146. George PT. A modified functional appliance for treatment of obstructive sleep apnea. *J Clin Orthodont* 1987; 21:171–175.
147. George PT. Mechanics of obstructive sleep apnea: A dentist's perspective. *Arch Otolaryngol Head Neck Surg* 1987; 113:1340.
148. Afzelius L-E, Elmqvist D, Hougaard K, et al. Sleep apnea syndrome: An alternative treatment to tracheostomy. *Laryngoscope* 1981; 91:285–291.
149. Martin RJ. Sleep-related respiratory disorders associated with daytime somnolence: Sleep apnea and hypoventilation syndromes. *In* RJ Martin (ed). Cardiorespiratory Disorders during Sleep. Mount Kisco, New York, Futura Publishing, 1984, pp 65–117.
150. Ikematsu T. Study of snoring, 4th report: Therapy. *J Jpn Oto-Rhino-Laryngol* 1964; 64:434–435.
151. Fujita S, Conway W, Zorick F, et al. Surgical correction of anatomic abnormalities in obstructive sleep apnea syndrome: Uvulopalatopharyngoplasty. *Otolaryngol Head Neck Surg* 1981; 89:923–934.
152. Simmons FB, Guilleminault C, Miles LE. The palatopharyngoplasty operation for snoring and sleep apnea: An interim report. *Otolaryngol Head Neck Surg* 1984; 92:375–380.

153. Moran WB, Orr WC. Diagnosis and management of obstructive sleep apnea: A multidisciplinary approach. *Arch Otolaryngol* 1985; 111:583–588.
154. Moran WB, Orr WC. Diagnosis and management of obstructive sleep apnea. Part II. *Arch Otolaryngol* 1985; 111:650–658.
155. Kimmelman CP, Levine SB, Shore ET, et al. Uvulopalatopharyngoplasty: A comparison of two techniques. *Laryngoscope* 1985; 95:1488–1490.
156. Simmons FB, Guilleminault C, Silvestri R. Snoring, and some obstructive sleep apnea, can be cured by pharyngeal surgery. *Arch Otolaryngol* 1983; 109:503–507.
157. Simmons FB, Guilleminault C, Miles LE. A surgical treatment for snoring and obstructive sleep apnea. *West Med J* 1984; 140:43–46.
158. Fujita S. UPPP for sleep apnea and snoring. *Ear, Nose Throat Surg* 1984; 63:73–86.
159. Fujita S, Conway WA, Zorick FJ, et al. Evaluation of the effectiveness of uvulopalatopharyngoplasty. *Laryngoscope* 1985; 95:70–74.
160. Conway W, Fujita S, Zorick F, et al. Uvulopalatopharyngoplasty. One-year follow-up. 1985; 88:385–387.
161. Kramer M, Anand VK, Schoen L, et al. Death associated with uvulopalatopharyngoplasty: A case report. *Sleep Res* 1985; 14:180.
162. Johnson JT, Sanders MH. Breathing during sleep immediately after uvulopalatopharyngoplasty. *Laryngoscope* 1986; 96:1236–1238.
163. Thawley SE. Surgical treatment of obstructive sleep apnea. *Med Clin North Am* 1985; 69:1337–1358.
164. Sanders MH, Johnson JT, Keller FK, et al. The acute effects of uvulopalatopharyngoplasty on breathing during sleep in sleep apnea patients. *Sleep* 1988; 11:75–89.
165. Scher AE, Thorpey MJ, Shprintzen RJ, et al. Predictive value of Mueller's maneuver in selection of patients with UPPP. *Laryngoscope* 1985; 95:1483–1487.
166. Katstantonis GP, Walsh JK. Somnofluoroscopy: Its role in the selection of candidates for uvulopalatopharyngoplasty. *Otolaryngol Head Neck Surg* 1986; 94:56–60.
167. Guilleminualt C, Hayes B, Smith L, et al. Palatopharyngoplasty and obstructive sleep apnea syndrome. *Bull Eur Physiopathol Respir* 1983; 19: 595–599.
168. Gislason T, Lindholm C-E, Almqvist M, et al. Uvulopalatopharyngoplasty in the sleep apnea syndrome. Predictors of results. *Arch Otolaryngol Head Neck Surg* 1988; 114:45–51.
169. Caldarelli DD, Cartwright R, Lilie JK. Severity of sleep apnea as a predictor of successful treatment by palatopharyngoplasty. *Laryngoscope* 1986; 96:945–947.
170. Schoen LS, Anand VK, Weisenberger S. Upper-airway surgery for treating obstructive sleep apnea. *Arch Otolaryngol Head Neck Surg* 1987; 113: 850–853.
171. Imes NK, Orr WC, Smith RO, et al. Retrognathia and sleep apnea: A life-threatening condition masquerading as narcolepsy. *J Am Med Assoc* 1977; 237:1596–1597.

172. Riley RW, Guilleminault C. Cephalometric analysis and flow-volume loops in obstructive sleep apnea patients. *Sleep* 1983; 6:301–311.
173. Riley RW, Powell NB, Guilleminault C. Inferior sagittal ostetomy of the mandible with hyoidmyotomy-resuspension: A new procedure for obstructive sleep apnea. *Otolaryngol Head Neck Surg* 1986; 94:589–593.
174. Riley RW, Powell NB, Guilleminault C, et al. Maxillary, mandibular, and hyoid advancement: An alternative to tracheostomy in obstructive sleep apnea syndrome. *Otolaryngol Head Neck Surg* 1986; 94:1591–1594.
175. Powell N, Guilleminault C. Mandibular advancement and obstructive sleep apnea syndrome. *Bull Eur Physiopathol Respir* 1983; 19:604–606.
176. Olsen KD, Kern EB, Westbrook PR. Sleep and breathing disturbance secondary to nasal obstruction. *Otolaryngol Head Neck Surg* 1981; 89: 804–810.
177. Zwillich CW, Pickett C, Hanson FN, et al. Disturbed sleep and prolonged apnea during nasal obstruction in normal men. *Am Rev Respir Dis* 1981; 121:158–160.
178. Heimer D, Scharf SM, Lieberman A, et al. Sleep apnea syndrome treated by repair of deviated nasal septum. *Chest* 1983; 84:184–185.
179. Olsen KD. The nose and its impact on snoring and obstructive sleep apnea. *In* DNF Fairbanks, S Fujita, T Ikematsu, FB Simmons (eds). Snoring and Obstructive Sleep Apnea. New York, Raven Press, 1987, pp 199–226.
180. Rubin AH, Eliaschar I, Joachim Z, et al. Effects of nasal surgery and tonsillectomy on sleep apnea. *Bull Eur Physiopathol Respir* 1983; 19:612–615.
181. Thach BT. Pediatric aspects of sleep apnea syndrome. *Ear Nose Throat J* 1984; 63:214–222.
182. Mangat D, Orr WC, Smith RO. Sleep apnea, hypersomnolence and upper airway obstruction secondary to adenotonsillar enlargement. *Arch Otolaryngol* 1977; 16:43–50.
183. Guilleminault C, Eldridge FL, Simmons FB, et al. Sleep apnea in eight children. *Pediatrics* 1976; 58:23–29.
184. Potsic WP, Pasquariello PS, Baranak CC, et al. Relief of upper airway obstruction by adenotonsillectomy. *Otolaryngol Head Neck Surg* 1986; 94: 476–480.
185. Mauer KW, Staats BA, Olsen KD. Upper airway obstruction and disordered nocturnal breathing in children. *Mayo Clin Proc* 1983; 58:349–353.
186. Orr WC, Martin RJ. Obstructive sleep apnea associated with tonsillar hypertrophy in adults. *Arch Intern Med* 1981; 141:990–992.
187. Lugaresi E, Coccagna G, Mantovani M, et al. Effects of tracheostomy in two cases of hypersomnia with periodic breathing. *J Neurol Neurosurg Psychiatr* 1973; 36:15–26.
188. Simmons FB, Guilleminault C, Dement WC, et al. Surgical management of airway obstructions during sleep. *Laryngoscope* 1977; 87:326–338.
189. Weitzman ED, Kahn E, Pollak CP. Quantitative analysis of sleep and sleep apnea before and after tracheostomy in patients with the hypersomnia-sleep apnea syndrome. *Sleep* 1980; 3:407–423.
190. Guilleminault C, Cummiskey J. Progressive improvement of apnea in-

dex and ventilatory response to CO_2 after tracheostomy in obstructive sleep apnea syndrome. *Am Rev Respir Dis* 1982; 126:14–20.
191. Olsen KD, Pearson BW. Sleep apnea tracheotomy. *Laryngoscope* 1984; 94:555–556.
192. Kenan PD. Complications associated with tracheostomy: Prevention and treatment. *Otolaryngol Clin North Am* 1979; 12:807–816.
193. Conway WA, Victor LD, Magilligan DJ Jr, et al. Adverse effects of tracheostomy for sleep apnea. *J Am Med Assoc* 1981; 246:347–350.
194. Simmons FB. Tracheostomy for obstructive sleep apnea: Indications and techniques. *In* Snoring and Obstructive Sleep Apnea. DNF Fairbanks, S Fujita, T Ikematsu, FB Simmons (eds). New York, Raven Press, 1987, pp 185–197.
195. Buckwalter JA, Sasaki CT. Effect of tracheotomy on laryngeal function. *Otolaryngol Clin North Am* 1984; 17:41–48.
196. Martin RJ. Sleep-related respiratory disorders associated with daytime somnolence: Sleep apnea and hypoventilation syndromes. *In* RJ Martin (ed). Cardiorespiratory Disorders During Sleep. Mt. Kisco, New York, Futura Publishing, 1984, pp 65-117.
197. Reite M, Jackson D, Cahoon RL, et al. Sleep physiology at high altitude. *Electroencephalogr Clin Neurophysiol* 1975; 38:463–471.
198. McNicholas WT, Carter JL, Rutherford R, et al. Beneficial effect of oxygen in primary alveolar hypoventilation with central sleep apnea. *Am Rev Respir Dis* 1982; 125:773–775.
199. White DP, Zwillich C, Pickett CK, et al. Central sleep apnea: improvement with acetazolamide therapy. *Arch Intern Med* 1982; 142:1816–1819.
200. Bradley TD, Brown IG, Zamel N, et al. Differences in pharyngeal properties between snorers with predominantly central sleep apnea and those without sleep apnea. *Am Rev Respir Dis* 1987; 135:387–391.
201. Sutton FD, Zwillich CW, Creagh CE, et al. Progesterone for outpatient treatment of Pickwickian syndrome. *Ann Intern Med* 1975; 83:476–479.
202. Lyons HA, Huang CT. Therapeutic use of progesterone in alveolar hypoventilation associated with obesity. *Am J Med* 1968; 44:881–888.
203. Rall TW. Central nervous system stimulants: the xanthines. *In* AG Gillman, LD Goodman, A Gillman (eds). The Pharmacological Basis of Therapeutics, 6th ed. New York, Macmillan, 1980, pp 592–607.
204. Kelly DH, Shannon DC. Treatment of apnea and excessive periodic breathing in the full-term infant. *Pediatrics* 1981; 68:183–186.
205. Shannon DC, Gotay F, Stein IM, et al. Prevention of apnea and bradycardia in low-birthweight infants. *Pediatrics* 1975; 55:589–594.
206. McMichan JC, Piepgras DG, Gracey DR, et al. Electrophrenic stimulation. *Mayo Clin Proc* 1979; 54:662–668.
207. Glenn WWL, Hogan JF, Loke JSO, et al. Ventilatory support by pacing of the conditioned diaphragm in quadriplegia. *N Engl J Med* 1984; 310: 1150–1155.
208. Glenn WWL, Gee JBL, Cole DR, et al. Combined central alveolar hypoventilation and upper airway obstruction. Treatment by tracheostomy and diaphragm pacing. *Am J Med* 1978; 64:50–60.
209. Hyland RH, Hutcheon MA, Perl A, et al. Upper airway occlusion induced by diaphragm pacing for primary alveolar hypoventilation: Im-

plications for the pathogenesis of obstructive sleep apnea. *Am Rev Respir Dis* 1981; 124:180–185.

210. Garay SM, Turino GM, Goldring RM. Sustained reversal of chronic hypercapnia in patients with alveolar hypoventilation syndromes. *Am J Med* 1981; 70:269–274.
211. Scharf SM, Feldman NT, Goldman MD, et al. Vocal cord closure. A cause of upper airway obstruction during controlled ventilation. *Am Rev Respir Dis* 1978; 117:391–397.
212. Ellis ER, Bye PTP, Bruderer JW, et al. Treatment of respiratory failure during sleep in patients with neuromuscular disease. *Am Rev Respir Dis* 1987; 135:148–152.

6

Nocturnal Asthma

Richard J. Martin, M.D.

Sleep-related asthma, which will be referred to as nocturnal asthma although it can be associated with sleep at any time of the day, is an intriguing problem that can be difficult to treat. The available information on this process, which is increasing yearly, will be discussed in detail, but as will become evident, an extensive fund of knowledge is not available. Since asthma in general is relatively easy to treat and severe problems occur uncommonly, two striking statistics that are not generally appreciated by the medical community reveal the severity of nocturnal asthma. Cochrane and Clark found that 68% of the adult asthmatic deaths occurred between midnight and 8:00 AM.[1] and Hetzel, et al. found that eight of 10 ventilatory arrests occurred between midnight and 6:00 AM.[2]

Nocturnal symptoms arising from bronchial asthma were realized as far back as 1698 by Floyer[3] and in 1882 by Salter,[4] but the exact incidence is unknown. Many authors feel that worsening of symptoms or decrements in airway function frequently occur in the asthmatic population during sleep. To determine the frequency of nocturnal asthma in a non-hospital-based population, Turner-Warwick[5] conducted a survey of 7729 asthmatic patients in the United Kingdom. Ninty-four percent responded that they awoke at least one night a month with symptoms of asthma. Seventy-four percent awoke at least one night a week, 64% at least three nights a week, and 39% awoke every night. Bagg and Hughes[6] also found morning decreases in peak expiratory flow rates in 30 of 40 stable asthmatics.

Martin RJ: Cardiorespiratory Disorders During Sleep, 2nd Edition. Futura Publishing Company, Inc., Mount Kisco, NY, © 1990.

Thus, the incidence of this potentially serious problem is higher than previously realized.

Mortality–Morbidity–Arousal Abnormalities

In 1971, 1198 deaths were attributed to asthma in England and Wales, 149 of which occurred in the greater London hospitals where Cochrane and Clark made their survey.[1] Forty-seven (32%) were in the age range of 35–64 on which the study was focused. Nine patients were excluded because other conditions may have been the cause of death. Also excluded were 15 because death occurred prior to hospital admission, two because patients were not admitted for acute asthma, and two case records were unobtainable. Although the population size was drastically reduced to 19 patients, important observations were made nevertheless.

Thirteen of the 19 patients (68%) died between midnight and 8:00 AM because of asthma. The remainder died at even intervals throughout the rest of the day. Of interest, only one patient was admitted to an intensive care unit and that was for a period of only two days. This patient died six days later on a general ward. Treatment would be important in considering the possible contributing factors to nocturnal death. Apparently a primary consideration as to the cause of death in this study was not on a lack of bronchodilator therapy, but rather the administration of sedatives. Fifteen of the 19 patients received sedation and 11 patients were given sedatives within 12 hours of death. In four patients, deterioration of their clinical condition rapidly followed sedative administration. However, in comparing this group to 19 surviving asthmatic patients, no difference could be found in the treatment programs. This raises the possibility of a patient subgroup that does not respond appropriately to sleep or sedation; that is, their arousal to important stimuli is blunted.

The possibility of a blunted arousal mechanism was studied in two adolescent males who had a history of severe nocturnal asthma that led to respiratory arrest.[7] These patients and control subjects were studied during sleep with leads for the measurement of sleep staging and a tight-fitting face mask attached to a pneumotachograph and an occlusion device for the measurement of arousal response time. Occlusion of the external airway was performed at end-expiration and released when alpha waves (arousal pattern) appeared on the electroencephalogram. Arousal from stage 2 sleep was the same between the controls and two patients (8.6 ± 4.9 SD seconds for the control vs. 8.4 ± 3.5 and 9.8 ± 1.8 for the two patients). The controls had a shorter time to arousal during stages 3–4 (8.8 ± 0.3 seconds vs. 20 ± 9.9 and 11.5 ± 0.3). Although there was greater variability during rapid eye movement (REM) sleep, again the controls tended to arouse more rapidly than the asthmatic patients (6.2 ± 3 seconds vs 9.8 ± 6 and 26.8 ± 20). This suggests that patients with severe nocturnal asthma may have a suppressed arousal response to bronchoconstriction and may not awaken until the process is quite severe. The possibility exists that suppressed arousal contributes to fatal nocturnal asthma.

Ballard et al.[8] determined the effect of sleep deprivation on the arousal response to induced bronchoconstriction during the next night's sleep. Airway resistance (measured on a breath-by-breath basis) was measured during sleep on each of two nights. One night was a "normal" sleep night and a second followed 24 hours of sleep deprivation. Nebulized methacholine via a mask was used to induce bronchoconstriction during sleep. Sleep following sleep deprivation produced a doubling in airway resistance before the subjects awoke complaining of chest tightness/wheezing compared to the "normal" sleep night. Thus arousal responses are depressed by prior sleep deprivation. In patients whose asthma is progressing over time, worsening sleep patterns probably develop that can lead to sleep deprivation and blunted arousal mechanisms.

In a 2 1/2 year survey of 1169 consecutive hospital admissions for asthma, a low percentage of respiratory arrests occurred as a result of asthma.[2] In nine patients, there were 10 successful resuscitations. Again, the crisis period was during the sleep hours between midnight and 6:00 AM; eight of the 10 respiratory arrests occurred during that 6-hour period. A feature common to all of these patients was the presence of large circadian swings in peak expiratory flow rates with an early morning fall. This early morning decrease was not limited to the patient with an impending respiratory arrest because it was seen in approximately 30% of all admissions. However, it correlated best with the risk of ventilatory arrest and also with sudden death out of all the variables analyzed. Also, unlike other signs on the examination, the circadian swings in peak flow did not show a relationship to the designation of acute or subacute asthma. The circadian change appears to be an individual characteristic.

Circadian Variation

All biologic functions have circadian rhythms associated with them. The respiratory unit is not different in this regard. In normals, peak expiratory flow rates are the highest at 4 PM and reach a nadir at 4 AM. This variation is approximately 5–8%. In asthmatics, this rhythm is followed, but the peak-to-trough variation can be much greater. When this variation approaches the 50% level, it is an important indicator of respiratory arrest and mortality.

To evaluate the effect of recumbency on circadian variation, five asthmatic patients remained in the sleeping position for over 24 hours.[9] With peak expiratory flow as the measure of change, it was determined that recumbency was not the factor producing the sleep-related fall found in this group on control days. This observation did not relate to the presence or absence of atopy. To further evaluate this phenomenon specifically in day versus night workers, an additional five asthmatic patients who worked night shifts were studied. The results showed that the circadian variation in peak flow was related to sleep rather than to the clock hour. In addition, it was found that when shifting from day work to night work and back again, the change in diurnal variation occurred rapidly and was complete by the end of the first new sleep cycle following the shift change. This rapid change in peak flow variation upon shift change is similar to the observed changes seen in the basic circadian rhythm, for example, body temperature.[10] Contrary to the peak flow changes, circadian variation in forced expiratory volume in one second in normal shift workers held a constant relationship to solar time.[11] However, it appears that none of these workers were asthmatic.

To further determine the effect of sleep on asthma, the effect of sleep interruption and sleep deprivation was investigated.[12] Twenty-one patients who had at least a 25% decrement in peak expiratory flow rates at 6:00 AM (in comparison to the highest recorded daytime value) were placed in the protocol. The study was divided into three parts to assess the effects of waking the patients once during the night or every 2 hours and the effect of total sleep deprivation. Seven of the 21 patients slept a control night and were then awakened at 2:00 AM for 15 minutes of activity before resuming sleep on the study night. In six of the seven patients, there was essentially no change in the 6:00 AM decrement in peak flow measurements, although interestingly in one patient the peak flow decrement was blocked by this nocturnal awakening. Overall there was no significant change in early morning peak flow resulting from the interruption of sleep at 2:00 AM. Another important point that this aspect of the study revealed was that the fall in peak expiratory flow was often well established by 2:00 AM with progressive deterioration to 6:00 AM.

Five different patients had measurement of peak flow rates every 2 hours during the night. The fall in this variable occurred between midnight and 2:00 AM in one patient, between 2:00 AM and 4:00 AM in three patients, and between 4:00 AM and 6:00 AM in another patient. Depending on the time the peak flow fell, these individuals were awakened one hour before this fall on subsequent nights for 15 minutes of exercise to determine if the 6:00 AM peak flow value would be improved. As before, no improvement in the peak flow decrement was seen.

Eleven patients took part in the last phase of this protocol. Initially, the peak expiratory flow was evaluated during the night to determine at what time the latest fall occurred; then on a subsequent night the patients were kept awake in the supine position until that time before being allowed to sleep. Two distinct groups emerged from this study. Six patients sustained virtually all of their nocturnal fall in peak flow rates while still awake. Five patients showed little or no fall while kept awake, but their usual fall ensued while asleep for the short interval before being awakened at 6:00 AM. This sleep interval lasted for less than 3 hours. Two patients from this group had a repeat deprivation night several days later and at that time most of the fall in peak flow rates occurred during wakefulness.

This study reveals two important points. The first is that arousal and exercise for 15 minutes does not alter the continuous drop in peak expiratory flow rates experienced throughout the night. The second is the question of whether sleep itself is the causative factor in the decremental changes of expiratory flow. Certainly one group of patients experienced the decreased flow rates while awake (electroencephalographic tracings were not used and the possibility, although slight, exists that the patients may have been in a drowsy state or in and out of sleep during the deprivation period), but this does not necessarily exclude any causal relationship between sleep and nocturnal asthma. The relationship, at best, is complex, and it would be difficult to construct experiments that could alter the time of sleep without affecting the phase of the peak expiratory flow rhythm (asthma) as well. As discussed previously, those same investigators showed that shift workers altered their peak flow responses to sleep time and not to solar time.

One investigation studied the relationship between sleep stages and "asthmatic episodes" in 12 adult patients with nocturnal symptoms.[13] The asthmatic episodes were conveyed by subjective means without the aid of any form of pulmonary function testing. There was a total of 35 subject nights in which 93 asthmatic incidents occurred. Except for the first hour or so of sleep, the incidences of these attacks were distributed fairly evenly throughout the night. This pattern did not depend upon the time of night the patients fell asleep or if adrenal corticosteroids were administered during the day. When relating these asthmatic incidents to sleep stages, it was shown that the percentage of episodes arising from each sleep stage approximated the percentage of sleep time spent in that period. Each patient was studied for at least two nights and on both nights considerable awake time was recorded because of the awakenings from the asthmatic incidents. When comparing the sleep patterns of six of these patients to an age-matched group, the mean sleep time was significantly less as a result of the frequent awakenings.

The results of this study do not support the notion that asthmatics' attacks are related either to sleep stages or to the time of the night. In addition, since dreaming is related to REM sleep, the theory that disturbing dreams are primarily responsible for precipitating asthmatics' symptoms is not supported. However, what is not evident from the study is the severity and duration of each episode. Thus, these factors may be related to sleep stages to some degree. The finding of marked awake time throughout the night supports the complaints of many patients that the inability to sleep well is a major problem.

The problem with the above studies is that the investigators needed to awaken the patients or have them spontaneously awaken. Recently, using the measurement of breath-by-breath airway resistance, asthmatic patients were allowed uninterrupted sleep while pulmonary function was being evaluated.[14] Normals and asthmatic subjects were studied both during "normal" sleep and during the night but kept awake in the recumbent position. In the asthmatic group there was a progressive and significant increase in airway resistance while awake during the night. However, on the sleep night, there was a more marked increase in resistance (Fig. 1a). This was independent of sleep stage. The normal subjects did not have an increase in airway resistance either during the awake or sleep nights (Fig. 1b). Thus, in asthma, there is a circadian rhythm to airway resistance (increased at night) that sleep potentiates. This potentiation of resistance is related to the duration one sleeps and not to sleep stages.

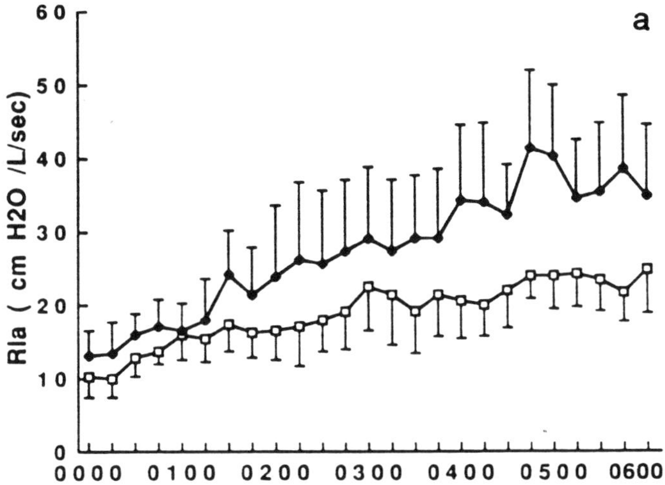

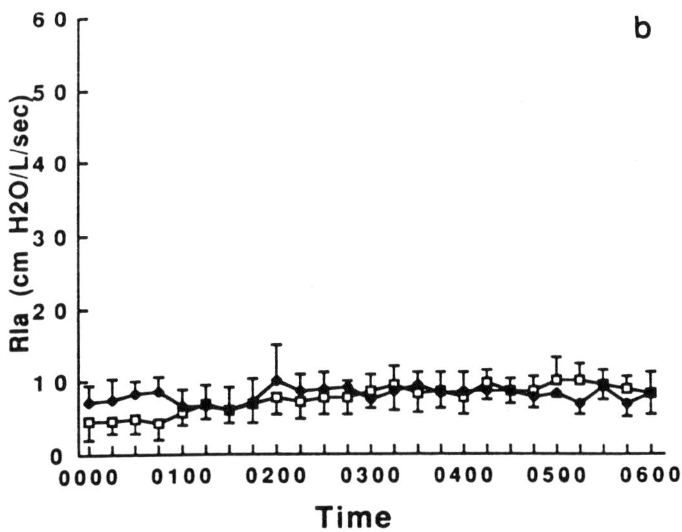

Figure 1 (a) Airway resistance measured throughout the night (awake, open squares; asleep, closed diamonds) in asthmatic subjects. There is a progressive increase in resistance awake from midnight to 6 AM that is significantly enhanced by sleep. Horizontal axis is clock time, vertical axis is resistance of the lower airways (Rla).

(b) As in Figure 1a, but the subjects are normals. No increases in resistance are seen awake or asleep. (From: reference 14, with permission.)

In an investigation of chronic stable asthmatic patients, the degree of oxygen desaturation associated with hypopneic or apneic-type breathing was greater during REM sleep.[15] This should not be confused with classical sleep apnea or with the findings discussed above of increasing lower airway resistance. This study was designed to relate oxygen desaturation during sleep to sleep staging and breathing irregularities in 10 adult asthmatics and 10 healthy age-matched subjects. Five of the 10 patients had a history of nocturnal symptoms. The results showed that both groups had similar total sleep time and duration of REM sleep and of non-REM sleep. However, the asthmatics spent more time in wakefulness and drowsiness than the matched control group. These patients also spent more time breathing irregularly (mean 52.1 minutes) than the controls (24.2 minutes, $P < 0.05$). The majority of irregular breathing was hypopneic in nature. Apneic periods were also present with the control group having 11 central apneic episodes, in the asthmatic group, 151 of 163 apneas were central. Of the other 12 apneas in the patient population, seven were obstructive and five were mixed. Most of the irregular breathing occurred during REM sleep for both groups. While the asthmatics spent more time with irregular breathing that the healthy subjects in all sleep stages, this difference was only significant during the stable wakefulness and drowsiness periods.

These investigators measured an important outcome of nocturnal periodic breathing, namely, oxygen desaturation. In the asthmatic individuals, there was a 9.7% (range 4%–18.9%) fall in saturation, while in the controls this was decreased by a mean of 4.3% (range 2%–6.2%). The four episodes of desaturation in the control group occurred during REM sleep. Two episodes were related to hypopneas, one occurred with apnea, and one with regular breathing. Sixteen of 28 episodes in the asthmatics occurred during REM sleep, nine in non-REM sleep, and three during wake–drowsiness periods. Eleven of these desaturation episodes were related to nonapneic irregular breathing, nine to apneas, and eight to regular breathing. When nonapneic desaturation occurs because of regular or irregular-type breathing, one must keep in mind that airway resistance may be increased, i.e., worsening of the asthmatic state. Indeed, these investigators measured expiratory time (prolongation reflects increasing airway resistance) in four of the asthmatics and found that during the desaturation episodes this variable was prolonged in three patients. Of interest, the oxygen desaturation did not correlate with a fall in forced expiratory volume in one second (FEV_1) from pre- to postsleep, but rather with the presleep saturation level.

Another study showed similar results in regard to sleep staging and nocturnal events.[16] Twelve adult patients with a history of nocturnal attacks were compared to age-, sex-, and weight-matched normals. In eight patients, nocturnal awakenings occurred, with 26 episodes recorded. The forced expiratory volume in one second decreased from a presleep value of 67% of predicted to 34.2% at the time of the attack. No awakenings due to asthma occurred in the first hour after sleep onset. Sleep efficiency was significantly altered in the asthmatics with nocturnal problems in comparison to the control subjects (76.5% ± 3.4 SEM vs. 92.8% ± 1.6, respectively, $P < 0.001$). The duration of sleep stages was not significantly different. Oxygen desaturation occurred only in the asthmatic patients with a mean duration of 27.3 seconds and a mean percent decrease from baseline of 6.5%. During REM sleep, oxygen desaturation was the most pronounced. The frequency of attacks was proportionally similar between REM sleep and non-REM sleep, but no awakenings occurred during stages 3 and 4.

The above studies are basically in agreement except for worsening of asthma as a function of sleep stages (Table 1); the airway resistance progressively increases during sleep. In addition, nocturnal awakenings in asthmatics occur more frequently in REM sleep, but oxygen desaturation and irregular breathing are worse during this stage. This rapid eye movement finding is not surprising because normals, sleep apnea patients, and chronic obstructive pulmonary

Table 1
Sleep Stages and Respiratory Patterns in Nocturnal Asthma

I. Sleep stages
   A. Increases in airway resistance during the night are related to duration of sleep and not sleep stages
II. Respiratory patterns
   A. Hypopneas and/or prolongation of expiration (reflecting increased airway resistance) are most frequent abnormalities
   B. Apneas—not frequent occurrences
      1. Central
      2. Upper airway obstruction
      3. Mixed

disease patients all have more cardiopulmonary abnormalities that are related to REM sleep (see appropriate chapters).

Causative Mechanisms of Nocturnal Asthma (Table 2)

Allergic Factors

Exposure to bedding or room allergens, particularly house dust, is a simple and attractive explanation for sleep-related asthma. This may be true in some cases,[17] but unfortunately, it is not an appropriate explanation for the vast majority. The frequency of nocturnal asthma in the hospital environment, which is essentially free of common environmental antigens, does not make an allergic etiology plausible. Alternatively, exposure to certain antigens during the day can result in delayed bronchospasm many hours later.[18–21] This might correspond to the nocturnal hours in some patients. Another type of external exposure to consider is the cyclic type of asthma which can occur after such variables as bronchial challenge tests.[22] In these situations, asthma not only occurs during the initial night after exposure but recurs over several nights without further exposure. This pattern may be brought about because the allergen remains in the bronchi or the airways become unstable and, then, in some manner, sleep plays a role in triggering the bronchospasm. This can occur by nocturnal reflex mechanisms, or chemical or humoral substances.

Preliminary results by Mohiuddin and Martin[23] suggest that the time of day a patient receives an antigen challenge by inhalation will determine if a late (delayed) asthmatic response will occur. That is,

Table 2
Potential Mechanisms of Nocturnal Asthma

Altered airway reactivity
Decreased catecholamines, cyclic AMP
Increased histamine levels
Airway secretions
Decreased cortisol
Airway cooling
Allergic factors (unusual)
Gastroesophageal reflux

most asthmatics develop an immediate response to an inhaled antigen to which they are sensitive. This is seen by a decrement in lung function, which is usually measured by the FEV_1. This response occurs within 15–20 minutes and dissipates within an hour. A second or late asthmatic response has been stated to occur in approximately 40% of these patients at 3–8 hours after the antigen challenge. As is customarily the case, the testing times have been done only during the day. It now appears that the time of day that the patient receives the antigen is very important in determining if a late asthmatic response will occur; that is, in three patients who only had an immediate response to the antigen challenge when given in the morning, there was both an immediate and delayed response to the challenge when given in the evening. This then led to severe nocturnal bronchoconstriction. If this information holds for the entire study, then the late asthmatic response may be an important aspect of nocturnal asthma.

Airway Secretions

Although asthmatics do not commonly complain of a productive cough as do patients with chronic bronchitis, secretions can still play a role in some patients with nocturnal asthma. At one extreme, autopsies have shown extensive mucus plugging of the airways in asthmatics.[2] In addition, animal studies have shown that the cough reflex mechanisms during sleep are suppressed, particularly during REM sleep.[24] With a suppressed clearance mechanism and potentially irritable airways, secretions may in some manner trigger or be involved in nocturnal asthma.

Not uncommonly, we see patients who develop upper respiratory infections and cough who tolerate the process better during the waking hours than during sleep. Upper respiratory infections can produce reflex bronchoconstriction, but this does not explain the observed awake-to-sleep difference. The exact role of secretions in this situation is not certain but is probably significant.

Asthma is a disease of the airways and this includes all airways, both intrathoracic and extrathoracic. Chronic sinusitis and/or postnasal drip are frequent problems in asthmatics. Not only will daytime symptoms improve as the sinus and discharge process is cleared, but nocturnal symptoms can dramatically improve. An example of this process is demonstrated by the following history. A 52-year-old female complained of progressive dyspnea and wheezing over a 6-month period. This was associated with postnasal drip and frequent nocturnal awakenings with worsening of breathing. The sinus films showed chronic pansinusitis, FEV_1 was 50% of predicted, and the ratio of FEV_1 to the forced vital capacity was 62%. After a program of inhaled and long-acting oral bronchodilators was initiated, her FEV_1 was 79% of predicted, but she still experienced "poor sleep." The morning FEV_1 was 50% of predicted. She was placed on an intensive program to clear nasal-sinus drainage, which included oral decongestants, saline nasal washes, and nasal steroids. Within several days she slept through the night and the morning FEV_1 was 75% of predicted.

The exact reason for worsening of symptoms in asthmatics because of sinus problems or extrathoracic secretions is not known. One possibility is a nasal or laryngeal irritation reflex producing bronchoconstriction. Another possibility is the difference between nasal breathing and mouth breathing in asthmatics. Exercise-induced bronchoconstriction is much greater with mouth breathing than nasal breathing.[25] Thus, if nasal congestion is present and the patient is mouth breathing, worsening of nocturnal symptoms may develop. A third possibility is that these secretions are aspirated, which can set off direct or reflex mechanisms worsening the asthma.

Gastroesophageal Reflux

The relationship between gastroesophageal reflux and nocturnal asthma is an intriguing topic. Obviously, in the recumbent position reflux would be potentiated. One usually relates this phenomenon to aspiration of gastric contents and direct irritability to the airways. However, the majority of asthmatic worsening may actually be due to reflex mechanisms. That is, the gastric contents irritate the esophageal mucosa and a reflex bronchoconstriction occurs. Both of these processes will be discussed.

Several surgical reports relate that gastroesophageal reflux with possible tracheobronchial aspiration is a trigger factor in asthma.[26–29] The predominant mechanism initiating the condition identified in these reported cases was an incompetent lower esophageal sphincter with or without an associated hiatal hernia. The medications that asthmatics are treated with, e.g., bronchodilators and steroids, tend to cause or potentiate the decreased tone in the gastroesophageal sphincter. The cause and effect of reflux asthma was stated to occur in several of these reports[26–28] when asthmatic symptoms were abolished following the surgical restoration of effective lower esophageal sphincter function.

In seeking the relationship between gastroesophageal reflux and asthma, Mays[30] compared 29 patients with severe asthma with 468 hospitalized nonasthmatic patients. Three of the asthmatic patients had lower lung field infiltrates of unknown origin, possibly related to aspiration. Using upper gastrointestinal radiography, 46% of the asthmatic patients had demonstrable reflux and 64% had hiatal hernia. Among the control patients only 5% had reflux and 19% hiatal hernias. The differences between the groups were significant. The high prevalence of hiatal hernia and reflux extended across the entire age spectrum of the asthmatic patients (20–68 years). In contrast, the peak incidence among control patients was the sixth decade. Since the asthmatic group was relatively small, these age incidences must be viewed cautiously.

Five asthmatics from the above study[30] had clinical symptoms compatible with the occurrence of reflux but had no demonstrable reflux on upper gastrointestinal series. Three of these five did have hiatal hernias. This brings up the point that gastrointestinal x-rays are very limited in truly detecting the incidence of reflux. Probably the best way to establish this process would be with esophageal probes that detect changes in pH values. Also, tracheal probes are one of the most sensitive methods to diagnose aspiration. Six of their patients had demonstrable reflux without historical evidence of clinical reflux, and three had hiatal hernias. Only five of the 29 asthmatics had no clinical or roentgenographic evidence compatible with reflux or hiatal hernia.

The relationship between asthma, reflux, and nocturnal symptoms is further supported by the study of Goodall et al.[31] Eighteen of 20 patients with nocturnal asthma completed a double-blind crossover study using cimetidine. The severity of reflux was graded using a symptom score of heartburn and regurgitation in addition to objective evaluation of upper gastrointestinal radiograph, fiberoptic endoscopy and biopsy, manometry, pH monitoring of the distal esophagus, and acid infusion testing. Significant improvement was seen in reflux and nighttime symptoms with cimetidine. Fourteen of the 18 patients felt that their chest symptoms had improved markedly during the period of cimetidine use.

In all probability, direct aspiration of gastric contents only plays an occasional role in nocturnal asthma. More likely, a vagal reflex mediated by esophageal receptors that are stimulated by reflux contents is the primary factor. In 15 patients with documented asthma and reflux, Mansfield and Stein[32] infused 0.1 N hydrochloric acid into the esophagus. There was both subjective and objective evidence of bronchoconstriction associated with this acid load. The bronchoconstriction improved after antacids relieved the symptoms.

In a similar study during sleep, Davis et al.[33] infused saline (control) and 0.1 N hydrochloric acid into the distal third of the esophagus. The asthmatic patients were divided into two groups based on the presence or absence of esophagitis as determined by the Bernstein test. The respiratory pattern was monitored continuously using an inductance vest. Saline infusion had no effect on the respiratory pattern. In patients with esophagitis, the acid infusion changes the respiratory pattern. These changes included: decreased mean expiratory flow (V_t/T_e), decreased ratio of inspiratory to total breath duration (T_i/T_{Tot}) and decreased inspiratory to expiratory timing (T_i/T_e). In addition, wheezing was auscultated. It was felt that acid in the esophagus alone triggered bronchoconstriction. This apparently occurs only in those patients who have preexisting esophagitis.

The above studies all point to a relationship between reflux and worsening of asthma. However, direct temporal measurements of lung function and low esophageal pH were not evaluated. Tan et al.[34] measured breath-by-breath airway resistance during sleep in asthmatic subjects with positive Bernstein tests. Acid infusion was done to lower the esophageal pH to less than 2. The mean lower airway resistance during the 30 minutes before acid infusion was 2.41 ± 0.78 cm H_2O/L/sec. This was not significantly different from that obtained during the 30 minutes of acid infusion (2.24 ± 0.48). These results suggest that gastroesophageal reflux does not trigger acute bronchoconstriction in patients with nocturnal asthma. Thus, this entire area needs further investigation to determine the exact relationship between reflux and asthma.

Increased Pulmonary Resistance during Sleep

An endogenous circadian rhythm is reflected in the smooth muscle tone of pulmonary airways in patients and normals.[35,36] In 11 hospitalized patients with reactive airway disease, the pulmonary resistance and thoracic gas volume (functional residual capacity) were measured every 3 hours around the clock.[35] The highest resistance occurred at 5:00 AM, and this was correlated with the highest thoracic gas volume. Both of these variables reflect airway narrowing and thus increased resistance. The increase in resistance started between 9:00 PM and midnight and progressively increased to 5:00 AM. The thoracic gas volume followed the same progression. This change in airway resistance was partially reversed by beta-sympathomimetics (metaproterenol) and parasympatholytics (Sch 1000).

Sullivan et al.[37] examined the effect of unanesthetized sleep on airway smooth muscle tone in dogs. This was an interesting experiment in which well-trained dogs breathed through an endotracheal tube via a permanent side-hole tracheostomy. In addition, the animals had exteriorized vagal loops to determine the effects of vagal stimulation to any observed changes. The tracheal smooth muscle tone was measured by the pressures generated in the inflated cuff of the endotracheal tube. During quiet wakefulness, the smooth muscle tone of the trachea was stable. As soon as sleep onset occurred and progressed through all of the non-REM stages, there was relaxation of the airway smooth muscle tone. This was reflected in the endotracheal balloon cuff pressure decreasing by 20–40 cm H_2O. A new, lower steady state developed during slow-wave (stages 3 and 4) sleep. In contrast, REM sleep was markedly different. The tracheal smooth muscle tone fluctuated markedly and erratically. The cuff pressure increased by as much as 90 cm H_2O. Neural control of this change in airway smooth muscle could be demonstrated by blocking the activity of the vagus nerve. This was done by cooling the exteriorized cervical vagal loops to a temperature that did not abolish resting awake tone. This partial vagal blockade decreased or abolished the fluctuations in tracheal smooth muscle tone during REM sleep. Therefore, in dogs, airway smooth muscle tone decreases in non-REM sleep and dramatically increases during REM sleep. This change in tone is related to variability in neural control of airway smooth muscle.

In an attempt to determine whether the changes that have been discussed are due to large or small airway deterioration, a group of 16 asthmatic patients with nocturnal symptoms was evaluated.[38] In this study, pulmonary flows, volumes, specific conductance diffusion, and helium-oxygen flow–volume curves were measured. The measurements were done at 6:00 AM and 2:00 PM on the same day. These measurement points represent the time (within 2 hours) where the low and high values for peak expiratory flows, respectively, have been reported. Twelve patients also had postbronchodilator measurement. A helium–oxygen combination is used to help delineate changes in the flow–volume loop from small and large airways. Helium is less dense than air but of similar viscosity. With helium, the maximal expiratory flow increases when obstruction is predominantly in large airways with low total cross-sectional area and turbulent flow. Lack of response to helium is attributed to obstruction principally in small airways with large total area and laminar flow.

At 2:00 PM, near-normal values for specific conductance with elevation in residual volume and low mid-expiratory flow rates were usually found. This is compatible with small airways obstruction. In seven patients this explanation was supported by the absence of a helium response. At 6:00 AM specific conductance was low, which suggests considerable large airway obstruction. The flow rates decreased significantly at 6:00 AM, similar to an acute attack, but without the degree of awareness these individuals would have to the same changes during the day. The response to inhaled bronchodilators at 6:00 AM is of interest. Eight of the 12 patients responded rapidly to the bronchodilators, but in four patients, little improvement was seen initially after bronchodilator. Both groups were similar by 2:00 PM. The patients in this latter group would appear to be the ones at high risk of severe nocturnal complications. That is, their pulmonary function was significantly decreased and they subjectively were not aware of it, nor did they respond to inhaled agents.

As stated previously, when breath-by-breath airway resistance is measured in asthmatic subjects, airway resistance increases progressively throughout the night.[14] This is true in the awake, recumbent position and markedly enhanced with sleep (Figure 1a,b).

Cortisol Levels

Two studies show that there is no direct relationship between plasma cortisol levels and peak expiratory flow rates. Barnes et al.[39] in five asthmatics showed that the circadian peak expiratory flow was highest at 4:00 PM and lowest at 4:00 AM, while the plasma cortisol level was highest at 7:00 AM and lowest at midnight; thus, no correlation existed. Soutar et al.[40] demonstrated in six asthmatics that the peak expiratory flow rates and plasma cortisol levels were the lowest during the night or in early morning. However, infusion of cortisol did not prevent the fall in peak flow in five of these patients. The continuous infusion of cortisol was gauged to deliver steroids in doses to prevent the observed nocturnal decrement. Large pharmacologic doses were not used. The observed increments in the lowest plasma corticosteroid level were 4.0–28.8 mg.

One patient in this study maintained his peak flow values after infusion of cortisol, which raises interesting possibilities. Is there variability from one night to the next in regard to the occurrence or degree of nocturnal asthma? All six of the patients in that study had constant nocturnal symptoms and decreases in peak flows prior to being placed into the protocol. Thus, it is unlikely that the objective finding would change from one night to the next. Another possibility is that there is a small subset of asthmatic patients who respond to reversal of the circadian cortisol level.

Catecholamine and Histamine Levels

There appears to be a temporal relationship between the nadir of circadian catecholamine and pulmonary function levels.[39,41] This low point for either urinary or plasma catecholamine levels is between 3:00 and 4:00 AM. This may be of importance as a fall in circulating epinephrine could directly reduce the stimulation of beta-adrenergic receptors in bronchial smooth muscle, inducing bronchospasm. In addition, an indirect effect of decreased circulating epinephrine is the release of histamine from mast cells because of diminished stimulation of beta-adrenergic receptors. This is important as histamine levels in venous plasma can correlate with the degree of bronchospasm.[42]

Barnes et al.[39] showed, in five asthmatic patients, that circadian changes in peak expiratory flow, circulating epinephrine, and cyclic AMP correlate positively with each other, but inversely with plasma histamine. As noted previously, there was not a significant correlation between peak expiratory flow and plasma cortisol levels. This suggests that release of histamine and perhaps other mediators from sensitized pulmonary mast cells could be due to the decrease in circulating nocturnal epinephrine. This, in turn, could produce bronchoconstriction. In addition, these investigators infused epinephrine in low doses and demonstrated decreased circulating histamine levels and improved peak expiratory flow rates. Interestingly, in normal subjects the circadian changes in plasma epinephrine occurred as in the asthmatics, but no significant rise in plasma histamine was observed.

Although the study of Barnes et al. was well done, the conclusion that circulating histamine is the cause of nocturnal airway obstruction cannot be drawn. Certainly, inhaled histamine is a potent bronchoconstrictor, whereas intravenously infused histamine is not.[43] Thus, other mediators may increase as histamine increases and may be the active substance(s). Several criteria[44] need to be observed before concluding that histamine is the causative agent of the decreased peak expiratory flow. These include artificial changes in catecholamine rhythm, producing immediate changes in the peak expiratory flow rhythm; natural changes in catecholamine rhythm, yielding changes in the expiratory flow rhythm at any time of the 24-hour cycle; and constant catecholamine levels, abolishing the circadian peak flow rhythm.

The exact cause of nocturnal exacerbation of asthma is far from understood. More than likely, a combination of multiple effects controls the airways of these susceptible patients. These processes would include the net effect of catecholamines, beta-adrenergic receptor responsiveness, mucociliary clearance, reflux mechanisms, vagal tone, corticosteroids, immunologic integrity, and arousal patterns. It appears that the circadian rhythms of all these factors are arranged to make the potential for nocturnal bronchoconstriction, respiratory failure, and death strong.

Airway Inflammation

To determine if inflammation plays a role in nocturnal asthma, Martin et al.[45] demonstrated that the total cell count in bronchial alveolar lavage fluid (BALF) is significantly higher at 4 AM in patients with nocturnal asthma compared to those without worsening of their asthma at night. Additionally, at 4 PM the BALF contents were similar in both groups. Comparing 4 PM and 4 AM, the nocturnal asthma group increased the cell count, whereas the other group did not. Neutrophils and eosinophils were the two cell populations that significantly increased from 4 PM to 4 AM in the nocturnal asthma group. Thus, the inflammatory cells appear to play a role in those asthmatics who markedly worsen their lung function at night by enhancing bronchial reactivity as discussed above.

Airway Cooling

Daytime studies have shown that a fall in body temperature of 0.7°C secondary to a short-duration cold exposure produces acute asthma attacks in the majority of asthmatic patients.[46,47] These investigators postulated that body cooling leads to vasoconstriction and cooling of the respiratory mucosa. This decrease in temperature of the mucosa consequently initiates bronchoconstriction in predisposed patients. This sequence of events was blocked when airway mucosa temperature was maintained by breathing warm, humidified air during body cooling.[48] Since body temperature can normally decrease by approximately 1°C during sleep,[49] this mechanism was recently tested to see if the nocturnal fall in pulmonary function could be reduced by breathing warm, humidified air.[50]

This study showed that the mean fall in temperature from baseline to awakening in seven asthmatics was significant. This decrement was unaffected by taking or withholding bedtime medications. The temperature drop was blocked by breathing warm humidified air (36.6°C before sleep, 36.6°C awakening). This air was delivered via a face tent at 37°C and 100% relative humidity. When breathing room air, FEV_1 decreased slightly, but significantly, from 2.9 L to 2.7 L ($P < 0.05$) and the forced expiratory flow between 25% and 75% fell from 2.4 L/s to 2.0 L/s ($P < 0.05$). When breathing warm humidified air, there was no significant change in morning pulmonary function. Using the heated air without regular evening medication did not prevent bronchoconstriction, but it was substantially reduced compared to room air breathing. Thus, these results suggest that nocturnal airway cooling may play a role in triggering sleep-induced asthma.

Bronchial Reactivity

As has been discussed extensively above, lung function worsens during the sleep-related hours. In the asthmatic patient, this would imply that bronchial reactivity must be changing during sleep. Martin et al.[51] demonstrated that the greater the overnight fall in peak expiratory flow rates, the larger the circadian change in bronchial reactivity. The bronchial reactivity was tested at 4 PM and 4 AM with marked increase in reactivity occurring at 4 AM. Those patients with the greater change in peak flow rates demonstrated such increased bronchial reactivity that their forced FEV_1 decreased by greater than 20% to inhaled normal saline alone. This effect was not seen at 4 PM.

The change in bronchial reactivity could affect the action of other factors that have been discussed above. The decrease in serum cortisol, circulating epinephrine, and cyclic AMP, as well as an increase in histamine, during the night[39] could have a direct effect on the airways as well as an interactive effect with bronchial reactivity. Similarly, cholinergic tone, which increases at night,[52] could affect bronchial responsivity and produce nocturnal effects. Gastroesophageal reflux[26–30] and airway cooling,[46–50] both of which may increase vagal tone, may induce nocturnal worsening of function in asthma, particularly when airway reactivity is increased. Finally, the demonstration that neutrophils and eosinophils in bronchoalveolar lavage fluid are increased at 4:00 AM in patients with nocturnal worsening of asthma, but not in those without nocturnal worsening,[45] suggests that airway inflammation may trigger the increase in bronchial reactivity.

Treatment

Reversible Factors

One should always approach the problem of treating nocturnal asthma by attempting to rule out any reversible causative factors. Investigation into the possibility of an extrinsic causative agent, particularly in the work environment, should be considered. Even if the patient is asymptomatic during the day, nocturnal exacerbation of asthma can be seen as a delayed effect. Another factor is the origin of secretions whether intra- or extrathoracic. If the asthmatic also has a degree of bronchitis or bronchiectasis, decreased clearance that is associated with sleep can worsen the problem. Bronchial hygiene, including postural drainage and percussion during the day and before sleep, has been beneficial in those occasional patients fitting this picture at our institution. As described above (see airway secretions), asthmatics commonly have sinusitis, nasal congestion, and accumulation of secretions in the posterior pharynx. This causes poor sleep and nocturnal asthma. Correcting this with oral decongestants, nasal steroidal preparations, and saline nasal washes can greatly improve the nocturnal asthma in this subset of patients. Rarely, a surgical procedure needs to be done to correct a particularly difficult-to-control sinus condition.

Reflux

Gastroesophageal reflux may or may not play an important role in nocturnal exacerbations. Certainly if the patient complains of "heartburn," retrosternal spasms, or a sour taste in the mouth when awakening in the morning, the clinical symptom complex is established. Occasionally a patient is not symptomatic but still has the problem. A trial of 6-inch wooden or brick blocks under the head of the bed (raising the head with pillows, etc., will not work) and bedtime antacids may give rapid relief. Another beneficial therapeutic intervention is the use of H-2 blockers. In our experience, as well as others,[31] these acid secretion blockers improve the symptoms of reflux and perhaps the related asthmatic problems. The dosage is variable, but the bedtime dosing should be the highest and, at times, it is all that is necessary. Surgery to solidify the gastroesophageal junction is rarely indicated.

If recurrent aspiration is documented, a more involved program needs to be undertaken. In addition to blocks under the head of the bed, no food or drink (except for medications) should be taken for several hours before bedtime. If further treatment is needed, a cricopharyngeal myotomy at times can alter the posterior pharyngeal anatomy to help prevent aspiration.

Bronchodilators

The majority of patients will not benefit from the above therapeutic interventions and will need some form of bronchodilator therapy. This may include simply maximizing a subtherapeutic program to ensure optimal bronchodilatory effects throughout the entire 24-hour day or additional maneuvers. These additional processes would be changes in the program of oral or inhaled agents. Inhaled agents are usually short-lived and do not give therapeutic effects throughout the entire night. However, an occasional patient may have difficulty only at the 2- to 3-hour mark after sleep onset. In this situation, optimal inhaled treatments at bedtime can improve the sleep period. This treatment should be given in doses just shy of producing tachycardia or tremors. It should be delivered via a compressor and not from a meter-dose container. This will ensure better delivery of the medication in the more difficult-to-treat asthmatics.

Proper Use of Theophylline—Chronopharmacology

Chronopharmacology, i.e., dosing medications where the maximum effect is needed, rather than a constant 24-hour blood level, is an important aspect in treating patients with nocturnal asthma. A recent publication[53] compared the efficacy of treating nocturnal asthma patients using once daily Uniphyl given at 7 PM (to get maximum serum theophylline concentration at 4–5 AM when nocturnal asthma is the worse) and twice daily Theo-Dur. Of interest, during the daytime hours, the serum theophylline concentration was significantly higher on Theo-Dur compared to Uniphyl, but the FEV_1 measurements were the same. At night, the theophylline levels were significantly higher on Uniphyl, and this improved the morning decrease in lung function. The bedtime to morning decrease in FEV_1 on Theo-Dur was 34.5% and on Uniphyl was 12.4%. The patients were also symptomatically better on the Uniphyl.

The entire area of chronopharmacology and drug absorption and metabolism at night needs extensive investigation. Asthma, as well as other disease processes, change during sleep and our attention needs to be directed to that time of the day.

Steroids

In order to minimize adrenal gland suppression and perhaps some other side effects of exogenous steroids, a short half-life steroid preparation is given in the morning when indicated. As mentioned in the Cortisol Level section above, a very small subset of patients may respond to nocturnal steroids. Giving a patient either a long-acting morning dose or a bedtime dose must be balanced against possible additional side effects. This form of therapy should be reserved for the patient who does not respond to any other interventions.

Warm Air

Breathing warm humidified air may produce considerable improvement in many asthmatics. Caution is needed as some asthmatics may have exacerbation of symptoms by either heat or humidification. Thus, this modality needs to be tested initially under supervision before the patient uses it at home. In over 30 patients tested at our center, none would use this form of therapy at home, even though improvement was seen in lung function.

Awaken for Treatment

Finally, there are patients who are apparently recalcitrant to any of the discussed therapeutic interventions. These individuals would appear to be at high risk of developing sleep-related respiratory failure or mortality. If the time of night where changes in gas tensions or pulmonary function can be established, these patients should be awakened 30–60 minutes prior to this for inhaled bronchodilator treatment. In some patients, this is very beneficial.

References

1. Cochrane GM, Clark TJH. A survey of asthma mortality in patients between ages 35 and 65 in the greater London hospitals in 1971. *Thorax* 1975; 30:300–315.
2. Hetzel MR, Clark TJH, Branthwaite MA. Asthma: Analysis of sudden deaths and ventilatory arrests in hospital. *Br Med J* 1977; 1:808–811.
3. Floyer J. A Treatise of the Asthma. London, R. Witkin and W. Inngs, 1698; pp 7–8.
4. Salter HH. Asthma: Its Pathology and Treatment, 1st American edition, 1882; p 33.
5. Turner-Warwick M. Epidemiology of nocturnal asthma. *Am J Med* 1988; 85(1B):6–8.
6. Bagg LR, Hughes DTD. Diurnal variation in peak expiratory flow in asthmatics. *Eur J Respir Dis* 1980; 61:298–302.
7. Hudgel DW, Kellum R, Martin RJ, et al. Depressed arousal response to airflow obstruction: A possible factor in near-fatal nocturnal asthma. *Am Rev Respir Dis* 1982; 125(S):202.
8. Ballard RD, Kelly PL, Tan WC, et al. Effects of sleep, before and after sleep deprivation, on ventilatory and arousal responses to induced bronchoconstriction. *Am Rev Respir Dis* 1988; 137(4):A54.
9. Clark TJH, Hetzel MR. Diurnal variation of asthma. *Br J Dis Chest* 1977; 71:87–92.
10. Bonjer FH. Physiological aspects of shift work. *Proc Int Congr Occup Health* 1960; 13:848–851.
11. Guberan E, Williams MK, Walford J, et al. Circadian variation of FEV_1 in shift workers. *Br J Ind Med* 1969; 26:121–125.

12. Hetzel MR, Clark TJH. Does sleep cause nocturnal asthma? *Thorax* 1979; 34:749–754.
13. Kales A, Beall GN, Bajor GF, et al. Sleep studies in asthmatic adults: Relationship of attacks to sleep stage and time of night. *J Allergy* 1968; 41:164–173.
14. Ballard RD, Saathoff MC, Patel DK, et al. The effect of sleep on nocturnal bronchoconstriction and ventilatory patterns in asthmatics. *J Appl Physiol* 1989; 67:243–249.
15. Catterall JR, Douglas NJ, Calverley PMA. Irregular breathing and hypoxaemia during sleep in chronic stable asthma. *Lancet* 1982; 1:301–314.
16. Montplaisir J, Walsh J, Malo JL. Nocturnal asthma: Features of attacks, sleep and breathing patterns. *Am Rev Respir Dis* 1982; 125:18–22.
17. Gervais P, Reinburg A, Gervais C, et al. Twenty-four-hour rhythm in the bronchial hyperreactivity to house dust in asthmatics. *J Allergy Clin Immunol* 1977; 59:207–213.
18. Davies RJ, Hendrick DJ, Pepys J. Asthma due to inhaled chemical agents: Ampicillin, benzyl penicillin, 6-amino penicillanic acid and related substances. *Clin Allergy* 1974; 4:227–247.
19. Siracusa A, Curradi F, Abbritti G. Recurrent nocturnal asthma due to tolylene diisocyanate: A case report. *Clin Allergy* 1978; 8:195–201.
20. Davies RJ, Green M, Schofield N McC. Recurrent nocturnal asthma after exposure to grain dust. *Am Rev Respir Dis* 1976; 114:1011–1019.
21. Gandevia B, Milne J. Occupational asthma and rhinitis due to western red cedar (*Thuja plicata*), with special reference to bronchial reactivity. *Br J Ind Med* 1970; 27:235–244.
22. Newman Taylor AJ, Davies RJ, Hendrick DJ, et al. Recurrent nocturnal asthma reactions to bronchial provocation tests. *Clin Allergy* 1979; 9:213–219.
23. Mohiuddin AA, Martin RJ. Circadian basis of the late asthmatic response. *Am Rev Respir Dis* 1989; (in press).
24. Sullivan CE, Murphy E, Kazan LF, et al. Waking and ventilatory responses to laryngeal stimulation in sleeping dogs. *J Appl Physiol: Respir Environ Exercise Physiol* 1978; 45:681–689.
25. Shturman-Ellstein R, Zeballos RJ, Buckley JM, et al. The beneficial effect of nasal breathing on exercise-induced bronchoconstriction. *Am Rev Respir Dis* 1978; 118:65–73.
26. Overholt RH, Voorhees RJ. Esophageal reflux as a trigger in asthma. *Dis Chest* 1966; 49:464–466.
27. Urschel HC Jr, Paulson DL. Gastroesophageal reflux and hiatal hernia. Complications and therapy. J Thorac Cardiovasc Surg 1967; 53:32–32.
28. Davis MV. Evolving concepts regarding hiatus hernia and gastroesophageal reflux. *Ann Thorac Surg* 1969; 7:120–133.
29. Babb RR, Notarangelo J, Smith VM. Wheezing: A clue to gastroesophageal reflux. *Am J Gastroenterol* 1970; 53:230–233.
30. Mays EE. Intrinsic asthma in adults: Association with gastroesophageal reflux. *J Am Med Assoc* 1976; 236:2626–2628.

31. Goodall RJR, Earis JE, Cooper DW, et al. Relationship between asthma and gastro-oesophageal reflux. *Thorax* 1981; 36:116–121.
32. Mansfield LE, Stein MR. Gastro-oesophageal reflux and asthma: A possible reflex mechanism. *Ann Allergy* 1978; 41:224–226.
33. Davis RS, Larsen GL, Grunstein MM. Esophageal acid infusion during sleep in asthmatic children with gastroesophageal reflux. *Am Rev Respir Dis* 1982; 125(S):190.
34. Tan WC, Ballard RD, Martin RJ, et al. The role of gastroesophageal reflux in nocturnal asthma. *Am Rev Respir Dis* 1988; 137:55.
35. Reinberg A, Gervais P. Circadian rhythm in respiratory functions with special reference to human chromophysiology and chromopharmacology. *Bull Physiopathol Respir* 1972; 8:663–675.
36. McDermott M. Diurnal and weekly cyclical changes in lung airways resistance. *J Physiol* 1966; 186:90–92.
37. Sullivan CE, Zamel N, Kozar LF, et al. Regulation of airway smooth muscle tone in sleeping dogs. *Am Rev Respir Dis* 1979; 119:87–99.
38. Hetzel MR, Clark TJH, Houston K, Physiological patterns in early morning asthma. *Thorax* 1977; 32:418–423.
39. Barnes P, Fitzgerald G, Brown M, et al. Nocturnal asthma and changes in circulatory epinephrine, histamine and cortisol. *N Engl J Med* 1980; 303: 263–267.
40. Soutar CA, Costello J, Ijuduola O, et al. Nocturnal and morning asthma. *Thorax* 1975; 30:436–440.
41. Todisco T, Grassi V, Sorbini CA, et al. Circadian rhythms of respiratory functions in asthmatics. *Respiration* 1980; 40:128–135.
42. Simon RA, Stevenson DD, Arroyave CM, et al. The relationship of plasma histamine to the activity of bronchial asthma. *J Allergy Clin Immunol* 1977; 60:312–316.
43. Brown R, Ingram RH Jr, Wellman JJ, et al. Effects of intravenous histamine on pulmonary mechanics in non-asthmatic and asthmatic subjects. *J Appl Physiol* 1977; 42:221–227.
44. Mills JN. Human circadian rhythms. *Physiol Rev* 1966; 46:128–171.
45. Martin RJ, Cicutto LC, Ballard RD, et al. Airway inflammation in nocturnal asthma. *N Engl J Med* (in press).
46. Chen WY, Horton DJ, Weiser PC. Airway obstruction induced by body cooling in asthmatics. *Physiologist* 1977; 20:16.
47. Chen WY, Horton DJ. Airways obstruction in asthmatics induced by body cooling. *Scand J Respir Dis* 1978; 59:13–20.
48. Horton DJ, Chen WY. Effects of breathing warm humidified air on bronchoconstriction induced by body cooling and by inhalation of methacholine. *Chest* 1979; 75:24–28.
49. Petersdorf RA. Disturbance of heat regulation. *In* MM Wintrobe, GW Thorn, RD Adams, et al. (eds). Harrison's Principles on Internal Medicine, 7th ed. New York, McGraw-Hill, 1974.
50. Chen WY, Chai H. Airway cooling and nocturnal asthma. *Chest* 1982; 81:675–680.
51. Martin RJ, Cicutto LC, Ballard RD. Factors related to the nocturnal worsening of asthma. *Am Rev Respir Dis* 1989; (in press).

52. Gaultier C, Reinberg J, Gerbeaux J, et al. Circadian changes in lung resistance and dynamic compliance in healthy and asthmatic children: Effects of two bronchodilators. *Respir Physiol* 1977; 31:169–182.
53. Martin RJ, Cicutto LC, Ballard RD, et al. Circadian variations in theophylline concentrations and the treatment of nocturnal asthma. *Am Rev Respir Dis* 1989; 139(1):475–478.

7

Respiration during Sleep and Cardiopulmonary Hemodynamics in Patients with Chronic Lung Disease

Eugene C. Fletcher, M.D.

A recent National Heart, Lung and Blood Institute (NHLBI) workshop summary statement on respiratory disorders of sleep by leading pulmonologists and sleep researchers from around the world extensively defined and discussed the pathophysiology and clinical aspects of respiratory disorders of sleep.[1] Not mentioned in this summary and position statement is the phenomenon of nonapneic nocturnal oxyhemoglobin desaturation (NOD), which, in terms of sheer numbers of patients, may be a far more common respiratory disorder of sleep than apnea, the main topic of the workshop. Furthermore, in a joint American College of Chest Physicians (ACCP)–NHLBI conference on oxygen therapy, succinct guidelines for the administration of continuous home supplemental oxygen have been stated.[2] Within this document, supplemental oxygen for chronic obstructive pulmonary disease (COPD) patients with nocturnal desaturation is recommended for patients "who develop Pa_{O_2} values of 55 mm Hg or less during sleep which is associated with hypoxic organ dysfunction." Yet there is little published evidence that NOD in patients with lung disease causes or contributes to cardiopulmonary dysfunction or is just a secondary manifestation of underlying lung and/or chest wall

Martin RJ: Cardiorespiratory Disorders During Sleep, 2nd Edition. Futura Publishing Company, Inc., Mount Kisco, NY, © 1990.

disease. Furthermore, there is no evidence that, if corrected by an expensive therapy such as supplemental oxygen, favorable long-term effects upon cardiopulmonary hemodynamics or, more importantly, improved patient longevity, will be realized. The purpose of this chapter is to give the reader insight into the phenomenon of NOD, its mechanism, prevalence, potential effects, if and when patients should be treated, and why treatment could be beneficial or have no effect at all.

Transient Hypoxemia in Chronic Lung and Thoracic Wall Disease

As early as 1958, investigators began to look at Sao_2 during sleep and discovered transient decrements to as low as 44% in COPD patients.[3,4] The combined use of continuous Sao_2 monitored by ear oximetry and sleep staging determined by electroencephalogram (EEG) allowed full appreciation of abnormal Sao_2 during sleep in patients with lung disease. One of the earliest studies to employ both ear oximetry and EEG monitoring during sleep[5] revealed transient drops in Sao_2 of as much as 36% beginning at baseline saturations of 73%–94%. This study separated NOD episodes into two types: those associated with abnormalities of breathing, such as apnea and hypopnea, and those not associated with obvious disordered breathing. Those episodes associated with apnea and hypopnea tended to be short (less than one minute) and showed less desaturation (a mean of 7.6%), and probably do not represent a serious threat to the cardiopulmonary integrity of the COPD patient.[6–8] However, 11 of 83 episodes of arterial NOD lasted longer than one minute (up to 30 minutes) and were associated with profound decreases in Sao_2.[5] For these, the mean maximum fall in Sao_2 was 22%, and all of the episodes lasting longer than 5 minutes occurred during REM sleep. An example of REM-related severe oxygen desaturation is seen in Figure 1. NOD has now been reported in other disease states with lung parenchyma or chest wall abnormalities associated with respiratory insufficiency. It has been described in asthma,[9] kyphoscoliosis,[10–12] diaphragmatic paralysis,[13,14] myotonic dystrophy,[15] cystic fibrosis,[16–19] childhood COPD,[20] and interstitial lung disease.[21,22] A recent article reviews NOD in a variety of restrictive lung conditions.[23]

The origin of longer, nonapneic NOD events is probably complex. Desaturations are believed to result from decreased alveolar

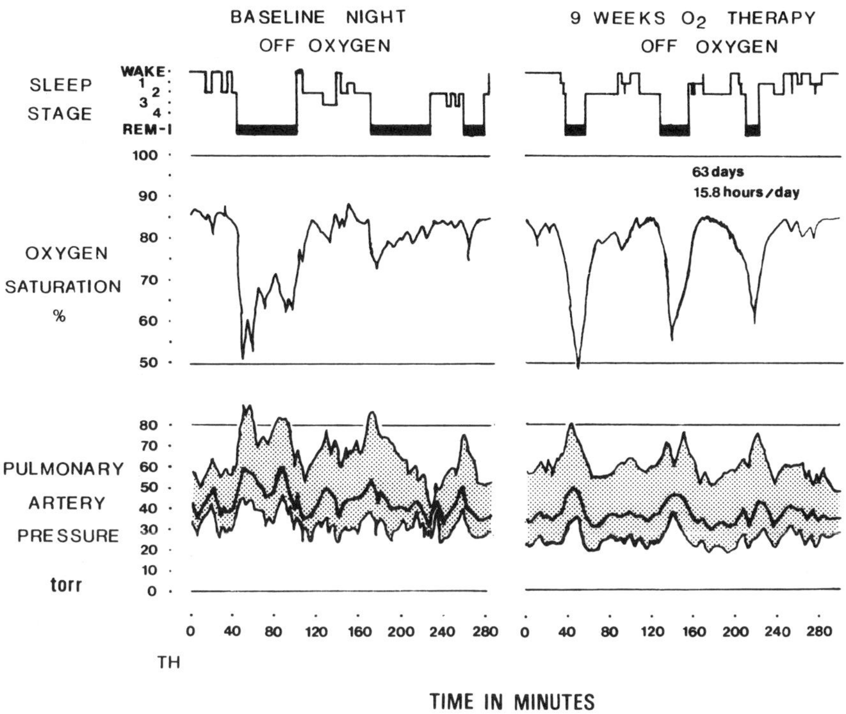

Figure 1. Example of marked nocturnal oxyhemoglobin desaturation (NOD) occurring during REM sleep in a patient with hypoxemic (daytime) COPD. The time course of the NOD coincides with onset and termination of REM sleep depicted by the solid bars (top panel). Increases in pulmonary artery pressure corresponding to the desaturations are observed in the bottom panels. Following nine weeks of home, nocturnal, low-flow oxygen, the NOD episodes and accompanying transient elevations of pulmonary artery pressure persist.

ventilation and worsening gas exchange. Semiquantitative measures of minute ventilation using visual observation,[24] nasal thermistor,[25] and pneumographs or related devices[26,27] have demonstrated alveolar hypoventilation as one cause of NOD during REM sleep. For example, both Hudgel et al.[27] and Fletcher et al.[28] have measured decreases in minute ventilation and tidal volume in COPD subjects from non-REM to REM sleep using a well-calibrated respiratory inductance plethysmograph. In seven NOD subjects (>10% fall in Sa_{O_2}) tidal volume and diaphragmatic EMG fell during periods of desaturation, mostly in REM sleep.[27]

However, hypoventilation alone does not account for the degree of desaturation seen during REM sleep. Three pieces of evidence point toward another mechanism. First, the small increase in $Paco_2$ from non-REM to REM sleep has been used as evidence both that alveolar hypoventilation occurs as well as evidence that hypoventilation alone cannot account for NOD, since larger rises in $Paco_2$ would be expected for the degree of hypoxemia.[24,28,29] Second, low-flow supplemental oxygen seems to readily eliminate NOD.[28,29] Third, several early authors, using a respiratory quotient of 0.82 to calculate alveolar–arterial oxygen gradient [(A–a)Do_2], showed deterioration of this parameter from non-REM to REM sleep.[24,30,31] They postulated that gas exchange abnormalities were contributing to the hypoxemia.

Since arterial oxygen tension (not content) is used to calculate (A–a)DO_2, comparison of gas exchange between non-REM and REM sleep using (A–a)Do_2 does not consider Pao_2 location on different portions of the oxyhemoglobin dissociation curve. Furthermore, breathing during REM sleep is erratic, with alternating periods of hypopnea and hyperpnea, and measuring respiratory quotient from expired gases is impossible.

Shedding additional light upon the mechanism of hypoventilation versus gas exchange during sleep, Fletcher et al.[28] examined both minute ventilation and venous admixture ($\dot{Q}_{\bar{v}a}/\dot{Q}_t$) during periods of desaturation. Pulmonary and radial artery catheters were used to sample simultaneous arterial and mixed venous blood during non-REM and REM sleep in seven COPD subjects. Using the van Slyke method to analyze O_2 and CO_2 content, alveolar oxygen tension (PAo_2), (A–a)Do_2, and $\dot{Q}_{\bar{v}a}/\dot{Q}_t$ were calculated. Minute ventilation was continuously measured during sleep using a respiratory inductive plethysmograph and cardiac output by thermodilution. The minute ventilation decreased by 26% during REM sleep and PAo_2 dropped significantly. $\dot{Q}_{\bar{v}a}/\dot{Q}_t$ showed a marked increase with the onset of NOD. The small drop in (A–a)Do_2 from non-REM to REM sleep did not reach statistical significance. A fall in the intrathoracic inspiratory pressure confirmed decreased respiratory effort. Cardiac output did not change with NOD, but arterial–venous content oxygen difference narrowed during desaturation. These findings support the theory of the mechanism of NOD to be a combination of alveolar hypoventilation and deterioration of gas exchange.

If abnormal gas exchange during sleep does contribute to NOD, then patients with the worst gas exchange while awake should be candidates for NOD. Fletcher et al. have recently examined upright baseline and steady-state exercise parameters of gas exchange in two groups of COPD patients.[32] All subjects had a mean daytime Pa_{O_2} above 60 torr but were divided according to the presence or absence of episodic NOD detected by formal polysomnographic sleep studies. Gas exchange, determined by measuring ventilation, expired gases, and arterial and venous blood gas tensions, and saturation was worse in the COPD patients with NOD than in those without. Specifically, NOD subjects showed worse awake $(A–a)D_{O_2}$ (40.8 vs. 21.5 torr) and $\dot{Q}_{\bar{v}a}/\dot{Q}_t$ (11.13% vs. 4.11%) than non-NOD subjects. During exercise, NOD subjects showed significant arterial CO_2 retention and absence of the expected decrease in V_d/V_t common with exercise in normals and also seen in the non-NOD control group. The rise in Pa_{CO_2} along with absence of the expected decrease in V_d/V_t during exercise indicates greater ventilation/perfusion ($\dot{V}/\dot{Q}$) mismatch in awake NOD patients.

In summary, the long episodes of NOD during REM sleep appear to be related to a combination of alveolar hypoventilation and deteriorating gas exchange. This is based upon measurement of minute ventilation and observations that carbon dioxide retention is minimal, NOD is easily reversed by low-flow supplemental oxygen without altering respiratory pattern, and parameters of gas exchange are worse during REM sleep in these patients. The patients with chronic lung disease that desaturate at night appear to have worse gas exchange abnormalities prior to sleep.

Pathophysiology of REM NOD

Since Aserinsky and Kleitman's original description of REM sleep, many phenomena affecting autonomic function and neuromuscular tone have been described.[33,34] Active neuronal inhibition of postural muscle activity may be looked upon teleologically as a protective mechanism to limit muscular activity during behaviorally active sleep. However, not only postural muscles undergo active neuronal blockade, but respiratory muscles as well, particularly those maintaining thoracic stability (intercostals and others) during inspiration.[35] In addition to diminished diaphragmatic activity manifested as decreased tidal volume during REM sleep, loss of intercostal muscle tone probably allows decreased thoracic gas volume.[36–38] Elevated FRC, a high closing volume, and preexisting gas exchange abnormalities in those with chronic lung disease make maintenance of sleeping $Sa{O_2}$ difficult during REM sleep (Fig. 2).[39] The decreased tidal volume combines with a fall in FRC, which in turns causes maldistribution of ventilation.[40] Such falls in FRC have been documented in infants,[36] adolescents and normal adults,[37,38,40,41] cystic fibrosis patients,[16,17] and in COPD patients.[27] This fall in FRC may have no effect upon sleep $Sa{O_2}$ in normals for two reasons. First, thoracic gas volume remains above closing volume, minimizing ven-

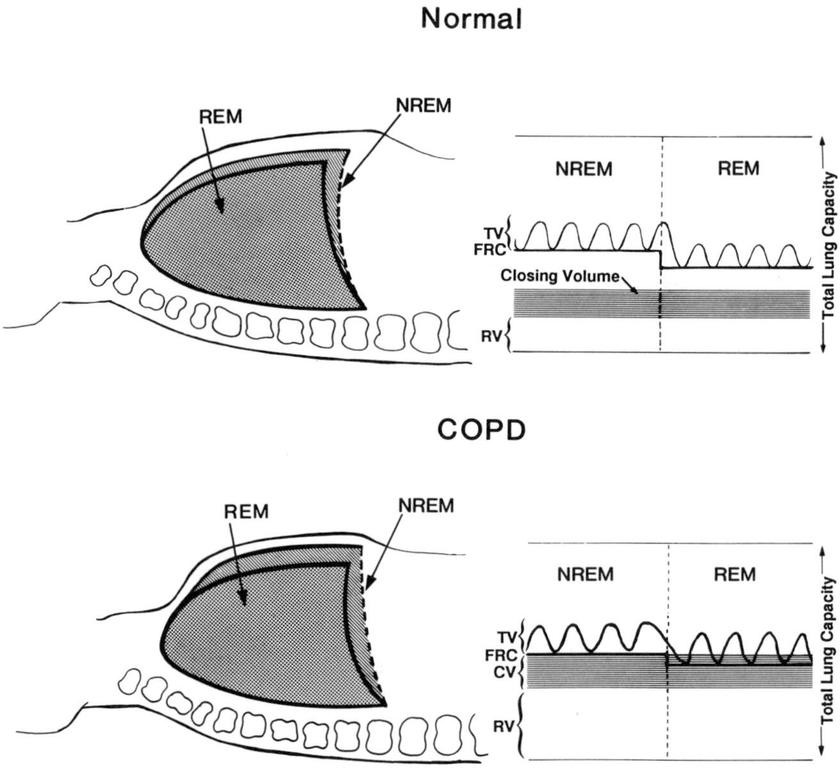

Figure 2. Schematic representation of the changes in functional residual capacity (FRC) leading to NOD. To normals breathing well above closing volume, a small decrease in FRC coinciding to decrease in skeletal muscle tone of REM sleep creates no change in $Sa{O_2}$. Most lung units remain above closing volume and well ventilated. To a patient with COPD, interstitial lung disease, or thoracic weakness or deformity, a fall in FRC may place many alveoli below closing volume. This may lead to maldistribution of ventilation or even microatelectasis in some areas, adding to the hypoxia from alveolar hypoventilation. (From: reference 39, with permission.)

tilation maldistribution. Second, normals have Pa_{O_2} levels high on the oxyhemoglobin dissociation curve, minimizing changes in SaO_2.

Why do some patients with chronic lung disease have NOD while others with apparently similar degrees of lung disease do not? First, preexisting $\dot{V}/\dot{Q}$ mismatch produces moderate awake and non-REM sleep hypoxemia, accounting for the observed differences in daytime Pa_{O_2} between NOD and non-NOD patients.[32] The presence of arterial hypoxemia before REM sleep onset may contribute directly to NOD because of the nonlinear shape of the oxyhemoglobin dissociation curve. The same drop in Pa_{O_2} beginning at the steep portion of the curve will allow a greater fall in Sa_{O_2} than one starting on the flat portion because of the shape of the curve. However, position on the curve alone does not explain NOD, as the majority of COPD patients with Pa_{O_2}'s between 60 and 80 do not show episodic NOD.[42] Second, at REM sleep onset, the generalized hypotonia with decreased FRC and decreased respiratory drive with low tidal volumes[27,28] and V_e[8,27,28] superimpose both alveolar hypoventilation and further ventilation maldistribution on lungs that already have alveolar units with low $\dot{V}/\dot{Q}$ ratios. Thus, mixed venous blood with a low P_{O_2} exerts a greater influence on end capillary oxyhemoglobin saturation. Those lung disease patients with preexisting gas exchange abnormalities who do not show REM sleep NOD presumably maintain adequate distribution of ventilation, a better V_e, a higher FRC, or all three during REM sleep.

Numerous other factors may contribute to REM hypoxemia. The presence of alveolar hypoventilation with a high alveolar CO_2 tension (PA_{CO_2}) may accentuate hypoxemia by lowering alveolar oxygen levels. Increased lower airway resistance such as that seen in nocturnal asthma[43] and increased upper airway resistance demonstrated in normals and apnea subjects[41,44] could disturb ventilation distribution. A depressed cough reflex and decreased mucociliary clearance causing pooling of secretions at night could further impair $\dot{V}/\dot{Q}$ matching.[45] Finally, depressed hypoxic and hypercarbic ventilatory responses during REM sleep could also contribute to REM hypoxemia.[46,47]

Clinical Significance of NOD

There are three important effects that NOD could have upon the clinical condition of the patient with obstructive, restrictive, or thoracic wall disease. First, many patients with COPD complain of disturbed sleep in the form of increased latency to sleep onset, frequent and early awakenings, and markedly shortened sleep periods. Second, severe hypoxemia associated with NOD could induce cardiac arrhythmias that might theoretically lead to nocturnal death. Finally, hypoxemia is associated with pulmonary hypertension and, possibly, recurrent NOD could lead to or aggravate chronic pulmonary hypertension. Of these possible complications, the most knowledge has been accumulated concerning pulmonary hypertension and will be discussed in greater detail.

Disturbed Nocturnal Sleep Quality

Next to fatigue and breathlessness, disturbed sleep in the form of sleep onset insomnia with frequent and early morning awakenings is one of the most common complaints of patients with COPD.[48] Many patients sleep for short periods at night and take frequent catnaps during the day. Several reports have documented disturbed EEG sleep architecture.[6,19,30,46,49,50] Leitch et al. report delayed sleep onset, prolonged and frequent periods of wakefulness, frequent stage shifts, and lowered sleep efficiency in 10 patients with COPD.[30] Several factors including retained secretions, increased nocturnal cough, medications, and hypercapnia/hypoxemia could all contribute to disturbed nocturnal sleep. The role of hypoxemia and supplemental oxygen in improving sleep quality is unsettled. Spier et al. found that although supplemental oxygen raised mean sleep and nadir Sao_2, it had no effect upon sleep quality.[19] Fleetham et al. found that arousals (40% of total) were related temporally to periods when Sao_2 was below baseline.[51] However, supplemental oxygen that raised Sao_2 to near-normal levels did not change any of the sleep parameters. Other authors find different results. One study showed a 52% sleep efficiency breathing room air for half the night and 80% sleep efficiency breathing supplemental oxygen for the other half.[52] Calverley et al. found that 2 L/min nasal oxygen during sleep improved mean nocturnal Sao_2, decreased sleep latency, and increased all stages of sleep.[53] With many variables that can cause disturbed sleep, oxygen is more likely to play a role in improving sleep when hypoxemia is present. It is unlikely that it will improve sleep in a patient not experiencing NOD. Further complicating this situation is a report that sleep deprivation (hence poor sleep) may cause a significant, albeit small, acute decrease in expiratory airflow from 1.06 L to 1.0 L in COPD patients deprived of one night of sleep.[54]

Cardiac Arrhythmias

The role of transient REM-related NOD in inducing cardiac arrhythmias and possibly sudden death is poorly understood, and few studies have been done to examine this question. One study has shown the incidence of death in COPD patients is higher at night, more so in the first hour of sleep and in the early morning hours where REM sleep is more uniformly experienced.[55] In that study, the rate of death was high among respiratory failure patients with hypoxemia and hypercarbia (those more likely to have REM NOD) but not those with hypoxemia without hypercarbia. The prevalence of COPD patients with cardiac arrhythmias has been noted to be higher than the general population. Two studies[56,57] show that about 70% of such patients exhibit either supraventricular (PACs) or ventricular arrhythmias (PVCs). Several studies have noted a diurnal variation in cardiac arrhythmias among COPD patients with the peak frequency occurring in the early morning, the most consistent period during which REM sleep occurs.[55–58] Some studies have examined the effect of supplemental oxygen on the frequency of cardiac arrhythmias. PVCs occurred about 25% less frequently during oxygen administration nights in a study by Flick and Block,[58] but this was not a statistically significant difference. There were episodes of ventricular tachycardia and idioventricular rhythm that occurred on the room air study nights only.[58] In one study, ST-T wave changes, rapid heart rate, and prolonged Qtc were more normal when bronchitic-type COPD patients slept with supplemental oxygen, but no relationship between these abnormalities and hypoxemia was established on the room air night.[59]

The only systematic study thus far examining PVCs during transient NOD in COPD patients was performed by Shepard et al.[60] PVCs occurred in 64% of 42 patients studied; 40% had complex ventricular arrhythmias. There was a 150% increase in PVCs in patients whose desaturation was below 80% (Fig. 3). It was concluded that hypoxemia, acidosis, elevated systemic pressure, elevated catecholamines, and elevated myocardial oxygen demands all contributed to the development of arrhythmias. The role of NOD in inducing nocturnal arrhythmias remains unanswered and a fruitful area for research.

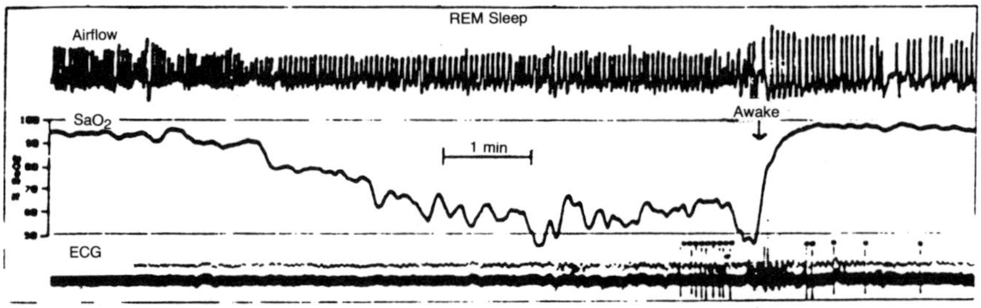

Figure 3. Airflow (top panel), ECG (bottom panel), and Sa_{O_2} during an episode of NOD in a patient with COPD. Premature ventricular complexes are seen during the end of the NOD episode and immediately upon waking, during recovery. (From: reference 60, with permission.)

Pulmonary Hypertension

Pulmonary artery pressure during sleep has been observed in a limited number of COPD patients using flow-directed pulmonary artery catheters.[26,61–63] Douglas et al.[26] observed prolonged elevation of pulmonary artery pressure during a REM-related desaturation in a single patient. Boysen et al.[62] monitored four patients (mean daytime Pa_{O_2} of 58 mm Hg) with Swan Ganz catheters in place. They observed transient increases in pulmonary artery pressure associated with falls in Sa_{O_2} resulting from both disordered breathing events and longer, REM related NOD. These falls and accompanying transient elevations in pulmonary artery pressure were ameliorated with oxygen. Fletcher and Levin have published data on the mechanism of pulmonary hypertension in patients with daytime hypoxemia and NOD and the effect of acute (overnight) versus chronic (6 weeks) use of nocturnal oxygen on cardiopulmonary hemodynamics.[63] Whole night sleep Sa_{O_2} was examined with subjects breathing room air ($N = 7$), 3 L/min oxygen ($N = 5$), and again breathing room air ($N = 7$) after 6–8 weeks of nocturnal O_2 use. Acute oxygen eliminated NOD and greatly ameliorated the transient elevations in pulmonary artery pressure (Fig. 4). Follow-up studies on room air after home O_2 therapy demonstrated the continued presence of NOD and pulmonary artery pressure elevations (Fig. 1) but a sustained reduction in total pulmonary resistance in four subjects. Because of many of the above observations, transient NOD has been proposed as a predecessor and possible etiologic factor in the development of pulmonary hypertension in patients with chronic lung disease.[64,65]

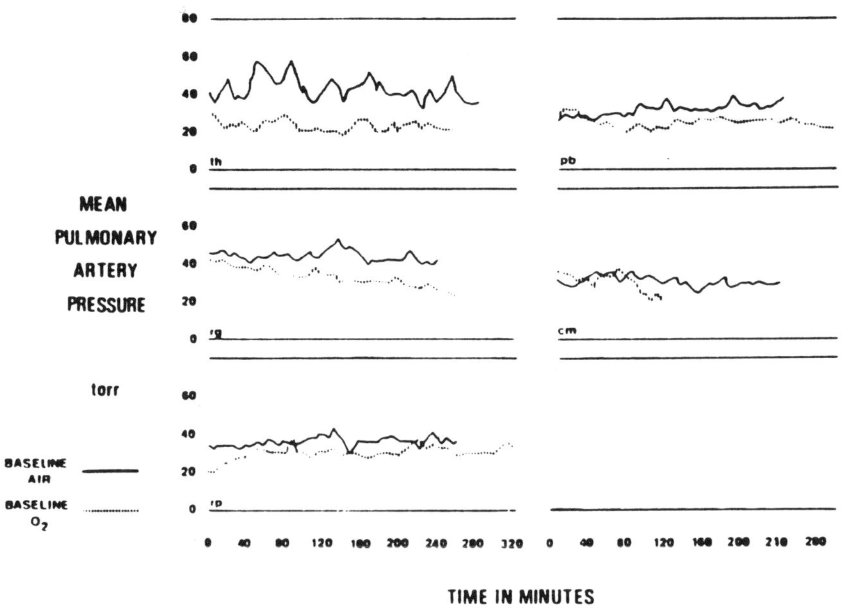

Figure 4. The acute effect of nocturnal supplemental oxygen administered to five patients with NOD but who were also hypoxemic (Pao_2 <55 torr) during the day. Solid line is one whole night mean pulmonary artery pressure (P_{pa}) continuously measured by indwelling right heart catheter. The broken line similarly measures P_{pa} during one whole night during administration of nasal supplemental oxygen at a rate of 4 L/min. Mean sleeping P_{pa} is substantially lowered in four of the five patients on the oxygen night. (From: reference 63, with permission.)

Recent attention has been given to the role of transient hypoxemia in the etiology of sustained pulmonary hypertension. It has been well demonstrated using the rat model that repetitive episodes of transient hypoxia can lead to many of the changes seen in chronic pulmonary hypertension. For example, exposing rats to hypoxic gas mixtures (Pao_2 55–60 torr) for 8 of 24 hours over 21 days causes elevation of right ventricular systolic pressure and an increase in the ratio of right ventricular weight to body weight.[66] Since administration of 100% O_2 to these animals did not immediately relieve the high systolic pressure, a mechanism other than acute hypoxic pulmonary vasoconstriction must explain the lasting changes of intermittent hypoxia.[67] Shorter periods of exposure to intermittent hypoxia (4 h/day, 24 exposures, alveolar Po_2 = 64 torr) have demonstrated increased right ventricular weight (33% increase) and red cell mass (44% increase), and after 75 exposures, elevation of pressure.[68] In these animals, the development of smooth muscle fibers in pulmonary vessels usually devoid of muscle may explain the more lasting effect of intermittent hypoxia. Age also affects mortality in these studies.[69]

The biochemical or cellular etiology of chronic pulmonary hypertension resulting from chronic hypoxia has not been delineated and includes such biochemical mediators as histamine, catecholamines, angiotensin II, or even a direct metabolic effect of hypoxia on pulmonary vascular smooth muscle.[70] Even less is known about the biochemical etiology of chronic pulmonary hypertension on the basis of intermittent hypoxia. Because the episodes of transient hypoxemia tend to be short and of minimal severity, a direct effect of hypoxia on vascular smooth muscle cell metabolism is possible but unlikely. A lingering biochemical, neurohumoral, or cell mediator of pulmonary vasoconstriction seems more likely. For example, transient hypoxemia in dogs ventilated acutely with hypoxic gases reduces bradykinin-converting enzyme activity to zero at a $Pao_2 < 26$ torr. Full activity returns 2 minutes after normoxia.[71] The same authors have noted similar changes in angiotensin-converting enzyme during induced hypoxia. Eicosanoids including arachidonic acid and its metabolites ([leukotrienes (leukotriene C_4)], thromboxanes, and prostaglandins) are potent vasoconstrictors.[70] Platelets as well as aggregated leukocytes can elaborate eicosanoids that can cause pulmonary vasoconstriction. Such cellular elements are known to adhere to damaged endothelium. For example, endothelial damage in the systemic circulation causes platelet deposition, which in turn invokes vascular smooth muscle growth through the release of a mitogenic factor.[72] A similar mechanism could be operative in the lung if vascular endothelium were damaged directly by transient hypoxemia or indirectly by enzymatic changes. Subsequent deposition of platelets could invoke hypertrophic responses in vascular smooth muscle that extend beyond the hypoxemic period. Johnson et al.[73] have demonstrated decreased platelet survival in hypoxemic COPD patients and correction with supplemental O_2. Platelet survival is a known indicator of endothelial integrity and damage.[72]

Experimental evidence of intermittent hypoxemia leading to sustained pulmonary artery pressure elevation in man is scant. Obstructive sleep apnea is a form of transient nocturnal hypoxemia associated with sustained pulmonary hypertension.[74] Repetitive apneas are accompanied by periodic, progressive elevations of pulmonary artery pressure that may not return to baseline upon wakefulness. Just as in COPD, the degree of hypertension is amplified by the presence of daytime hypoxemia.[75] The fact that the intermittent hypoxemia may lead to reversible pulmonary hypertension is demonstrated by lowering of pulmonary artery pressure in such patients following tracheostomy.[76–78] Again, as in animal models of transient hypoxia, the biochemical (or other) mediator of chronic pulmonary hypertension is unknown.

If untreated, pulmonary hypertension and cor pulmonale resulting from hypoxemia portend a bad prognosis in patients with chronic lung disease. Once cor pulmonale with hypoxemia was diagnosed in patients with COPD, the 5-year mortality (modified by age and FEV_1) ranged from 15% to 80%.[79–81] The use of O_2 in patients with hypoxemic COPD has improved survival figures.[82,83] Thus, the role of transient NOD in causing or aggravating chronic pulmonary hypertension becomes an important question. It has been demonstrated that continuous home oxygen may actually lower pulmonary artery pressure in severely hypoxemic COPD patients ($Pa_{O_2} < 55$ torr)[84,85] whereas O_2 used less than 17 hours per day may be ineffective.[86,87] These studies have been directed toward a population of COPD patients with levels of daytime hypoxemia known to be associated with persistent pulmonary hypertension.[88] No studies have addressed prevention of pulmonary hypertension by the initiation of oxygen at an earlier stage of disease, for example, in patients with NOD who do not have severe daytime hypoxemia.

One reason for the inability to address this issue is the time required to observe the development of pulmonary hypertension as well as the absence of precise correlations between pulmonary artery pressures and clinical measures of pulmonary function. The severity of pulmonary hypertension varies only roughly with the clinical severity of the lung disease as well as the degree of hypoxemia and hypercapnia.[88] Longitudinal increments in pulmonary artery pressure have been difficult to demonstrate prospectively. Burrows et al.[88] and Boushy and North[89] were able to detect only small yearly incremental rises in pulmonary artery pressure in subjects followed 7 years or 18–38 months, respectively. Weitzenblum et al.[90] showed an increase from 15.1 to 18.3 mm Hg ($P < 0.001$) over a 60-month period in 53 COPD subjects with a normal pulmonary artery pressure. In 32 subjects whose mean pulmonary artery pressure was above 20 mm Hg, pressure increased from 27.7 to 31.0 mm Hg ($P < 0.05$) over the same period. A more recent study by the same authors has shown a

0.5 mm Hg/year increase in pulmonary artery pressure over a 5- to 12-year period in 90 COPD patients.[91] Schrijen et al.[92] found no significant increase in resting pulmonary artery pressure in either group over a 3-year period.

Evidence of a Link between NOD and Daytime Pulmonary Hypertension

Before supplemental oxygen can be efficaciously prescribed to help ameliorate progression of pulmonary hypertension in chronic lung disease patients with NOD, it must be determined whether or not there is an association between abnormal waking cardiopulmonary hemodynamics and NOD in patients with mild daytime hypoxemia. Such evidence has begun to appear. Fletcher et al.[93] examined gas exchange, pulmonary function, red cell mass, radionuclide cardiac ejection fraction, and supine hemodynamics in 36 patients with lung disease and NOD using the following criteria of desaturation: a supine awake and non-REM Sao_2 of $\geq$ 90% interrupted by a 5-minute or longer fall below this level, reaching a nadir Sao_2 of 85% or lower (Fig. 5). These data were compared to those from 13 subjects with similar symptoms and objective measures of pulmonary dysfunction but without evidence of NOD during sleep.

The two groups did not vary with respect to age, spirometry, lung volumes, or DLco. The NOD subjects had a significantly lower resting daytime Pao_2 (70.0 versus 82.4 torr) than non-NOD subjects. This appeared to be due to differences in gas exchange between groups [higher $(A\text{–}a)Do_2$ (28.1 versus 19.1 torr) yet similar alveolar oxygen tensions and $Paco_2$]. The NOD subjects had a higher hemoglobin (15.2 vs. 14.4 g/100 ml, $P < 0.05$) and RBC mass/kg (27.5 vs. 25.2 ml/kg, $P < 0.05$) than non-NOD subjects. Resting room air mean pulmonary artery pressure and pulmonary vascular resistance were higher in the NOD versus non-NOD group (23.3 vs. 20.4 mm Hg and 172 vs. 102 dyne/sec/cm^{-5}, respectively, $P < 0.05$) (Fig. 6). The relative differences in mean pulmonary artery pressure and pulmonary vascular resistance were sustained breathing hypoxic (F_io_2 = 0.13) and hyperoxic (F_io_2 = 0.9-1.0) gases. Of the 36 NOD patients, 27 had pulmonary hypertension (defined as a pulmonary artery pressure > 20 mm Hg) at the time of initial catheterization. The mean pulmonary artery pressure of these 27 subjects was 25.3 ± 3.72 mm Hg.

Two hypotheses are compatible with these data. First, it is pos-

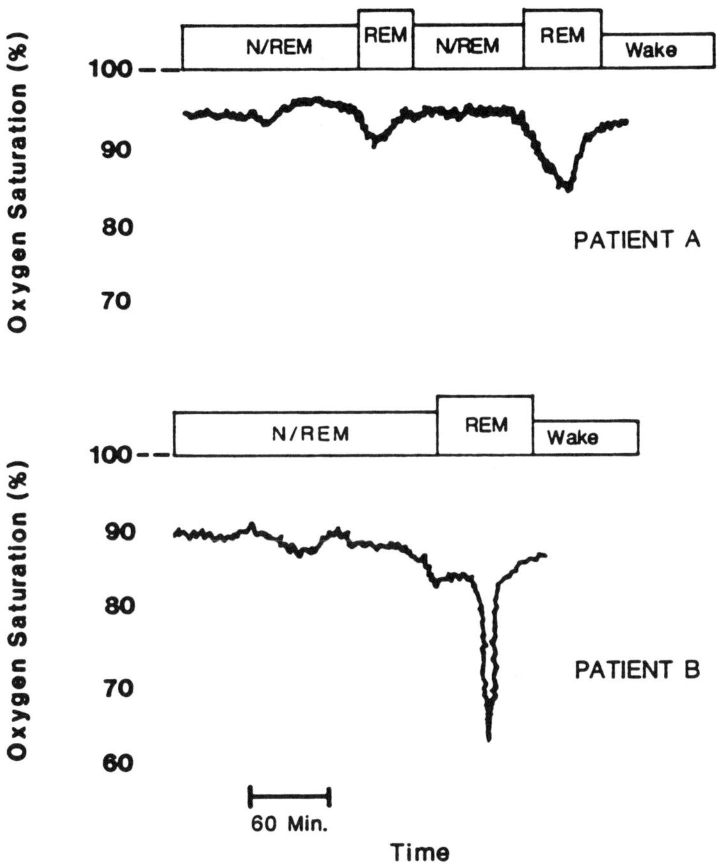

Figure 5. Whole night tracings of Sao_2 in two patients with COPD and daytime Pao_2 levels greater than 60 torr but NOD associated with REM sleep. These represent extremes (mildest to most severe) seen in 36 patients in references 32, 42, and 93. See text for explanation. (From: Reference 42, with permission.)

sible that the groups differ because of functional characteristics of the lung parenchyma that cause worse $\dot{V}/\dot{Q}$ matching, hypoxemia, and a greater propensity toward NOD. The recurrent NOD and accompanying transient elevation of pulmonary artery pressure could then lead to daytime pulmonary hypertension through hypoxic vasoconstriction and previously mentioned biochemical mechanisms. Second, differences in daytime Pao_2 could indicate structural or anatomic differences between the groups that adversely affect both $\dot{V}/\dot{Q}$ relationships as well as pulmonary hemodynamics. It is generally agreed, in part because of the shape of the oxyhemoglobin dissociation curve, that the lower the Pa_{O_2} at sleep onset, the more likely that REM desaturation will occur. Thus, by the second hypothesis, REM desaturation could be a marker for structural lung abnormalities, rather than a cause of abnormal hemodynamics. Separation of these two possibilities hinges on the difference in daytime Pa_{O_2} between the two groups. If the groups had equal daytime Pa_{O_2}'s (implying equivalent gas exchange and structural similarities) as well as equivalent pulmonary function tests, it could be argued that persistent hemodynamic differences resulted from functional (chronic vasoconstriction with vascular smooth muscle hypertrophy) rather than structural (vessel destruction or obliteration) changes to the vasculature.

To gain further insight into these two possibilities, 13 of the 36 NOD subjects who most closely matched the 13 non-NOD subjects were selected by computer on the basis of age, FEV_1, and daytime Pa_{O_2}.[93] Using these three parameters, the matched groups were equivalent in age, spirometry, lung volumes (plethysmography),

Figure 6. (facing page) Comparison of various supine cardiopulmonary hemodynamic variables in 36 patients with chronic lung disease and NOD (——), 13 patients with lung disease without NOD (. . . .), and 13 subjects from the NOD group matched to the 13 non-NOD subjects for age, FEV_1, and Pa_{O_2} (-•-•-) (93). Conditions of data collection are: center points: breathing room air (F_iO_2 = 0.21), points to the left of center: breathing hypoxic gas (F_iO_2 ~ 0.13), and points to the right of center: breathing hyperoxic gas (F_iO_2 ~ 1.0). Upper left panel: mean Sa_{O_2} and mean Sv_{O_2} under each condition of F_iO_2 for all NOD and all non-NOD subjects. Upper right panel: cardiac output all NOD and non-NOD subjects. Middle left panel: pulmonary vascular resistance, all NOD, all non-NOD, and 13 matched NOD subjects. Middle right panel: mean systemic artery pressure, all NOD and all non-NOD subjects. Lower left panel: systolic and diastolic pulmonary artery pressure, all NOD and non-NOD subjects. Lower right panel: mean pulmonary artery for all NOD, all non-NOD, and 13 matched NOD subjects, and capillary wedge pressure for all NOD and non-NOD subjects. Vertical brackets represent one standard deviation from the mean. Numerical values beside closed circles with arrows pointing to adjacent closed circles are *P* values comparing 36 NOD versus 13 non-NOD subjects under the same F_iO_2's using *t* tests for paired data. A straight horizontal bracket means there is a significant difference between F_iO_2 values for all parameters above the bracket. The curved brackets apply only to the single parameters directly below them. The absence of a *P* value and bracket means there is no difference between the parameters at different F_iO_2s. (From: reference 93, with permission.)

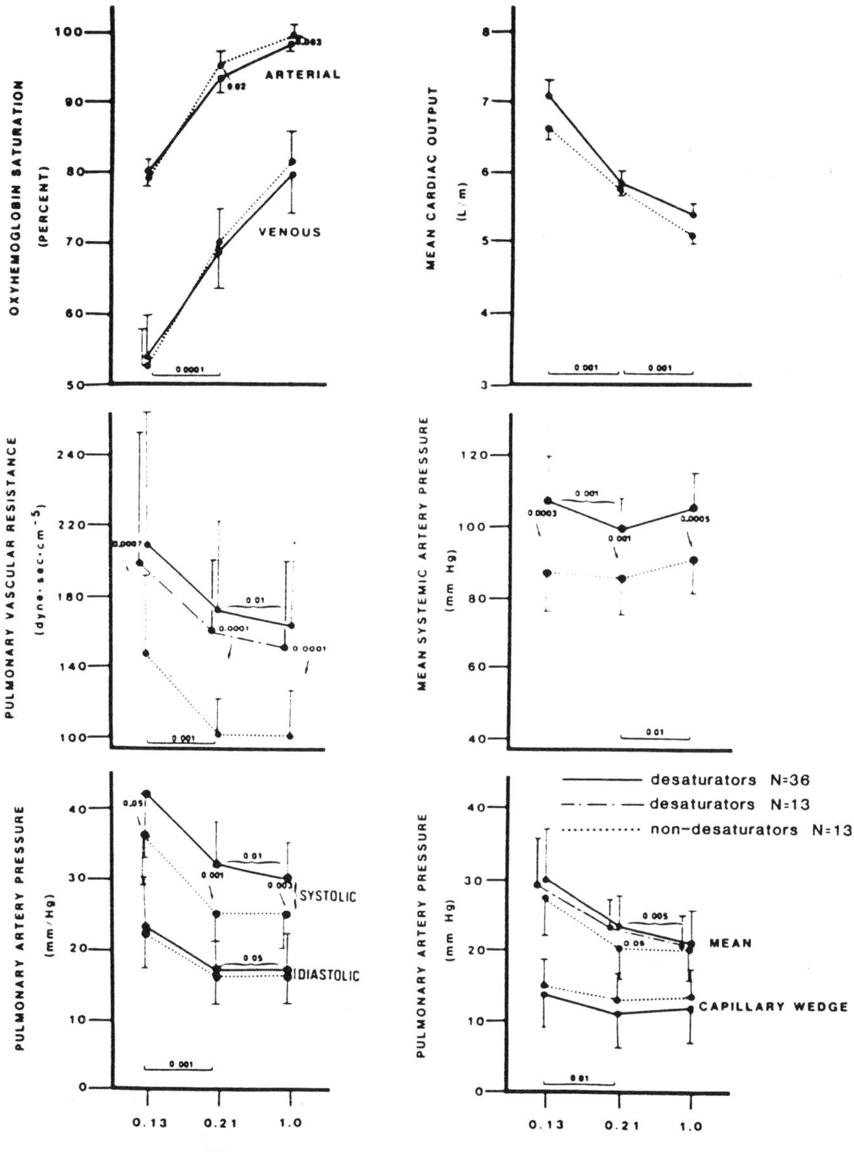
OXYHEMOGLOBIN SATURATION (PERCENT)
ARTERIAL
VENOUS
MEAN CARDIAC OUTPUT (L/m)
PULMONARY VASCULAR RESISTANCE (dyne·sec·cm⁻⁵)
MEAN SYSTEMIC ARTERY PRESSURE (mm Hg)
PULMONARY ARTERY PRESSURE (mm/Hg)
SYSTOLIC
DIASTOLIC
PULMONARY ARTERY PRESSURE (mm Hg)
desaturators N=36
desaturators N=13
non-desaturators N=13
MEAN
CAPILLARY WEDGE
FIO2
0.13
0.21
1.0

DLco, and daytime Pa_{O_2}. Thus, there was no basis on which to infer a difference in the structure of the pulmonary parenchyma. Yet, differences between groups in variables marking hematopoietic effects of hypoxemia persisted. Although the mean pulmonary artery pressure for the 13 matched NOD subjects did not differ from the 13 non-NOD subjects (22.6 vs. 20.4 mm Hg, respectively), pulmonary vascular resistance remained higher (160 vs. 102 dyne/sec/cm^{-5}; $P < 0.0004$) in the NOD group (Fig. 6). Thus it would appear that even with equivalent levels of daytime oxygenation, NOD patients have worse resting pulmonary hemodynamics than non-NOD patients with equivalent daytime Pa_{O_2} levels.

This study also sheds further light upon the role of "NOD" versus "differing levels of daytime hypoxemia" between NOD and non-NOD subjects in producing abnormal cardiopulmonary hemodynamics. Group levels for pulmonary artery pressure and pulmonary vascular resistances could not be differentiated on the basis of daytime Pa_{O_2} or mean whole night sleep Sa_{O_2} because of the overlap in the latter two variables between the two groups (Fig. 7A,B). However, the mean sleep nadir Sa_{O_2} and classification into non-NOD versus NOD clearly distinguished higher (NOD) and lower (non-NOD) pulmonary vascular resistance at a cutoff of 125 dyne/sec/cm^{-5} (Fig. 7C). Belonging to the non-NOD group and a nadir sleep Sa_{O_2} of 86% or above insured a PVR of below 125 dyne/sec/cm^{-5} in 11/12 (92%) non-NOD subjects. If the mean nadir sleep Sa_{O_2} fell below 85%, there was a 32/36 (91%) chance that resting supine daytime PVR would be above 125 dyne/sec/cm^{-5}. This separation on the basis of nocturnal Sa_{O_2} but not daytime Pa_{O_2} may indicate that NOD plays a more important role in sustained changes in pulmonary hemodynamics than does the daytime resting Pa_{O_2} level.

Because differences in resting supine pulmonary artery pressure in the above study were small, it appeared logical to stress cardiopulmonary hemodynamics using exercise to bring out even greater differences between NOD and non-NOD subjects with chronic lung disease (Fig. 8). Using a fiberoptic, flotation catheter, cardiopulmonary hemodynamics were examined during supine rest, upright rest, and exercise gas exchange in 16 NOD and 10 non-NOD subjects.[32] The groups were again selected on the basis of the above sleep desaturation criteria.[42] All subjects had an average (over 6 months) daytime Pa_{O_2} above 60 torr but were divided according to the presence or absence of episodic NOD detected by sleep studies. Resting supine mean pulmonary artery pressures were significantly different (20.3 ±

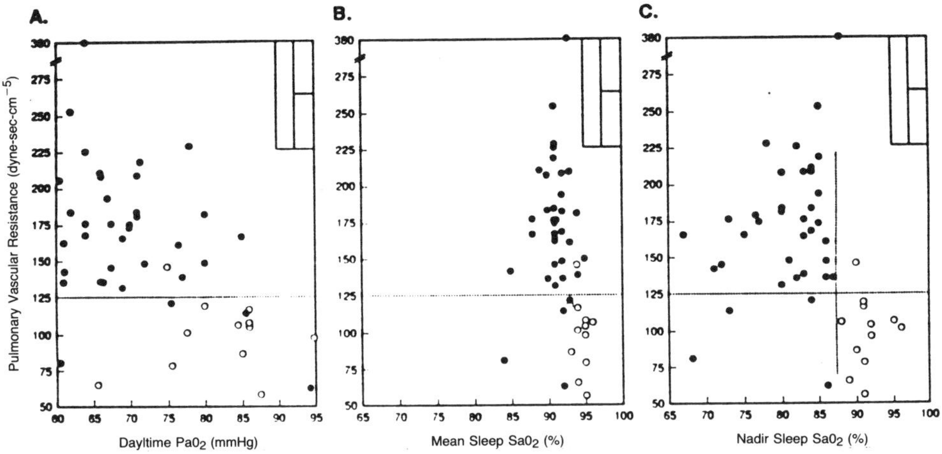

Figure 7. Pulmonary vascular resistance (PVR) versus three parameters of oxygenation in 36 NOD and 12 non-NOD patients.[93] PVR was measured in the supine position using invasive techniques. (A): PVR versus mean daytime Pao_2 as determined from three blood gases drawn in a sitting or semirecumbent position over a 6-month period prior to right heart catheterization. Whereas inclusion in NOD versus non-NOD groups allows a reasonable separation of PVR levels at 125 dyne/sec/cm^{-5} (32/36 NOD above this level), substantial overlap of daytime Pao_2 levels does not allow separation of PVR based upon this variable. (B) PVR versus mean sleep Sao_2 as determined from the mean of two whole night ear oximeter tracings (during polysomnography). Overlap of mean whole night sleep Sao_2 values does not permit differentiation of PVR levels. (C) PVR versus nadir sleep Sao_2 levels for all subjects. For nadir Sao_2, a cutoff at 85% shows good separation of PVR levels at 125 dyne/sec/cm^{-5}. If the patient's mean nadir sleep Sao_2 remained above 85%, there was only a 1/12 chance that PVR would be above this level. If the mean nadir sleep Sao_2 fell below 85%, there was only a 1/9 chance that PVR would be below 125 dyne/sec/cm^{-5}. This separation on the basis of nocturnal nadir Sao_2 may indicate that NOD plays a more important role in sustained changes in pulmonary hemodynamics than does daytime resting Pao_2 level.

4.4 mm Hg non-NOD vs. 23.8 ± 4.9 mm Hg NOD). While both groups showed increase in pulmonary artery pressure during exercise, resting and exercise systolic pulmonary artery pressure and mean exercise pulmonary artery pressure (52.3 vs. 42.3 mm Hg, $P < 0.02$) were significantly higher in the desaturators (Fig. 9). Pulmonary capillary wedge almost doubled in both groups from rest to exercise values, but right atrial pressure increased by the same amount, and

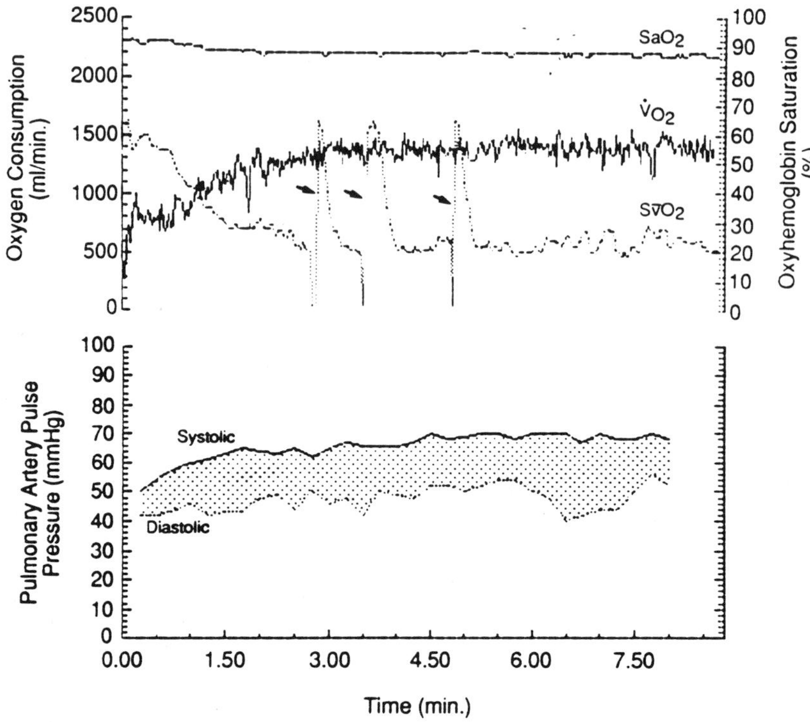

Figure 8. Pulmonary artery pressure (P_{pa}) response to a fixed load (steady state) in a NOD subject with COPD and a daytime resting Pao_2 above 60 torr.[32] Breath-by-breath Vo_2 reaches a plateau at about 3 minutes. Sao_2 falls from 91% to 88% shortly after onset of exercise. Svo_2 falls to approximately 22% by the third minute and remains stable. Artifactual increase in Svo_2 results from inflation of the balloon and wedging of the catheter tip (→). The response is abnormal in that P_{pa} climbs during exercise. (From: reference 32, with permission.)

Figure 9. (facing page) Pulmonary hemodynamic and oxyhemoglobin saturation changes from upright rest (closed circles, left) to upright ergometer exercise (closed circles, right) in NOD (solid line) and non-NOD (broken line) subjects. * or NS above the exercise points indicate statistical significance between baseline upright and exercise values (*t* test for paired data). The "†" between curves indicates lack of significance in the percent change from baseline to exercise between the two groups. The NS or *P* value at either side of the vertical brackets indicates significance level between groups for that condition. Upper left: there is no overall change in Sao_2 during exercise in either group. The Svo_2 drops significantly and nearly equally in both groups. Upper right: the increase in cardiac output is roughly the same in both

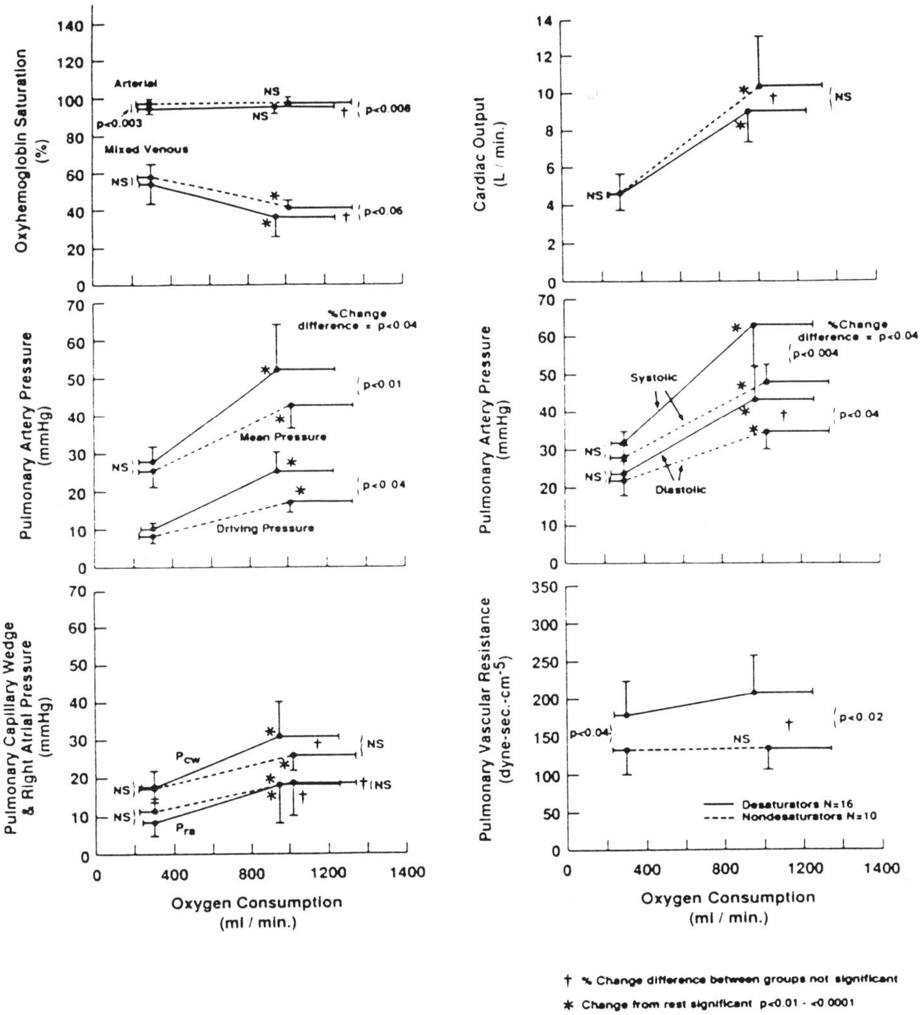

(Continued from facing page)
groups. Middle left: the increase in P_{pa} is greater in NOD than in non-NOD subjects. Pulmonary driving pressure is not different at baseline upright but is during exercise. Middle right: the increase in systolic and diastolic P_{pa} is greater in the non-NOD subjects. Lower left: although there appears to be a significant increase in P_{cw} during exercise in both groups, these changes do not differ between groups. Lower right: PVR is different between NOD and non-NOD subjects both at upright rest and during exercise. There was no significant difference between groups in V_{O_2} or V_{CO_2} at rest or exercise. (From: reference 32, with permission.)

increase in P_{cw} because of an "auto-PEEP" phenomenon could not be ruled out. Pulmonary vascular resistance did not change during exercise for either group but was higher in desaturators than nondesaturators at upright rest and exercise. Arterial desaturation during exercise was not predictive of NOD since non-NOD as well as NOD subjects showed such desaturation.

Since parameters of pulmonary function do not vary between groups in the two studies by Fletcher et al.,[32,93] it would appear that NOD may play an active role in determining pulmonary artery pressure. The similarity in DLco between the two groups (which may correlate with parenchymal destruction and loss of pulmonary vasculature) also points more to a functional (pulmonary artery constriction in response to hypoxemia) rather than anatomic (arterial obliteration secondary to parenchymal destruction) difference between groups. However, the final answer to this question lies in the outcome of the prospective studies of nocturnal supplemental oxygen versus sham in COPD patients now being conducted in Europe and in the US. If supplemental oxygen limits the progression of pulmonary hypertension while it progresses in the sham group, it is unlikely that lung structural differences in these groups account for the difference in resting pressures.

Diagnosis, Importance, and Prevalence of NOD

Since no daytime parameter of blood gas or pulmonary function is predictive of NOD, the only reliable way of detecting it is to study the patient with lung or thoracic wall disease in the sleep laboratory or, at minimum, to obtain an oximeter screen. Attempts at relating the presence of NOD to daytime blood gases, FEV_1, clinical severity of disease, symptoms, age, body weight, sex, exercise desaturation, and ventilatory control have failed to come up with a distinct feature or combination of features that would permit diagnosis of NOD, thereby avoiding polysomnography. It is stated that the worse the COPD and the lower the awake Pao_2, the more likely the patient is to show NOD, but this may not be predictive in individual patients and the correlation with pulmonary function is generally poor.[94,95] It is also stated that the bronchitic or "type B" COPD patient is more likely to desaturate than the eucapnic and normoxic "pink puffer."[8,26,53,96,97] Douglas et al.[26]

found transient NOD in all 10 "blue bloaters" and in neither of two pink puffers. Flenley et al.[96] found frequent REM NOD in all of 15 blue bloaters with pulmonary hypertension and polycythemia, whereas eight pink puffers had infrequent desaturation. The significance of these findings is questionable due to the difficulty of pigeonholing COPD patients into these categories. Blunted ventilatory response to hypercapnia and hypoxia are additional determinants of the "blue and bloated" syndrome[97] and therefore might also be predictive of NOD. Several publications[7,97–100] have suggested that blunted ventilatory responses to CO_2 and hypoxia may be markers of NOD in patients not clinically classifiable as blue bloaters or pink puffers. The relationship between ventilatory control and desaturation is further muddied by the change in chemosensitivity that may occur during sleep, independent of awake chemosensitivity, which is when most of the above studies were done.

A recent attempt to apply results of multiple routine variables failed to elicit a combination that would reliably predict NOD in patients with less severe hypoxemia ($Pao_2 > 60$ torr).[42] There were no differences between NOD and non-NOD groups when comparing anthropomorphic data and various parameters of pulmonary function. Awake Pao_2 in the NOD subjects was lower and $Paco_2$ higher than in the non-NOD subjects. Stepwise logistic regression using 18 clinical parameters showed the combination of a high $Paco_2$, low Pao_2, and a history of chronic bronchitis to be related to NOD. However, the overlap precluded clinical use of this approach as a screen for NOD.

Two recent studies have questioned the importance of NOD in determining cardiopulmonary hemodynamics and the clinical relevance of making this diagnosis on the management and longevity of COPD patients.[95,101] Using noninvasive contrast echocardiography, Himelman et al.[101] discovered evidence of cor pulmonale (high peak pulmonary systolic pressures, increased right to left ventricular volume ratios, or thickened right ventricular wall) in 75% of 33 COPD patients with Pao_2s above 55 mm Hg. Nocturnal desaturation, defined as a 4% drop from baseline was discovered in six subjects with nadir sleep Sao_2s ranging from 85% to 69%. These authors were unable to demonstrate a correlation between nadir nocturnal desaturation and degree of pulmonary hemodynamic dysfunction. It does not state, but is presumed, that all six of the desaturators had evidence of cor pulmonale. This lack of correlation should be interpreted with caution since the level of dysfunction within the whole group was severe (mean FEV_1 = 1.0) and the prevalence of cor pulmonale high at 75%. This could easily have been on the basis of pulmonary parenchymal destruction (emphysema) rather than related to transient nocturnal or relative daytime hypoxemia since both mechanisms can contribute to abnormal pulmonary hemodynamics. In addition, no polysomnography was performed (Sao_2 tracings only), and the presence and duration of REM sleep could not be confirmed.

A recent study by Connaughton et al.[95] examined whether "sleep studies contribute to the management of patients with severe COPD." These authors found that daytime Sao_2 correlated well with nocturnal mean and nadir Sao_2 and forced vital capacity (FVC). Furthermore, in patients treated with home supplemental oxygen, there was no difference in survival between groups with "excess nocturnal hypoxia" versus those without. They concluded that daytime Sao_2 or FVC was just as good a predictor of survival as knowledge of nocturnal Sao_2. Two important points should be noted. First, there was a wide range of Pao_2 (hence Sao_2) levels in the two participating centers (53 ± 10 and 58 ± 11 mm Hg), and one could naturally expect high correlations between daytime and nocturnal Sao_2 levels just as Sao_2's measured at 9:00 AM should correlated strongly with Sao_2 measured at 5:00 PM on the same day. Secondly, more than half the subjects had resting daytime Sao_2 levels below 90% or near a Pao_2 of 55 mm Hg. From data of the NOTT[82] and British supplemental oxygen trials[83] one would expect a higher mortality in the majority of the group based upon the presence of daytime hypoxemia alone. It must be agreed that knowledge of sleep saturation would probably not change therapy or predict prognosis in a broad range of hypoxemic ($Pao_2 < 55$–60 torr) COPD patients since supplemental oxygen will be indicated in these patients based upon the results of home oxygen studies.[82,83] One should not, on the basis of this study,[95] rule out the benefit of discovering sleep hypoxemia to those with higher daytime Pao_2 but transient NOD.

Low-flow oxygen during sleep corrects hypoxemia[26,29,30,63] and greatly ameliorates the elevation in pulmonary artery pressure that otherwise develops during hypoxemia. Since patients with a resting daytime $Pao_2 < 55$ torr will be candidates for continuous home oxygen therapy, NOD will already be treated, reducing the urgency for further studies on efficacy of oxygen therapy in this setting. Thus, future studies of incidence, pathogenesis, cardiopulmonary hemodynamics, natural history, methods of detection, and treatment of transient, REM sleep-related NOD should be directed toward the subset of chronic lung disease patients who would not otherwise qualify for home supplemental oxygen: those with a daytime $Pao_2 \geq 60$ torr. The ultimate goal should be to determine the natural history of NOD and the possible benefit from treatment with oxygen or other agents.

In determining the clinical importance of NOD, an important question arises as to the prevalence of NOD among chronic lung disease patients with a Pao_2 in the range that would not otherwise receive home supplemental oxygen. Statistical analysis has been compiled on 152 such patients studied during formal polysomnography.[42] All had a daytime $Pao_2 \geq 60$ torr (Fig. 5). Nine subjects were disqualified by the discovery of sleep apnea (greater than five obstructive apneas per hour of sleep) and eight because they could not sleep in the laboratory setting. Twenty seven percent of the remaining 135 subjects showed NOD.

During the course of this study, three patients showed reversible NOD. Two of these underwent initial polysomnography on the day of discharge following 10-day and 14-day hospitalizations for acute exacerbations of COPD. At the time of study, the patients were free of wheezes on quiet respiration and were judged to be clinically stable. Another outpatient using oral theophylline and an inhaled beta-2 agonist was also studied during what he termed to be his "usual state of health." Physical exam on the day following polysomnography showed marked expiratory wheezes and a course of corticosteroids resulted in improved airflow and clinical symptoms. All three of these subjects showed NOD to 85% or below during REM sleep on their initial sleep study. Each was screened 2–4 weeks later in preparation for inclusion in a long-term nocturnal oxygen protocol and did not show evidence of NOD. The patient who cleared with a short course of steroids, when restudied 3 months after the initial screen (while off steroids), again showed no evidence of NOD. Thus, it is important to note that NOD may be a reversible phenomenon in some patients.

Treatment of NOD

Any discussion of the treatment of NOD must be prefaced by the question: "if it is not known that NOD has a detrimental effect upon pulmonary hemodynamics, or that therapy alters hemodynamics, should we treat it?" At this point, it can only be said that hemodynamics are worse in NOD patients with chronic lung disease and, therefore, the potential exists for altering hemodynamics. Only long-term follow-up studies will provide answers to this and other questions about sleep quality and mortality.

Based upon the data published to date, it would appear that therapy should certainly be directed toward those patients with a daytime Pao_2 less than 55 mm Hg and perhaps to those with a Pao_2 between 55 and 60 mm Hg. This is particularly true in those who have physical, electrocardiographic, or roentgenographic signs of right-sided heart failure or unexplained polycythemia. Where more sophisticated noninvasive (sonicated contrast-enhanced Doppler, echocardiography, rest or exercise radionuclide cardiography) methods of assessing cardiopulmonary hemodynamics are available, additional information may aid the clinician in deciding if NOD should be searched for and treated. When the daytime Pao_2 is above 60 mm Hg and pulmonary hypertension is suspected, some form of nocturnal Sao_2 monitoring may be in order, keeping in mind that if NOD is found, efficacy of treatment is still not proven.

As most practitioners are aware, formal polysomnographic sleep studies are quite expensive and burdensome to the patient. Many clinicians have resorted to simple overnight oximetry to detect NOD. There are a great many pitfalls to this technique, and at this time the author cannot recommend such a screening method to rule NOD in or out. A "normal" whole night Sao_2 tracing (e.g., Sao_2 continuously above baseline awake or 90%) does not rule out NOD since the absence of EEG monitoring does not allow the clinician to know if the patient experienced REM sleep, the stage when NOD would be most likely to occur. Therefore, the physician might wrongly assume that the patient has normal nocturnal Sao_2. A more likely error is that multiple dips in Sao_2 may be observed that appear very much like NOD but in reality are artifacts caused by malpositioning of the oximeter earpiece (partial slippage or laying on the earpiece) or slippage or excessive pressure on finger pulse oximeter monitors. So many artifact and false positives have been produced in over 250 COPD patients studied in the author's laboratory that oximetry monitoring without polysomnography has been abandoned.

Medroxyprogresterone Acetate

Medroxyprogesterone acetate (MPA) is believed to be centrally acting respiratory stimulant that has been shown to lower $Paco_2$ in some patients with alveolar hypoventilation.[102] Skatrud et al. found that MPA improved hypoxemia and hypercarbia in five of 17 COPD patients.[103] This improvement persisted at 4 weeks of therapy. Using a double-blind controlled trial, Dolly and Block found that although waking arterial blood gases improved in 19 patients, the effect upon sleep Sao_2 was not significant at the end of one month.[104] Considering the frequent side effects of MPA and the fact that many authors have reported failure of ventilatory stimulation with long-term use in alveolar hypoventilators, it appears unlikely that this form of therapy will be useful in COPD patients with NOD.

Almitrine Bismesylate

Almitrine bismesylate has been used extensively in Europe and successfully in many trials in the United States to improve oxygenation and decrease hypercarbia. It is a peripheral chemoreceptor agonist, which in single-[105] and multiple-dose studies[106–108] has improved both awake and sleeping Sao_2. Longer-term studies up to 6 months[109] have also showed improved daytime and nocturnal oxygenation. Goethe et al. recently demonstrated an increase in Pao_2 by 8.1 ± 2.1 mm Hg and a decrease in $Paco_2$ by 3.0 ± 0.7 mm Hg in nine patients in a double-blind, placebo ($N = 11$) controlled trial over one year.[110] Almitrine improved sleep Sao_2 in five patients in whom sleep studies were done.

Use of this drug for patients with abnormal cardiopulmonary hemodynamics is questionable because of the demonstrated acute elevations of pulmonary artery pressure both in animals, and in humans with COPD. MacNee et al.[106] treated 10 bronchitics with almitrine and demonstrated an 11 mm Hg increase in mean pulmonary artery pressure at rest from 22 to 33 mm Hg. This increase was also seen in five patients treated chronically (3 months) whose mean pulmonary artery pressure increased from 17 off drug to 23 mm Hg on drug at rest, and from 35 to 42 mm Hg during exercise.

Supplemental Oxygen

Low-flow supplemental oxygen between 2 and 4 L/min has been amply shown in numerous studies to completely reverse or greatly ameliorate NOD and the accompanying transient elevations in pulmonary artery pressure during sleep.[26,29,62,63] Chronic administration of oxygen during sleep has been demonstrated to lower mean sleep pulmonary artery pressure in some NOD patients.[63] However, discontinuation of the oxygen allows immediate return of NOD with the associated pulmonary hypertension.

The current guidelines for the administration of continuous home supplemental oxygen in patients with COPD are based upon successful demonstration of prolongation of life in two well-controlled prospective studies.[82,83] For the most part, these guidelines are aimed at a population that will already have demonstrable pulmonary hypertension,[88] which, recognized after the onset of right heart failure, portends a bad prognosis.[111,112] In her recent review of the structural changes in pulmonary hypertension, Dr. Lynne Reid states that "By the time a patient presents with symptoms, the structural changes are so important that reversal of a constrictor (hypoxemic) component is only palliative."[113] Some ongoing studies are attempting to address the prevention of pulmonary hypertension by initiating oxygen at an earlier stage of disease, but thus far no results are available and the decision by the clinician to use supplemental oxygen must remain judgmental.

As mentioned in the first paragraph of this chapter, the ACCP-NHLBI national conference on oxygen therapy[2] has recommended oxygen therapy during sleep for patients "who develop Pa_{O_2} values of 55 mm Hg or less during sleep which is associated with hypoxic organ dysfunction." In the study by Fletcher et al. employing invasive measurement of pulmonary hemodynamics, all the subjects[93] met or exceeded this level of sleep hypoxemia. Furthermore, 27/36 or 75% met the second criteria by having well-documented (although unsuspected) pulmonary hypertension at right heart catheterization (mean pulmonary artery pressure of 25.7 mm Hg). If all physicians detected and followed the consensus recommendation of this nationally recognized group of clinical investigators, an additional 1.8 million patients with COPD could be placed on home oxygen at a cost of over $2.2 billion without clear evidence of potential benefit. It therefore behooves the clinican to carefully consider the economic ramifications of diagnosing and treating nocturnal oxyhemoglobin desaturation until such time as information on the efficacy or lack thereof is available. In the meantime, a conservative approach to COPD patients with suspected nocturnal oxyhemoglobin desaturation is warranted.

References

1. Weil JV, Cherniack NS, Dempsey JA, et al. NHLBI workshop summary; Respiratory disorders of sleep: Pathophysiology, clinical implications, and therapeutic approaches. *Am Rev Respir Dis* 1987; 136:775–761.
2. Fulmer JD, Snider GL. ACCP-NHLBI national conference on oxygen therapy. *Chest* 1984; 86:234–247.
3. Robin ED. Some interactions between sleep and disease. *Arch Intern Med* 1958; 102:669–675.
4. Trask CH, Cree EM. Oximeter studies on patients with chronic obstructive emphysema, awake and during sleep. *N Engl J Med* 1962; 266:639–642.
5. Wynne JW, Block AJ, Hemenway J, et al. Disordered breathing and oxygen desaturation during sleep in patients with chronic obstructive lung disease (COLD). *Am J Med* 1979; 66:573–579.
6. Arand DL, McGinty DJ, Littner MR. Respiratory patterns associated with hemoglobin desaturation during sleep in chronic obstructive pulmonary disease. *Chest* 1981; 80:183–190.
7. Littner MR, McGinty DJ, Arand DL. Determinants of oxygen desaturation in the course of ventilation during sleep in chronic obstructive pulmonary disease. *Am Rev Respir Dis* 1980; 122:849–857.
8. Catterall JR, Douglas NJ, Calverley PMA, et al. Transient hypoxemia during sleep in chronic obstructive pulmonary disease is not a sleep apnea syndrome. *Am Rev Respir Dis* 1983; 128:24–29.
9. Calverley PMA, Catterall JR, Shapiro C, et al. Cor Pulmonale in asthma. *Br J Dis Chest* 1983; 77(3):303–307.
10. Mezon BL, West P, Israel J, et al. Sleep breathing abnormalities in kyphoscoliosis. *Am Rev Respir Dis* 1980; 122:617–621.
11. Guilleminault C, Kurland G, Winkle R, et al. Severe kyphoscoliosis, breathing and sleep. *Chest* 1981; 79:626–630.
12. Simonds AK, Parker RA, Branthwaite MA. Effects of protriptyline on sleep related disturbances of breathing in restrictive chest wall disease. *Thorax* 1986; 41:586–590.
13. Amis TC, Ciofetta G, Hughes JMB, et al. Regional lung function in bilateral diaphragmatic paralysis. *Clin Sci* 1980; 59:485–492.
14. Efthimiou J, McLelland J, Round J, et al. Diaphragm paralysis causing ventilatory failure in an adult with rigid spine syndrome. *Am Rev Respir Dis* 1987; 136:1483–1485.
15. Coccagna G, Mantovani M, Parchi CL, et al. Alveolar hypoventilation and hypersomnia in myotonic dystrophy. *Neurol Neurosurg Psychiatry* 1975; 38:977–984.
16. Francis PWJ, Muller NL, Guiwitx D, et al. Hemoglobin desaturation. Its occurrence during sleep in patients with cystic fibrosis. *Am J Dis Child* 1980; 134:734–740.
17. Muller NL, Francis PW, Gurwitz D, et al. Mechanism of hemoglobin desaturation during rapid-eye-movement sleep in normal subjects and in patients with cystic fibrosis. *Am Rev Respir Dis* 1980; 121:463–469.

18. Stokes DC, McBride JT, Wall MA, et al. Sleep hypoxemia in young adults with cystic fibrosis. *Dis Child* 1980; 134:741–743.
19. Spier S, Rivlin J, Hughes D, et al. The effect of oxygen on sleep, blood gases and ventilation in cystic fibrosis. *Am Rev Respir Dis* 1984; 129: 712–718.
20. Gaultier C, Praud JP, Clement A, et al. Respiration during sleep in children with COPD. *Chest* 1985; 87:168–173.
21. Bye PT, Issa F, Berthan-Jones M, et al. Studies of oxygenation during sleep in patients with interstitial lung disease. *Am Rev Respir Dis* 1984; 129:27–32.
22. Perez-Padilla RR, West P, Lertzman M, et al. Breathing during sleep in patients with interstitial lung disease. *Am Rev Respir Dis* 1985; 132:224–229.
23. George CF, Kryger MH: Sleep in restrictive lung disease. *Sleep* 1987; 10(5):409–418.
24. Koo KW, Sax DS, Snider GL. Arterial blood gases and pH during sleep in chronic obstructive pulmonary disease. *Am J Med* 1975; 58: 663–670.
25. Wynne JW, Block AJ, Hunt LA, et al. Disordered breathing and oxygen desaturation during daytime naps. *Johns Hopkins Med J* 1978; 143:3–7.
26. Douglas NJ, Calverley PM, Leggett RJ, et al. Transient hypoxemia during sleep in chronic bronchitis and emphysema. *Lancet* 1979; 1:1–4.
27. Hudgel DW, Martin RJ, Capehart M, et al. Contribution of hypoventilation to sleep oxygen desaturation in chronic obstructive pulmonary disease. *J Appl Physiol: Respir Environ Exercise Physiol* 1983; 55:669–677.
28. Fletcher EC, Gray BA, Levin DC. Nonapneic mechanisms of arterial oxygen desaturation during rapid-eye-movement sleep. *J Appl Physiol Environ Exercise Physiol* 1983; 54:632–639.
29. Goldstein RS, Ramcharan V, Bowes G, et al. Effect of supplemental nocturnal oxygen on gas exchange in patients with severe obstructive lung disease. *N Engl J Med* 1984; 310:425–429.
30. Leitch AJ, Clancy LJ, Leggett RJ, et al. Arterial blood gas tensions, hydrogen ion, and electroencephalogram during sleep in patients with chronic ventilatory failure. *Thorax* 1976; 31:730–735.
31. Flick MR, Block AJ. Continuous in vivo monitoring of arterial oxygenation in chronic obstructive lung disease. *Ann Intern Med* 1977; 86:725–730.
32. Fletcher EC, Luckett RA, Miller T, et al. Exercise hemodynamics and gas exchange in COPD patients with chronic obstructive pulmonary disease sleep desaturation and a daytime Pao_2 above 60 torr. *Am Rev Resp Dis* 1989; 140:1237–1245.
33. Aserinsky E, Kleitman N. Regularly occurring periods of eye motility, and concomitant phenomena, during sleep. *Science* 1953; 118:273–274.
34. Aserinsky E, Kleitman N. Two types of ocular motility occurring in sleep. *J Appl Physiol* 1955; 8:1–10.
35. Jouvet M. Neurophysiology of the states of sleep. *Physiol Rev* 1967; 47: 117–177.
36. Henderson-Smart DJ, Read DJ. Reduced lung volume during behavioral active sleep in the newborn. *J Appl Physiol* 1979; 46:1081–1085.

37. Tabachnik E, Muller NL, Bryan AC, et al. Changes in ventilation and chest wall mechanics during sleep in normal adolescents. *J Appl Physiol* 1981; 51:557–564.
38. Tusiewicz K, Moldofsky H, Bryan AC, et al. Mechanics of the rib cage and diaphragm during sleep. *J Appl Physiol* 1977; 43:600–602.
39. Fletcher EC. Sleep, breathing, and oxyhemoglobin saturation in chronic lung disease. *In* EC Fletcher (ed). Abnormalities of Respiration During Sleep: Diagnosis, Pathophysiology, and Treatment. Orlando, Florida, Grune & Stratton, 1986.
40. Hudgel DW, Devadatta P. Decrease in functional residual capacity during sleep in normal humans. *J Appl Physiol: Respir Environ Exercise Physiol* 1984; 57:1319–1322.
41. Hudgel DW, Martin RJ, Johnson B, et al. Mechanics of the respiratory system and breathing pattern during sleep in normal humans. *J Appl Physiol: Respir Environ Exercise Physiol* 1984; 56:133–137.
42. Fletcher EC, Miller J, Divine GW, et al. Nocturnal oxyhemoglobin desaturation in COPD patients with arterial oxygen tensions above 60 mm Hg. *Chest* 1987; 92:604–608.
43. Martin RJ. Nocturnal asthma. *In* RJ Martin (ed). Cardiorespiratory Disorders during Sleep. Mt Kisco, New York, Futura Publishing, 1984, pp 119–145.
44. Orem J. Control of the upper airways during sleep and the hypersomnia-sleep apnea syndrome. *In* J Orem, CD Barnes (eds). Physiology in Sleep. New York, Academic Press, 1980, pp 273–213.
45. Bateman JRM, Pavia D, Clarke SW. The retention of lung secretions during the night in normal subjects. *Clin Sci Mol Med* 1978; 55:523–527.
46. Fleetham JA, Bradley CA, Kryger MH, et al. The effect of low flow oxygen therapy on chemical control of ventilation in patients with hypoxemic COPD. *Am Rev Respir Dis* 1980; 833–840.
47. Berthan-Jones M, Sullivan CE. Ventilatory and arousal responses to hypoxia in sleeping humans. *Am Rev Respir Dis* 1982; 125:632–639.
48. Kinsman RA, Yaroush RA, Fernandez E, et al. Symptoms and experiences in chronic bronchitis and emphysema. *Chest* 1983; 83:755–761.
49. Brezinova A, Catterall JR, Douglas NJ, et al. Night sleep of patients with chronic ventilatory failure and age matched controls: Number and duration of the EEG episodes of intervening wakefulness and drowsiness. *Sleep* 1982; 5:123–130.
50. Fletcher EC, Martin RJ, Monlux RD. Disturbed EEG sleep patterns in chronic obstructive pulmonary disease. *Sleep Res* 1982; 11:186.
51. Fleetham J, West P, Mezon B, et al. Sleep, arousals, and oxygen desaturation in chronic obstructive pulmonary disease. *Am Rev Respir Dis* 1982; 126:429–433.
52. Kearley R, Wynne JW, Block AJ, et al. The effect of low flow oxygen on sleep disordered breathing and oxygen desaturation. *Chest* 1980; 78:682–685.
53. Calverley PMA, Brezinova V, Douglas NJ, et al. The effect of oxygenation on sleep quality in chronic bronchitis and emphysema. *Am Rev Respir Dis* 1982; 126:206–210.

54. Phillips BA, Cooper KR, Burke TV. The effect of sleep loss on breathing in COPD. *Chest* 1987; 91:29–32.
55. McNicholas WT, Fitzgerald MX. Nocturnal deaths among patients with chronic bronchitis and emphysema. Br Med J 1984; 289:878
56. Holford FD, Mithoefer TC. Cardiac arrhythmias in hospitalized patients with chronic obstructive pulmonary disease. *Am Rev Respir Dis* 1973; 108:879–885.
57. Kleiger RE, Senior RM. Longterm electrocardiographic monitoring of ambulatory patients with chronic airway obstruction. *Chest* 1974; 65: 483–487.
58. Flick MR, Block AJ. Nocturnal vs. diurnal cardiac arrhythmias in patients with chronic obstructive pulmonary disease. *Chest* 1979; 75:8–11.
59. Tirlapur VG, Mir M. Nocturnal hypoxemia and associated electrocardiographic changes in patients with chronic obstructive airway disease. *N Engl J Med* 1982; 306:125–130.
60. Shepard JW Jr, Garrison MW, Grither DA, et al. Relationship of ventricular ectopy to nocturnal oxygen desaturation in patients with chronic obstructive pulmonary disease. *Am J Med* 1985; 78:28–34.
61. Coccagna G, Lugaresi E. Arterial blood gases and pulmonary and systemic arterial pressure during sleep in chronic obstructive pulmonary disease. *Sleep* 1978; 1:117–124.
62. Boysen PG, Block JA, Wynne JW, et al. Nocturnal pulmonary hypertension in patients with chronic obstructive pulmonary disease. *Chest* 1979; 76:536–542.
63. Fletcher EC, Levin DC. Cardiopulmonary hemodynamics during sleep in subjects with chronic obstructive pulmonary disease: the effect of short and long term oxygen. *Chest* 1984; 85:6–14.
64. Flenley DC. Clinical hypoxia: causes, consequences, and correction. *Lancet* 1978; 1:542–546.
65. Block AJ, Boyson PG, Wynne JW. The origins of cor pulmonale, a hypothesis. *Chest* 1979; 75:109.
66. Nattie EE, Bartlett D Jr, and Johnson K. Pulmonary hypertension and right ventricular hypertrophy caused by intermittent hypoxia and hypercapnia in the rat. *Am Rev Respir Dis* 1978; 118:653–658.
67. Ressl J, Urbanova D, Widimsky J, et al. Reversibility of pulmonary hypertension and right ventricular hypertrophy induced by intermittent high altitude hypoxia in rats. *Respiration* 1974; 31:38–46.
68. Widimsky J, Urbanova D, Ressl J, et al. Effect of intermittent altitude hypoxia on the myocardium and lesser circulation in the rat. *Cardiovasc Res* 1973; 7:798–808.
69. McGrath JJ, Prochazka J, Pelouch V, et al. Physiological response of rats to intermittent high altitude stress: effects of age. *J Appl Physiol* 1973; 34:289–293.
70. Fishman AP. Pulmonary circulation. *In* AP Fishman, AB Fisher (eds). Handbook of Physiology; Section 3: The Respiratory System; Volume 1, Circulation and Nonrespiratory Function. Bethesda, Maryland, American Physiological Society, 1985, pp 93–165.
71. Stalcup SA, Lipset JS, Legant PM, et al. Inhibition of converting enzyme

activity by acute hypoxia in dogs. *J Appl Physiol Respir Environ Exercise Physiol* 1979; 46:227–234.
72. Harker LA, Ross R, Glomset J. Role of the platelet in atherogenesis. *Ann NY Acad Sci* 1976; 275:321–330.
73. Johnson TS, Ellis JH Jr, Steele PP. Improvement of platelet survival time with oxygen in patients with chronic obstructive airway disease. *Am Rev Respir Dis* 1978; 117:255–257.
74. Weitzenblum E, Krieger J, Apprill M, et al. Daytime pulmonary hypertension in patients with obstructive sleep apnea syndrome. *Am Rev Respir Dis* 1988; 138:345–349.
75. Bradley TD, R Rutherford, Grossman RF, et al. Role of daytime hypoxemia in the pathogenesis of right heart failure in the obstructive sleep apnea syndrome. *Am Rev Respir Dis* 1985; 131:835–839.
76. Tilkian A, Guilleminault C, Schroeder J, et al. Hemodynamics during sleep-induced apnea. *Ann Intern Med* 1976; 85:714–719.
77. Coccagna G, Mantovani M, Brignani F, et al. Tracheostomy in hypersomnia with periodic breathing. *Bull Physiopathol Respir* 1972; 8:1217–1227.
78. Motta J, Guilleminault C, Schroeder JS, et al. Tracheostomy and hemodynamic changes in sleep-induced apnea. *Ann Intern Med* 1978; 89:454–458.
79. Williams JF, Behnke RH. The effect of pulmonary emphysema upon cardiopulmonary hemodynamics at rest and during exercise. *Ann Intern Med* 1964; 60:824–842.
80. Damsgaard T, Kok-Jensen A. Prognosis in severe chronic obstructive pulmonary disease. *Acata Med Scand* 1974; 196:103–108.
81. Traver GA, Cline MG, Burrows B. Predictors of mortality in chronic obstructive pulmonary disease. *Am Rev Respir Dis* 1979; 119:895–902.
82. Nocturnal Oxygen Therapy Trial Group. Continuous or nocturnal oxygen therapy in hypoxemic chronic obstructive lung disease. *Ann Intern Med* 1980; 93:391–398.
83. Medical Research Council Working Party. Long term domiciliary oxygen therapy in chronic hypoxic cor pulmonale complicating chronic bronchitis and emphysema. *Lancet* 1981; 1:681–686.
84. Weitzenblum E, Sautegeau A, Ehrhart M, et al. Long-term oxygen therapy can reverse the progression of pulmonary hypertension in patients with chronic obstructive pulmonary disease. *Am Rev Respir Dis* 1985; 131:493–498.
85. Timms RM, Khaja FU, Williams GW. Hemodynamic response to oxygen therapy in chronic obstructive pulmonary disease. *Ann Intern Med* 1985; 102:29–36.
86. Stark RD, Finnigan P, Bishop JM. Daily requirement of oxygen to reverse pulmonary hypertension in patients with chronic bronchitis. *Br Med J* 1972; 3:724–728.
87. Stark RD, Finnegan P, Bishop JM. Long-term domiciliary oxygen in chronic bronchitis with pulmonary hypertension. *Br Med J* 1973; 3:467–470.
88. Burrows B, Kettel LJ, Niden AH, et al. Patterns of cardiovascular dysfunction in chronic obstructive lung disease. *N Engl J Med* 1972; 286: 912–918.

89. Boushy SF, North LB. Hemodynamic changes in chronic obstructive pulmonary disease. *Chest* 1977; 72:565–570.
90. Weitzenblum E, Loiseau A, Hirth C, et al. Course of pulmonary hemodynamics in patients with chronic obstructive pulmonary disease. *Chest* 1979; 75:656–662.
91. Weitzenblum E, Mammosser M, Ehrhart M. Evolution and prognosis of pulmonary hypertension in chronic obstructive pulmonary diseases. *Herz* 1986; 11:147–154.
92. Schrijen F, Uffholtz H, Polu J, et al. Pulmonary and systemic hemodynamic evolution in chronic bronchitis. *Am Rev Respir Dis* 1978; 117: 25–31.
93. Fletcher EC, Luckett RA, Miller T, et al. Pulmonary vascular hemodynamics in chronic lung disease patients with and without oxyhemoglobin desaturation during sleep. *Chest* 1989; 95:157–166.
94. Demarco FJ, Wynne JW, Block AJ, et al. Oxygen desaturation during sleep as a determinant of the "blue and bloated" syndrome. *Chest* 1981; 79:621–625.
95. Connaughton JJ, Catterall JR, Elton RA, et al. Do sleep studies contribute to the management of patients with severe COPD? *Am Rev Respir Dis* 1988; 138:341–344.
96. Flenley DC, Cloverly PM, Douglas NJ, et al. Nocturnal hypoxemia and long-term domiciliary oxygen therapy in "blue and bloated" bronchitics. Physiopathologic correlations. *Chest* 1980; 77:305–307.
97. Mathews AW. The relationship between central carbon dioxide sensitivity and clinical features in patients with chronic airway obstruction. *Q J Med* 1977; 182:179–195.
98. Fleetham JA, Mezon B, West P. Chemical control of ventilation and sleep arterial oxygen desaturation in patients with COPD. *Am Rev Respir Dis* 1980; 122:583–589.
99. Goethe B. Effect of chemosensitivity on arterial oxygen saturation during sleep. *Am Rev Respir Dis* 1979; 119:119.
100. Tatsumi K, Kimura H, Kunitimo F, et al. Sleep arterial oxygen desaturation and chemical control of breathing during wakefulness in COPD. *Chest* 1986; 90:68–73.
101. Himelman RB, Struve SN, Brown JK, et al. Improved recognition of cor pulmonale in patients with severe COPD. *Am J Med* 1988; 84:891–898.
102. Tyler JM. The effect of progesterone on the respiration of patients with emphysema and hypercapnia. *J Clin Invest* 1960; 39:34–41.
103. Skatrud JF, Dempsey JB, Iber C, et al. Correction of CO_2 retention during sleep in patients with chronic obstructive pulmonary diseases. *Am Rev Respir Dis* 1981; 124:260–268.
104. Dolly R, Block AJ. Medroxyprogesterone and COPD; effect on breathing and oxygenation in sleeping and awake patients. *Chest* 1983; 84:394–398.
105. Powles ACP, Tuxen DV, Pugsley SO, et al. The effect of almitrine on sleep hypoxemia in patients with chronic airflow limitation. *Am Rev Respir Dis* 1984; 129:A66.
106. MacNee W, Connaughton JJ, Hayhurst MD, et al. The effects of almitrine on pulmonary artery pressure and right ventricular performance in chronic bronchitis and emphysema. *Respiration* 1984; 46:157–158.

107. Kurtz D, Weitzenblum E, Drieger J, et al. Sommeil et desaturation nocturne de patients atteints de bronchopneumonpathies chroniques obstructives. *Rev Mal Respir* 1985; 2(suppl 1):S45–S52.
108. Prefaut C, Bourgouin-Karaouni D, Ramonatxo M, et al. Blood gases and pulmonary haemodynamic followup during a one year double blind bismesilate almitrine therapy in COPD patients. *Am Rev Respir Dis* 1985; 131(2):A71.
109. Connaughton JJ, Douglas NJ, Morgan AD, et al. Almitrine improves oxygenation when both awake and asleep, in patients with hypoxia and CO_2 retention due to chronic bronchitis and emphysema. *Am Rev Respir Dis* 1985; 132:206–210.
110. Goethe B, Cherniack NS, Bachand RT, et al. Long-term effects of Almitrine Bismesylate on oxygenation during wakefulness and sleep in COPD. *Am J Med* 1988; 84:436–444.
111. Kawakami Y, Kishi F, Yamamoto H, et al. Relation of oxygen delivery, mixed venous oxygenation, and pulmonary hemodynamics to prognosis in chronic obstructive pulmonary disease. *N Engl J Med* 1983; 308: 1045–1049.
112. Lindsay DA, Read J. Pulmonary vascular responsiveness in the prognosis of chronic obstructive lung disease. *Am Rev Respir Dis* 1972; 105: 242–250.
113. Reid LM. Structure and function in pulmonary hypertension—new perceptions. *Chest* 1986; 89:279–288.

8

Neuromuscular and Skeletal Abnormalities with Nocturnal Respiratory Disorders

Richard J. Martin, M.D.

At times, in medicine, a problem seems unusual until the appropriate questions and investigations are made on a large population of patients. As stressed in previous chapters, the better the history and work-up, the more patients that we are able to find with sleep apnea, nocturnal asthma, and nocturnal cardiac problems. The same is true for neuromuscular and skeletal problems (Table 1). Obviously, without ample knowledge of the involved nocturnal respiratory pathophysiology, appropriate treatment modalities cannot be designed. This is particularly important in patients with neuromuscular abnormalities, as pulmonary complications are the most common cause of morbidity and mortality.

Any patient with a central nervous system disorder, a primary myopathy, a neuropathy, or bony abnormality involving the thoracic cage should be asked appropriate questions related to nocturnal respiratory problems, and if the potential for a problem exists, formal studies should be done. As will become evident, even simple daytime therapeutic intervention, such as respiratory muscle training, can dramatically improve the nocturnal respiratory pattern and oxygen saturation. This, in turn, improves the quality of life and could possibly prevent future morbidity and mortality due to respiratory disorders.

Martin RJ: Cardiorespiratory Disorders During Sleep, 2nd Edition. Futura Publishing Company, Inc., Mount Kisco, NY, © 1990.

Table 1.
Neurologic and Skeletal Disorders Associated with Nocturnal Cardiorespiratory Abnormalities

Dysfunction of autonomic nervous system
Cerebral vascular abnormalities
Brain-stem lesions
Spinal cord process
Muscular dystrophies
Increased intracranial pressure
Seizures
Myasathenia gravis
Klein-Levin syndrome
Kyphoscoliosis

In dealing with the neuromuscular system, a simple relationship between the chemical control of breathing and the ability of the muscles to receive the output signal or produce the force to maintain ventilation should be the working principle. However, as will be outlined, the relationship is not a simple one and other factors may be involved. This chapter will discuss the broad categories of neuromuscular and skeletal problems, as well as specific entities, in an attempt to clarify the relationship between the control of ventilation and the ability of the muscles to perform the involved work.

Dysfunction of Autonomic Nervous System

Three groups of patients with autonomic dysfunction have been investigated for abnormal cardiopulmonary patterns during sleep (Table 2). These groups are made up of those with familial or acquired dysautonomia, diabetes mellitus, and the Shy-Drager syndrome. Familial dysautonomia is a rare, recessive genetic disorder presenting in childhood. The anatomic process is an absence of unmyelinated nerve fibers in the peripheral and autonomic nerves. Features of this disease include absence of the fungiform papillae of the tongue, defective lacrimation, vasomotor instability, including blotching of the skin, relative pain insensitivity, motor incoordination, and absence of deep tendon reflexes.[1] The acquired form may be secondary to the remote effects of a neural tumor. Dysphagia may be the presenting symptom, which can lead to repeated aspiration pneumonia and a high mortal-

Table 2.
Autonomic Dysfunction and Respiratory Sleep Disorders

I. Categories
   A. Dysautonomia
      1. Familial
      2. Acquired
   B. Diabetes mellitus
   C. Shy-Drager syndrome
II. Daytime
   A. Signs and symptoms may be mild or absent
   B. Classical sleep apnea picture occurs but is infrequent
III. Sleep-related cardiorespiratory disturbances
   A. Apneas, hypoventilation
   B. Marked fluctuations in heart rate and blood pressure is not seen due to autonomic dysfunction
   C. Arousal response is poor and hypoxic seizures or death can occur

ity rate. In diabetes, both the sympathetic and parasympathetic pathways of the autonomic nervous system are involved. Thus problems of orthostatic hypotension, decreased sweating, impotency, delayed gastric emptying, which can lead to reflux and aspiration, small- and large-bowel problems, and bladder distension due to large residual urine may arise.[2] The Shy-Drager syndrome is a progressive disorder of unknown etiology involving generalized autonomic and nervous system defects. Severe orthostatic hypotension occurs with this disorder as well as with other autonomic problems. As the disease progresses, some patients develop a Parkinson-like illness with hypokinesia, rhythmic postural tremor, and rigidity. Others manifest a cerebellar-type incoordination.[3]

Dysautonomia

A reported case of a patient with dysautonomia exemplifies the nocturnal problems that can develop.[4] Eventually there was a postmortem diagnosis of a ganglioneuroma originating in the lumbar sympathetic ganglia. Abnormalities in the brain were confined to the brain stem and consisted of complete loss of neurons with severe fibrillary gliosis in the region of the Edinger-Westphal nuclei, the locus ceruleus, and the reticular formation bilaterally. In a classic example of nocturnal breathing disorders, the family noted a normal awake respiratory pattern but shallow or no respiration during sleep. With this periodic breathing, the patient became cyanotic and developed clonic seizure activity. Phenobarbital was prescribed as an anticonvulsant, which only prolonged the apneic spells and seizures. Eventually daytime somnolence developed. On admission to the hospital, diffuse dysautonomic changes of dilated, nonreactive pupils, decreased tearing and sweating, abnormal temperature control, and poorly functioning cardiovascular reflexes were noted. Polysomnographic evaluation revealed frequent obstructive and central apneas. The bradycardia–tachycardia pattern typically associated with the apneas was absent due to the abnormal cardiac reflex mechanism (see Chapter 4). Endotracheal intubation and positive-pressure breathing initially alleviated the sleep-related periodic breathing, but negative-pressure ventilation after extubation only served to potentiate the obstructive-type apnea. This would be expected because when tone in the upper airway is decreased, an increase in negative intrathoracic pressure will pull the pharyngeal structures into apposition. Naloxone and aminophylline were tried without success. The patient had a tracheostomy, but even with this intervention, progressive daytime somnolence and nighttime hypoxia continued. Ventilation assistance helped, but one night the ventilator became disconnected and the patient died during sleep.

This case report is of great interest in that pathologic abnormalities were found in areas of the brain stem that are associated with respiratory control and arousal. Thus, not only were central apneas present, but poor upper airway control resulted in obstructive apneas (see Chapter 4). Since only nocturnal respiratory abnormalities were present, this suggests that sleep eliminated the beneficial conscious respiratory control. Definite abnormalities were seen in the reticular formation that could affect arousal. Indeed, the arousal system was so poor that seizures frequently occurred and ultimately sleep-related death ensued.

The relationship of the retroperitoneal sympathetic tumor to the dysautonomia and sleep apnea is interesting. In the patient's serum, cytotoxic antineuroblastoma immunoglobulin was found. "Remote" nervous system effects of a neuroblastoma include cerebellar ataxia, infantile polymyoclonus–opsoclonus syndrome, mental retardation, and a myasthenia-like syndrome,[5–7] but a definite toxic substance has not yet been isolated. It is intriguing to postulate that in all sleep-related respiratory disorders, there is an abnormal chemical circulating substance. This would help to explain why anatomic abnormalities are not always seen.

Another study[8] showed that nonapneic, irregular breathing occurred in two young patients with familial dysautonomia. In one of the patients, who presented with frequent cyclical vomiting, the irregular nocturnal pattern was associated with a drop in the esophageal pH, suggesting that reflux played a role in potentiating the pattern. However, the other patient's irregular pattern occurred without any fall in the esophageal pH level. The respiratory irregularities consisted of short hypopneas, skipped breaths, and pauses or abrupt termination of inspiration, producing a reduction in inspiratory time. Although the disordered breathing occurred frequently during the night, there was no excessive daytime somnolence or nighttime snoring noted.

Diabetes Mellitus

Unexpected cardiorespiratory arrests have occurred in diabetic autonomic neuropathy patients mainly associated with anesthesia or pneumonia.[9–11] This would suggest that there are problems in ventilatory control in these patients. Nocturnal respiratory disorders could also be common.

Rees et al.[12] studied eight patients with diabetes mellitus of at least three years' duration who had evidence of autonomic neuropathy. A matched group of diabetic patients without neuropathy were similarly evaluated during sleep. The matching was appropriate and included sex, age, weight, and insulin requirements. Diabetic complications were more common in the neuropathy group. During sleep, three of the eight autonomic neuropathy patients had more than 30 apneic episodes (range 32–73). In two patients, the apneas were mainly central in nature, while the third patient had predominantly obstructive episodes. The longest episode lasted 108 seconds. The bradycardia–tachycardia commonly occurring with apneas was seen only with the very long obstructive-type episodes and only to a minimal degree. The minimum heart rate found was 57 per minute with the maximum tachycardia of 96 per minute. This may reflect decreased autonomic innervation to the heart. The other five neuropathy patients and the eight control patients had fewer than 15 nocturnal apneic episodes. None of the 10 patients studies complained of daytime hypersomnolence or knew of any abnormal sleep problems.

In another study,[8] four normal-weight diabetics with autonomic dysfunction and without daytime somnolence were evaluated during sleep. Two of the four had a history of mild snoring. All four patients had some form of periodic breathing during sleep. Two patients had obstructive apneas at a rate of 9 and 11 per hour associated with minimal oxygen desaturation to the upper 70% or lower 80% range. One patient had six central apneas per hour with the longest at 52 seconds and an oxygen saturation of 84%. The fourth diabetic had nonapneic hypopneas (pauses, skipped breaths) associated with reflux and decreased esophageal pH. As in other patients with autonomic dysfunction, little change in heart rate was noted with the abnormal breathing patterns.

Shy-Drager Syndrome

At least one case of Shy-Drager syndrome with irregularities in the awake and sleep respiratory pattern has been reported, with the ultimate outcome of respiratory arrest and death.[13] Briskin et al.[14] monitored three patients with Shy-Drager syndrome who presented with symptoms of obstructive sleep apnea. Two of the three also underwent overnight hemodynamic monitoring. All three patients had significant daytime hypersomnolence, and apneas were observed during sleep. One subject required nocturnal resuscitation on two occasions because of respiratory arrest. All three patients had normal hypercapnic ventilatory responses, and two had normal hypoxic ventilatory responses. The third patient's response to hypoxia was severely blunted. One patient died in his sleep before the institution of nocturnal polysomnographic and hemodynamic monitoring.

The polysomnographic evaluation showed that both patients averaged over 430 apneic episodes, over 70% of which were obstructive. The rate of the apneas was 75 and 79 per hour. The sleep staging was abnormal, showing marked decreases in stages 3 and 4 with almost total absence of REM sleep.

The hemodynamic monitoring was essentially normal during wakefulness. Neither of the patients responded appropriately to maneuvers to increase or decrease the heart rate during sleep. Heart rates only slightly cycled during the apneas between 60 and 90 beats per minute. Both showed wide swings in pulmonary artery pressures during the obstructive apneas similar to sleep apnea patients, but the expected systemic arterial pressure elevations were severely blunted.

The arterial oxygen tension fell to the mid-30 mm Hg range during apneas and oscillated between 40 and 60 mm Hg during the course of sleep.

Before tracheostomy was performed in these two patients, one died during sleep. After tracheostomy, the remaining patient's clinical status improved dramatically as far as daytime somnolence, confusion, and disorientation. On repeated testing, central apneic episodes increased and four and a half months after tracheostomy he died during sleep.

An additional four reported patients with Shy-Drager syndrome also had predominantly upper airway obstruction during sleep.[8] Three of the four had severe daytime hypersomnolence and, again, cardiac response to the apnea was blunted.

It is not surprising that patients with dysfunctioning of the autonomic nervous system would have problems in the control of breathing, i.e., sleep apnea. This is because the autonomic nervous system links peripheral receptors and central outputs for breathing control. However, in the few reported patients who have had daytime chemical control of breathing studies (ventilatory responses to hypoxia and hypercapnia), the responses are usually normal. In these individuals, sleep may produce marked alteration in the control mechanisms and arousal responses (see Chapters 2 and 4). Perhaps these patients have even greater blunting of the arousal system than the sleep apneic patients who have an intact autonomic system. As a result, heart rate and systemic blood pressure do not fluctuate greatly in this patient population. Alpha-wave electroencephalogram activity, which connotes arousal at the end of the apnea, occurs uncommonly in these patients. The role of baroreceptor stimulation or lack thereof may also be important.

It needs to be stressed that respiratory sleep disorders occur and can be extremely serious and life-threatening in patients who exhibit autonomic dysfunction. Occasionally daytime somnolence is not present, either because of a lack of severe oxygen desaturation or a minimal number of apneas (Chapter 4). These findings are independent of the patients' ages or the causes of the autonomic nervous system disease process.

Cerebral Vascular Abnormalities

The problems of nocturnal cardiorespiratory problems as sequelae of cerebral vascular events is not well documented in the literature. Information relative to sleep changes in intracranial pressure, cerebral blood flow, arterial blood gas alterations, respiratory patterns, and cardiac output would be beneficial in the management of these patients. Some clinical information does exist on post-cerebral-infarct respiratory patterns.

Cheyne-Stokes respiratory pattern is specifically defined as short pauses alternating with a longer respiratory phase where the depth and frequency of respiration increase incrementally from the pause and gradually diminish toward the end (Fig. 1). There is a diamond-shaped respiratory phase alternating with no respirations. This is seen in patients with neurologic injuries, usually where bilateral lesions exist in the basal ganglia or deep in the cerebral hemispheres.[15,16]

In patients with neurologic or cardiovascular disease, Cheyne-Stokes respiration was observed during wakefulness and during non-REM sleep.[17] During REM sleep, the pattern was essentially oblated. In certain of these patients, it was clear that sleep onset occurred only with the decrement or pause portion of the respiratory cycle, while the crescendo portion caused awakening, and the patient was irritated and manifested great annoyance from repeated sleep arousals. These patients were often given sedatives by the attending physicians for agitation.

In comparing 34 patients with Cheyne-Stokes respiration to 59 patients with hypersomnolence and sleep-linked respiratory periodicity, Schwartz and Eprinchard found several differences.[17] For the Cheyne-Stokes group, the mean age and the arterial oxygen tension were higher, while the carbon dioxide tension and hematocrit were lower than in the other group. There was additionally a much higher percentage of women in the Cheyne-Stokes group.

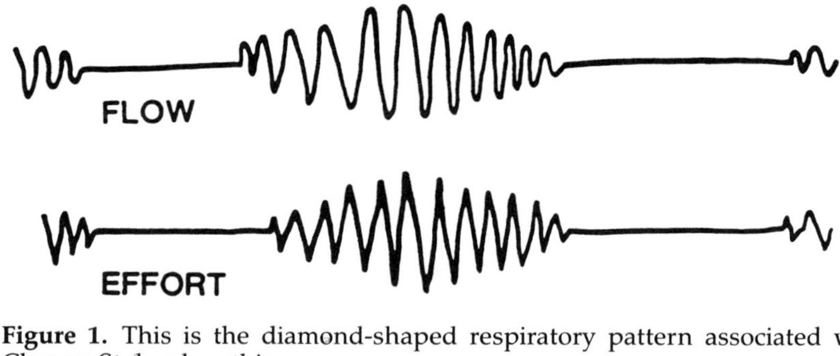

Figure 1. This is the diamond-shaped respiratory pattern associated with Cheyne-Stokes breathing.

Although apneas and hypopneas are similar to Cheyne-Stokes respiration, there are many facets that are strikingly different. Similarities include lengthening of the periodic breathing as non-REM progresses and a worsening of the respiratory pattern with weight gain or the administration of sedatives. In this author's experience, Cheyne-Stokes breathing can be greatly improved or stopped by intravenous aminophylline, while the other types of respiratory abnormalities remain unchanged. Additional differences include the opposite influence of REM sleep with a worsening of the pattern in apneic or hypopneic states, while the Cheyne-Stokes pattern is rarely seen during this sleep stage. There is a tendency toward hypocapnia with Cheyne-Stokes and hypercapnia with apneas/hypopneas. Also, during wakefulness the Cheyne-Stokes pattern can commonly be seen while apneas and hypopneas are not.

Power et al.[18] reported a case of a 63-year-old woman who complained of persistent sleep arousal for 10 years following a cerebral infarct. The infarct left her with a left-sided hemiplegia and pseudobulbar palsy. Computed axial tomography confirmed the presence of a large cerebral infarct on the right side involving the parietal, temporal, and frontal lobes. A left-sided cerebellar defect was also noted. The nocturnal respiratory pattern showed almost continuous episodes of Cheyne-Stokes respiration during light and slow-wave non-REM sleep. Combining data from two polysomnographic evaluations, Cheyne-Stokes respiration occupied 88% of light sleep (stages 1 and 2) and 83% of slow-wave sleep (stages 3 and 4). Whereas periodic breathing is usually worse during REM sleep, in this study, a regular respiratory pattern was seen over 98% of the REM period. Severe episodic oxygen desaturation was not associated with the Cheyne-Stokes breathing. The oxygen saturation did fluctuate slightly between 88% and 95% throughout sleep. The heart rate remained between 75 and 85 beats per minute with rate changes of only four beats per minute during the irregular breathing.

A disturbed sleep pattern was seen with fragmented sleep linked to the periods of Cheyne-Stokes breathing. This arousal pattern differs from other arousals related to abnormal breathing because it did not occur at the termination of the respiratory pause. The arousals occurred with either the rising or falling portion of the respiratory cycle. The majority of arousals occurred during light sleep (98%), even though the abnormal breathing pattern was equally spaced throughout non-REM sleep.

If this patient's abnormal breathing pattern occurred with the onset of her stroke (all nocturnal complaints were temporally linked to that time), then a neuroanatomic separation of the neurons that control respiration in REM and non-REM sleep is present (see Chapters 2 and 4 for full discussion). It would be interesting to evaluate patients with localized lesions to help clarify this issue. Also, in congestive heart failure where Cheyne-Stokes respiration is thought to be due to decreased circulation time and, as a result, a delayed responsiveness to hypo/hypercapnia, this breathing pattern should be seen during all sleep stages. However, this concept remains to be tested.

Acute respiratory failure and apnea have been reported with both bilateral[19] and unilateral[20] medullary infarction. In addition, typical symptoms of sleep apnea may develop rapidly or slowly progress over several months from the insult.[21] The polysomnographic study can show upper airway obstruction, central apneas, and hypopneas with severe oxygen desaturation. Tracheostomy, or nasal continuous positive airway pressure was shown to be of benefit. Additionally, over time, the measured mouth occlusion pressure reflecting neural output to the respiratory muscles improved.[22] This probably represents elimination of the severe nocturnal hypoxic insult to the brain, resulting in better integration of functioning (Chapter 4). These reports exemplify the importance of obtaining a full nocturnal evaluation and not assuming that the apneas are central because of a brain-stem abnormality.

The mechanisms involved in the production of the obstructive apnea syndrome with medullary infarction can only be postulated. It is likely that multiple factors are involved. An infarction to that area may result in weakness of the pharyngeal and palatal muscles. As discussed extensively in Chapter 4, there is loss of tone in all oropharyngeal structures during sleep, and if other contributing circumstances exist, obstructive apnea will be present. In this setting, the weakness of this muscle group potentiates sleep-related problems. The presence of palatal weakness, as seen in medullary infarcts, is an indication of involvement of the nucleus ambiguous and/or its efferent outflow. It is important to note that pharyngeal abductors may be weakened as they are also innervated by this area. Therefore, it is very reasonable to assume that upper airway obstruction, central apneas, and/or primary alveolar hypoventilation can occur after insults to the brain stem.

Spinal Cord and Brain-Stem Lesions

Surgery and Injury

Any high spinal cord surgery has the potential of adversely affecting respiration by decreasing the respiratory rate, volume, and effort during wakefulness or sleep. This potential can occur acutely and/or after a period of time.[23–29] The amount of respiratory impairment after percutaneous cervical cordotomy for pain can vary in severity depending on the extent of the spinal cord lesions. The majority of cases only demonstrated functional impairment with testing. Dysfunction is greater with a bilateral cordotomy and when high levels of analgesia are obtained. Ventilatory support is needed, particularly during sleep. At times, the respiratory pattern reverts back to normal. Surgery involving the anterior cervical spine can produce sleep-related apneas that improve over time. Postoperatively, the patients who have nocturnal apneas develop daytime confusion. If the condition is recognized, treatment can be successful, but if not, patients have been known to die in their sleep. Additionally, patients with cervical spine fractures can develop obstructive sleep apnea after injury.[30,31] These case reports exhibit the important role that afferent pathways play in the ventrolateral cervical spinal cord in regulation of respiration. Patients must be closely observed whenever damage to the pathway occurs.

Poliomyelitis

Although poliomyelitis is now rarely seen, sequelae still exist in patients who were stricken by this disease in prior years. As early as 1958, abnormalities in the central regulation of respiration were reported and the role of sleep was implicated in potentiating the respiratory abnormalities.[31] Abnormalities in respiratory control can be worsened by other factors, including weight gain or parenchymal lung disease. Therefore, any patient with a past history of poliomyelitis should be considered at risk to develop respiratory abnormalities during sleep.

Guilleminault and Motta[32] studied five patients between 1970 and 1976 for excessive daytime sleepiness who had poliomyelitis a minimum of 16 years prior to the onset of daytime sleepiness. All of the patients were male and had some bulbar musculature involvement at the time of the initial poliomyelitis bout. All were socially active and were employed in demanding professions. The daytime hypersomnolence began only one to three years prior to their being studied.

Awake pulmonary function studies showed a restricted pattern in all five subjects. The maximum voluntary ventilation was uniformly reduced. Arterial blood gases were slightly altered with minimal hypoxemia in all and hypercapnia in two.

All of the patients had three types of apneic episodes during sleep with a mean of 96 apneas per hours (range 80–109). There were 52% central apneas, 32% mixed, and 16% obstructive apneas. The longest apneas occurred during REM sleep. Large swings in oxygen saturation occurred in all patients with the lowest mean saturation of 72% during REM sleep. In one patient, systemic and pulmonary artery pressures were monitored and showed patterns of normal tension or hypertension in relation to normal breathing or apnea with hypoxia.

These poliomyelitis patients demonstrated that a centrally placed lesion can affect not only the central respiratory output (central apneas), but also the control of the upper airway mechanism (upper airway obstruction). Since the respiratory center neurons in the medulla are in close proximity to the neurons of the upper airway muscular control, a lesion in a general area could certainly affect two specific areas.

The reason for the long latent period from the acute bout of poliomyelitis to symptoms of nocturnal problems is unknown. The natural history of patients with sleep apnea in the absence of neurological disorders is also unknown but is most likely very slowly progressive. All neurologic patients with potential respiratory center abnormalities should be considered at risk for the development of sleep-related respiratory abnormalities.

These patients were treated with chest cuirass ventilators (negative pressure around the chest). As could be predicted, the upper airway obstructive episodes worsened. If the rate of the respirator was low enough, this became clinically insignificant, and the patient tended to improve. In one patient, the respirator became disconnected at night resulting in very severe apneas and hypoxemia. Whether this rapid worsening of respiratory function was due to a rapid progression of his respiratory control problems, change in carbon dioxide set point due to the ventilator, or a change in arousal patterns is not known. If this form of therapy is used, appropriate alarm systems are necessary.

Amyotrophic Lateral Sclerosis

Amyotrophic lateral sclerosis is a chronic progressive disease of the nervous system of unknown etiology. Pathologic characterization consists of motor neuron degeneration in the spinal cord with involvement of the lower brain stem and often the Betz cells in the motor cortex. Clinically, there is disturbance in motility reflecting dysfunction of both the lower and upper motor neurons.

Eleven patients with amyotrophic lateral sclerosis were studied during sleep to determine if abnormalities exist in this population.[33] There were six males and six females with an age range of 53–77 years (mean age of 56). Eight of these patients had more central apneas during the night than a control population, but this was not statistically significant. Three patients had central or obstructive apneas or a combination of the two for at least 20% of the night. The apneas occurred only during REM sleep in one patient, while in the other two, the periodic breathing occurred during both phases. Changes in oxygen saturation were not mentioned in this study.

Abnormal breathing during sleep in amyotrophic lateral sclerosis would not be surprising considering the pathology involved. Involvement of the hypoglossal nucleus is an early sign, resulting in a slurring dysarthria and weakness of tongue movement. As the disease progresses, the tongue atrophies and may lie immobile on the floor of the mouth. The palatal and pharyngeal musculature becomes weak, resulting in aphagia, nasal speech, and regurgitation of liquids. This weakness would tend to potentiate upper airway obstruction during sleep. Weakness of the respiratory muscles and possibly a decreased neural drive to respiration would then potentiate hypoventilation and/or central apneas.

This discussion of the spinal cord and brain-stem lesions could also apply to many other entities involving pathology in the same areas. It is important that detailed history of nocturnal respiratory patterns and daytime symptoms be obtained in these patients. The history should be taken not only from the patient but also from other family members or friends. If indicated, a sleep study should be done with careful follow-up of any prescribed treatments.

Muscular Dystrophies

Muscular dystrophies are inherited myopathies characterized primarily by progressive, severe weakness. An abnormality such as a missing or structurally abnormal protein, e.g., an enzyme or a structural protein, has generally not been found in the muscular dystrophies. Although pathological and biochemical abnormalities can be detected in muscle tissue, there is no clear evidence of any neural abnormality in traditional terms. Classifications of the dystrophies are based on clinical and genetic analysis, but no classification is entirely satisfactory.

The highest morbidity and mortality associated with muscular dystrophy is related to the respiratory system. Frequently, as the disease progresses, respiratory muscle weakness and daytime hypercapnia and hypoxemia develop. Initially, in the upright position, gas exchange may still be normal because of the gravitational forces on the abdominal contents and diaphragm. However, when the patient lies down, this force is lost and paradoxical respiratory movement (on inspiration, chest wall out and abdomen in, the diaphragm is moving upward) and abnormal arterial blood gases develop. On further examination, during sleep when increasing muscle hypotonia develops, hypoxemia and/or hypercapnia may also occur. This was shown to be the case in a group of muscular dystrophy patients. In those individuals whose supine blood gases were normal, the sleep oxygen and carbon dioxide tensions changed in a manner similar to normals. When abnormal blood gases were present in the supine position, a pronounced further deterioration occurred during sleep with a fall in the arterial oxygen tension below 45 mm Hg and a carbon dioxide level exceeding 70 mm Hg.[34]

As more muscular dystrophy patients are evaluated for nocturnal respiratory abnormalities, the following case reports will probably be considered typical. In a 45-year-old male with Limb-Girdle disease, Skatrud et al.[35] documented severe REM-related oxygen desaturation. This patient was diagnosed as having muscular dystrophy from the age of 36. At 43, he began to note supine and left lateral decubitus dyspnea and throbbing nocturnal headaches. His wife noted the development of progressive daytime somnolence and nocturnal apneic episodes 7 months before admission. Nocturia and dependent edema occurred two months before evaluation. Diaphragmatic excursion was not detected by percussion, and paradoxical inward movement of the abdomen occurred during inspiration in the supine, but not upright, position. The patient's pulmonary function tests showed a restrictive pattern that worsened in the supine position. He had carbon dioxide retention with a level of 52 mm Hg. Nearly complete diaphragmatic paralysis was documented using transdiaphragmatic pressures. The maximal transdiaphragmatic pressure was only 1.3 cm H_2O at total lung capacity compared with 30–40 cm H_2O in normal subjects.

The sleep study showed that there was a regular breathing pattern without apnea or periodicity during slow-wave sleep (no comment made about stages 1 or 2). Breathing frequency was decreased compared to that during wakefulness (16 versus 22 breaths/min) and qualitative measurements of rib cage and abdominal excursion were decreased. Oxygen saturation was 5% lower during sleep (90% vs. 95%) than awake. In contrast, during REM sleep, numerous repetitive episodes of oxygen desaturation were associated with further decreased rib cage and abdominal excursions. Apneas did not occur during these episodes. The mean number of desaturations per night was 49 with a mean duration of 46 ± 14 seconds and a mean desaturation of 17 ± 7%. The lowest oxygen desaturation was 55%. Bradycardia accompanied episodes of severe hypoventilation.

In this patient, the mechanism of severe sleep hypoxemia during REM sleep can be related to the inhibition of the intercostal and accessory muscles. This type of inhibition has been described in normals during REM sleep. The rib cage contribution to tidal volume during REM sleep decreased from 43% to 19%.[36] This is associated with a decrease in intercostal electromyographic activity. Thus, in patients with weakened diaphragmatic and/or accessory respiratory muscles, inhibition of these muscles to any greater degree will produce significant oxygen desaturation due to hypoventilation and probably ventilation-to-perfusion mismatching as well as shunting of blood.

These authors tried nocturnal oxygen but stated that the patient complained of worsening morning headaches. A chest cuirass (negative-pressure ventilator) improved the patient's status. There were fewer oxygen desaturation levels, and they were of shorter duration. The lowest level of desaturation was 80%.

Martin et al.[37] described the use of inspiratory muscle training to improve both the day and night respiratory patterns and oxygen levels in a patient with acid maltase deficiency. In this report, a 42-year-old male was diagnosed as having progressive muscular dystrophy at 36 years of age. Extensive studies were done because of worsening of his daytime and nighttime pulmonary symptoms. His pulmonary symptoms began 4 years prior to evaluation when he complained of increasing shortness of breath, which rapidly progressed to dyspnea upon minimal exertion. A year later, he was placed on nocturnal oxygen because of noncardiac shortness of breath during the night. Within another year, there was a history of restless sleep with snoring and fatigue in the morning. His respiratory symptoms of shortness of breath progressed until he needed to pause during spoken sentences to "gasp for air." Nocturnal dyspnea progressed even on supplemental oxygen and despite elevation of the head of his bed.

One year prior to inspiratory muscle training, polysomnographic evaluation was performed with room air. The study showed prolonged periods of hypopneic breathing resulting in significant oxygen desaturation with a nadir of 54%. During the study, 24 minutes were spent with an oxygen saturation level between 80% and 90%, and it fell below 80% for 10 minutes. In contrast to the previously discussed report, this type of pattern and desaturation occurred during all stages of sleep, but REM sleep was still the most severely involved.

Because of significant and progressive pulmonary dysfunction that worsened in the supine position with paradoxical respiration (Fig. 2a,b), inspiratory muscle training was instituted using the recently developed techniques of breathing against resistors for 15 minutes twice a day.[36] Since the patient showed diaphragmatic fatigue using a resistor of 6 cm H_2O/L/sec, he started on this resistor for 6 weeks. After that time, his endurance run improved, showing diaphragmatic fatigue occurring on a resistor of 21 cm H_2O/L/sec. This resistor was used for five weeks, after which he could perform an endurance run of 10 minutes on a 46 cm H_2O/L/sec resistor, which he continued to use at home.

Once inspiratory muscle training was implemented, progressive improvement in pulmonary function, arterial blood gases, muscle strength, and endurance tests occurred. In addition, the patient was able to sleep in the supine position and no longer required nocturnal oxygen. The repeat polysomnographic study showed marked improvement in the respiratory pattern and oxygen saturation level. Comparing this study with the original one, the time spent in non-REM sleep and REM sleep was equivalent. This similarity is important because REM sleep can produce more periodic-type breathing. There was only 8 minutes of oxygen desaturation with the lowest value of 85% during the respiratory muscle training study.

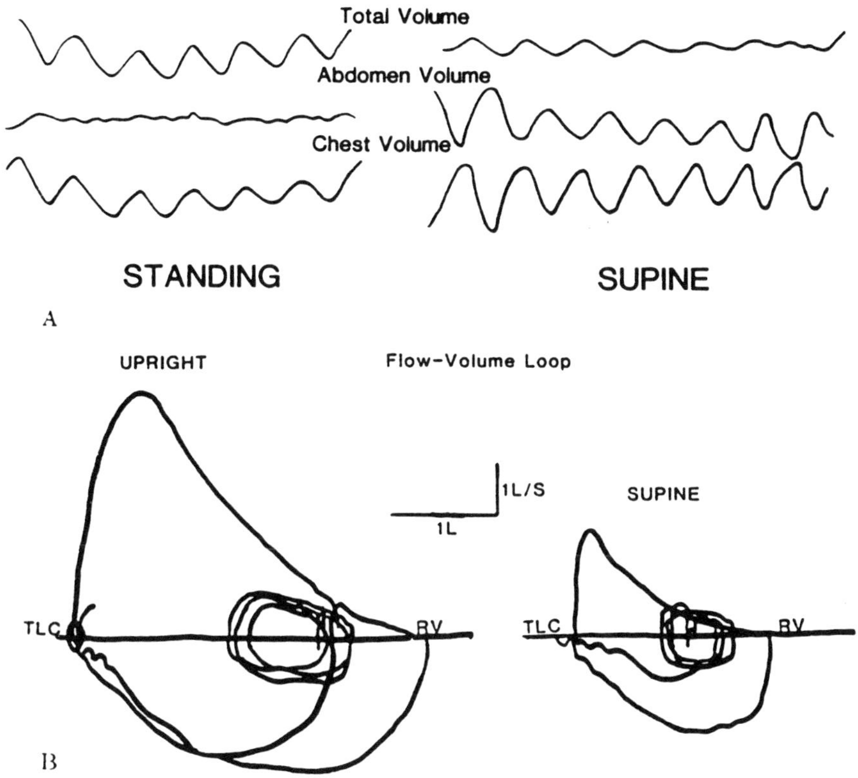

Figure 2. (a) The use of an inductance vest enables the measurement of chest wall and abdominal contributions to the total volume moved in a given breath for a patient with acid maltase deficiency muscular dystrophy. In the upright position, very little of the total volume is supplied by the abdominal component connoting the possibility of a weak diaphragm. In the supine position, without the aid of gravity, there is paradoxic breathing; that is, the chest and abdomen are moving in opposite directions during respiration, which decreases the total volume moved. (b) Flow–volume loop in upright and supine position. Worsening of flows and volumes in the supine position are noted here as a consequence of muscle weakness demonstrated in (a).

Although peripheral muscle training has been attempted in patients with muscular dystrophy without much success, this case represents the possibility of improving the respiratory muscles with endurance training. The daytime benefit was obvious as evidenced in the patient's ability to talk comfortably and to accomplish activities without shortness of breath. The marked improvement in the nocturnal pattern of respiration and oxygenation can be explained by the improvement in respiratory muscle strength and endurance. Prior to training, in the awake, supine position, he had very little muscle reserve for ventilation. This was seen in the paradoxical breathing pattern. Once he fell asleep, particularly during REM sleep, there was a further loss of muscle tone.[36] This can result in oxygen desaturation by hypoventilation, causing hypercapnia, and by producing areas of shunting because of very low tidal volumes.

Other forms of muscular dystrophy also cause nocturnal respiratory disorders with oxygen desaturation. A 22-year-old patient with Duchenne's dystrophy, which progressed to the point that the patient was wheelchair bound, was referred for postprandial dyspnea. This was secondary to eating meals too large for his pulmonary reserve and diaphragmatic weakness. With the increased intra-abdominal area secondary to the meal, the diaphragm was pushed further cephalad, thus compromising the pulmonary reserve. In reviewing his case, the hemoglobin level was noted to have increased from 14.5 g to 17 g over a 2-year period. In addition, the arterial carbon dioxide tension was elevated over the same period of time from 36 mm Hg to 43 mm Hg, with a fall in the oxygen tension from 75 mm Hg to 62 mm Hg. Both inspiratory and expiratory muscle weakness were present. Although neither the patient nor the family felt that any nocturnal respiratory abnormalities were present, the patient underwent a polysomnographic study because of the increasing hemoglobin level. It was thought that either nonapneic oxygen desaturation was occurring during sleep or that upper airway obstruction was present because of weakened oropharyngeal muscles. The sleep study showed nonapneic, hypopneic oxygen desaturation to the 40% level. This low level occurred during REM sleep, while during non-REM sleep, the desaturation was in the 55%–60% range. On 2 L of oxygen via nasal prongs, all oxygen desaturation was blocked. This patient was also instructed in progressive inspiratory muscle training.[38] After 3 months, subjective daytime symptoms of fatigue and shortness of breath subsided and nocturnal oxygen desaturation without supplemental oxygen was minimized to a low level of 81%. The awake carbon dioxide level was now 39 mm Hg. Buchsbaum et al.[39] described two muscular dystrophy patients (Duchenne's and congenital myopathy) who had daytime alveolar hypoventilation and nocturnal worsening. One patient developed cerebral edema secondarily to carbon dioxide retention, while pulmonary hypertension was evident in both of the patients. The patient with congenital myopathy (an adult) was treated with a negative-pressure ventilator. Her daytime symptoms were reversed, and there was improvement in blood gases and pulmonary hypertension. Within 18 months following this therapy, her usual daily activity could be resumed without restriction and she returned to college.

Smith et al.[40] studied 14 patients with Duchenne muscular dystrophy. Despite their lack of sleep-related symptoms and normal daytime arterial blood gas measurements, significant sleep related hypopnea and/or apnea occurred in all of the patients. These respiratory abnormalities were associated with marked oxygen desaturation. Thus, awareness of this problem can lead to prophylatic intervention and reduction in morbidity and perhaps mortality.

Myotonic Dystrophy

Myotonic muscular dystrophy is characterized by muscular wasting, myotonia, endocrine dysfunction, cataracts, psychological problems, and cardiopulmonary and gastrointestinal abnormalities. A separate section under the muscular dystrophies is being devoted to myotonic dystrophy because of the known high frequency of cardiopulmonary problems that are easily exacerbated during sleep (Table 3). As will become apparent, the respiratory dysfunction is both a central process as well as one involving the peripheral respiratory muscles.

The cardiac abnormalities[41–50] are a result of myocardial muscle involvement, which is identical to changes found in voluntary muscles.[47,48] Electrocardiographic abnormalities occur in approximately 60%–70% of these patients. Common alterations are left axis deviation, prolonged PR interval, decreased amplitude of the P waves, intraventricular conduction defects, ST segment changes, and atrial arrhythmias. Atrial fibrillation and flutter are the most common of the atrial disturbances, but the ventricular rate is usually controlled because of a high degree of atrioventricular block. Cardiac enlargement, left ventricular failure, and sudden death have been described; although this is uncommon, it can occur during sleep.

Somnolence and lethargy were first reported in patients with myotonic dystrophy by Thomasen.[51] Then in 1954, 1955, 1959, and 1964, multiple cases of alveolar hypoventilation, pulmonary hypertension, and heart failure were described.[52–55] Several of these patients were described as having daytime somnolence, cyanosis, and periodic breathing. It is important to note that the elevation in carbon

Table 3.
Myotonic Dystrophy

I. Cardiac involvement
   A. Arrhythmias, sudden death
   B. Same muscle pathology as seen in skeletal muscles
II. Central nervous system defect
   A. Abnormal response to hypoxic and hypercapnia
   B. If respond normally to hypoxia and hypercapnia, still respond abnormally to sedation, anesthesia or sleep
III. Sleep-related problems
   A. Narcolepsy-like process
      1. Responds to ritalin
   B. Apneas, hypoventilation causing significant oxygen desaturation
   C. Respiratory muscle weakness causing hypoxemia and hypercapnia
   D. Arrhythmias

dioxide tension tended to be reversible on command. In other words, the respiratory muscles were strong enough to reverse the hypercapnia and secondary hypoxemia if the patient voluntarily hyperventilated. Additionally, carbon dioxide ventilatory response curves were much more depressed than in a group of nonmyotonic muscular dystrophy patients who had more respiratory dysfunction as measured by complete pulmonary function tests.[54] These data suggest that a central respiratory abnormality does occur in this disease.

In support of the concept that there is a central depressant effect on the respiratory center in myotonic dystrophy is the high incidence of complications that occur when these patients are submitted to anesthesia. In one study of 25 myotonics, five had profound or prolonged respiratory depression during the operation and a further four died in the immediate postoperative period.[56] Gillam et al.[57] used a relatively normal pulmonary function group of myotonic patients with normal ventilatory responses to carbon dioxide and compared their response to a small dose of thiopentone to a normal control group. The myotonic group showed an exaggerated response by having a higher percent decrease in minute ventilation and more drowsiness or narcosis. This suggests that even relatively normal (as far as the respiratory system) muscular dystrophy patients have an ongoing abnormality in respiratory control that is brought out by mild insults and probably first appears clinically during sleep.

It was not until the mid-1970s that the respiratory sleep pattern was investigated in this group of patients. Coccagna et al.[58] described a 50-year-old patient who had hypersomnia since childhood with muscle involvement for only three years. The patient stated that he required an excessive amount of sleep since adolescence, and his wife confirmed that most of his free time was spent sleeping. He would also fall asleep during meals and at his job on an assembly line. There was no history of cataplexy or sleep paralysis. The patient was cyanotic and had erythrocytosis and a restrictive pattern on pulmonary function tests with blunted ventilatory responses to carbon dioxide. Arterial gas analysis during wakefulness showed marked hypoxia and hypercapnia.

The nocturnal sleep pattern was highlighted by several episodes of REM onset sleep following prolonged and numerous awakenings. During sleep the respiratory pattern became substantially more irregular then during wakefulness. Long periods occurred where breathing gradually shallowed, culminating in the onset of central apneas. The apnea lasted up to 20 seconds. During REM sleep, the shallow respiratory excursions and apneas were more prolonged and, at times, upper airway obstructions were noted.

Hemodynamic monitoring was performed on this patient. In the awake state, the systemic arterial pressure was normal (137/70 mm Hg), but the pulmonary artery pressure was greatly elevated (72/40 mm Hg, mean 51). The arterial oxygen tension was 44 mm Hg, and the carbon dioxide level was 62 mm Hg. During sleep, the systemic pressure rose slightly through non-REM sleep and to 150/79 during REM sleep (normally the blood pressure falls during non-REM sleep and is variable during REM sleep, Chapter 2). The pulmonary artery pressure also had the highest recording during REM sleep: 94/58. These values were correlated with falls in oxygen tensions (28 mm Hg) and elevation in carbon dioxide (80 mm Hg).

The patient was treated for 1 month with intermittent positive-pressure breathing. There was improvement in both the day/night systemic and pulmonary artery pressures as well as oxygen and carbon dioxide levels. The hematocrit fell from 65% to 54%. However, daytime somnolence was still present and sleep-onset REM continued. The respiratory pattern was improved, but apneas still occurred, particularly during REM sleep. Unfortunately, the patient refused any long-term follow-up.

This patient exemplifies several important points in regard to cardiorespiratory function and hypersomnia in myotonic dystrophy. The abnormalities that are present in the blood gases are related both to the primary muscle involvement and a central deficiency in respiratory control. The patient had restricted pulmonary function studies typical of respiratory muscle weakness, and the chest radiograph was normal except for elevated diaphragms. The hypoxemia and hypercapnia were out of proportion to the amount of lung restriction and worsened during sleep (hypopneic, apneic breathing), connoting a hindered respiratory center. The elevation in pulmonary artery and systemic pressures worsened or improved as the corresponding changes in blood gas tension occurred.

The origin of hypersomnia in this entity is interesting. The initial hypothesis is related to hypercapnia causing a carbon dioxide narcosis. As seen in this case, the hypersomnolence persisted as the carbon dioxide level was corrected. Another hypothesis is a primary central disturbance of sleep regulation. This helps to explain the abundance and sleep-onset of REM sleep that is seen in this case as well as in other reports. Perhaps these patients have a variation of narcolepsy. We have given a similar patient ritalin and seen improvement in her daytime somnolence.

Guilleminault et al.[59] studied six young male adult myotonic patients who had excessive daytime somnolence but minimal restrictive respiratory pattern and normal or minimal alteration in arterial blood gases. Only one patient had REM-onset sleep. In four patients, the apneic index was normal. Two had 16 and 36 apneas per hour. These latter two patients had obstructive, mixed, and central apneas with 59% and 64% being obstructive/mixed in nature. The major nocturnal hypoxemia occurred in the two patients during apneic episodes with arterial oxygen tension decreasing to 40 mm Hg from the mid-80 range. The other patients also had significant decrements in oxygen tension, presumably secondary to hypopneic type of breathing. Hemodynamic variables of systemic and pulmonary artery pressures rose as the oxygen level fell. Twenty-four-hour Holter electrocardiographic monitoring showed that arrhythmias were more prevalent during sleep but not related to any specific sleep stage.

In this interesting series of cases, there was only mild clinical involvement of muscle dysfunction, yet all had excessive daytime somnolence. In addition, only two had significant apneas during sleep that would explain this somnolence. It is intriguing that in this young, normal-weight population, one third of the patients had severe nocturnal apneas. The other four patients had decrements in oxygen tension of at least 16 mm Hg. This, again, reveals that there is a central process in myotonias that is causing abnormalities in gas exchange during sleep, while during the waking hours, they are clinically stable.

Other reports have appeared suggesting either a central process and/or a peripheral mechanism in myotonic patients who have hypersomnolence and respiratory abnormalities during sleep.[60–62] An additional awake study of mild myotonic patients stressed a mechanical factor in the pathogenesis of respiratory insufficiency.[63] Very little has been written on the treatment of such disorders. We reported on improvement in both the nocturnal respiratory pattern and daytime somnolence after therapeutic interventions.[64]

In this series,[64] three females with myotonia who complained of daytime somnolence and fatigue underwent polysomnographic evaluations before and during treatment. The age range was 14–38 years. One patient had a sister with myotonic dystrophy who had died during sleep. This individual was reported by teachers to have stopped breathing in class at school. Two patients had cardiac pacemakers because of significant daytime rhythm disturbances. Treatment with a carbonic anhydrase inhibitor, dichlorphenamide, used as a respiratory stimulant, was initiated. The sleep abnormalities are shown in Table 4.

The apneas in all three patients were central except in patient 2, who had four obstructive and two mixed apneas. Nonapneic desaturation was considered to be a fall in the oxygen saturation level as measured by ear oximetry of greater than 4% from awake, supine levels. This nonapneic oxygen desaturation was a result of hypopneic breathing. The nadir level of desaturation in these patients was 78% before treatment and 89% after treatment. In addition to the improve-

Table 4.
Sleep Abnormalities Pre- and Post-Treatment with Dichlorphenamide

	Nonapneic desaturations (N)		*Apneas (N)*		*Total sleep time with periodic breathing (min)*	
Patient	Pre-Tx	Post-Tx	Pre-Tx	Post-Tx	Pre-Tx	Post-Tx
1	140	18	5	3	55	7
2	49	25	91	15	28	5
3	128	0	14	5	36	1

ment in nocturnal respiratory sleep patterns and saturation, the daytime symptoms of somnolence, nap taking, and fatigue diminished in all three patients resulting in an overall improvement in their quality of life.

Follow-up at 1 year showed continued improvement in the symptoms of two of the three patients. We discontinued medication in one patient, and she developed the same nocturnal patterns that were seen before treatment. Treatment was reinstituted with resolution of the abnormalities once again. In another patient who later manifested return of daytime somnolence, REM-onset sleep was found to be present. Although symptoms of narcolepsy were not present, she was treated with ritalin. Improvement was seen in the somnolence. The improvement seen in the symptoms and breathing during sleep after the use of a central respiratory stimulant supports the belief that a central process is prominent in this disease. In addition, a general stimulant, such as ritalin, improved the somnolence in one patient.

Increased Intracranial Pressure

Neurologic patients with increased intracranial pressure secondary to trauma or other entities are at a risk to develop cardiopulmonary abnormalities. Certainly if the intracranial pressure is too high, mechanical ventilation is necessary to lower the carbon dioxide level in order to decrease cerebral blood flow and intracranial pressure. This section will briefly review the area of sleep and/or coma and intracranial pressure.

Since 1960, the measurement of intracranial pressure has become routine practice in neurosurgery when indicated.[65] Cooper and Hulme studied the relationship between intracranial pressure and sleep in patients with raised pressures. They found that the pressure rose during REM sleep[66] and stage 2 sleep.[67] These findings have been seen in other types of patients (normal pressure hydrocephalus and cerebral atrophy).[68–70] The significant rise in intracranial pressure has been attributed to variations in cerebral blood flow,[71] neurogenic reflex, and cerebral vasoconstriction or increased brain metabolism.[72] The pressure has been observed to rise less steeply during the transition from wake to sleep and stage 1 sleep.[73]

Munari and Calbucci evaluated intracranial pressure changes and electroencephalograms in 16 brain-injured patients (ages 8–37 years) with coma of varying intensity and in 32 patients without raised pressures or altered consciousness.[74] These authors confirmed the increase in intracranial pressure during stages 1, 2, and REM sleep as well as decrease in pressure during stages 3 and 4 sleep. They felt that there was a similarity between sleep and coma. When patients fall asleep or the coma deepens, there is a resulting rise in intracranial pressure. Conversely, at the moment of awakening from sleep or from a coma, the pressure falls.

Seizures

Seizures during sleep, as in wakefulness, produce alterations in respiration and gas exchange. Conversely, respiratory abnormalities, such as apnea during sleep, can lead to seizures secondary to severe hypoxia. Thus, suspected seizure activity during sleep needs to be fully investigated.

Wyler and Wegmuller[75] reported on a 26-year-old male who has had seizures since the age of 1 1/2 years. The seizures worsened at the age of 18 and were also associated with hallucinations and a nocturnal history of waking up choking. The patient had been treated with a variety of anticonvulsant medications. Both awake and sleep electroencelphalograms demonstrated spike epileptiform discharges from the temporal areas bilaterally. Although this article states that the patient had "central apneas" (no oxygen saturation values given), a tracheostomy was performed to relieve the apneas. The apneas subsided and his daytime sleepiness and day and night seizures diminished. This would strongly suggest that the apneas were obstructive in nature. The seizures may have improved because of diminished sleep deprivation[76] and/or by improvement in the oxygen saturation.

Other Disorders

The prevalence of abnormal cardiopulmonary patterns during sleep in neurologic entities is not established. Intermittent case reports suggest that a good sleep and respiratory history should be taken in all neurologic abnormalities. This section will briefly consider a couple of these problems.

Myasthenia gravis is a disease characterized by muscle weakness or easy muscle fatigue. It is important to note that in the respiratory system, there is a predilection to the cranial muscles, so the symptoms of difficulty in chewing, dysarthria, and dysphagia would suggest the possibility that obstructive apneas could develop during sleep. Spire et al.[77] found that two of eight myasthenia patients had 10 or more apneas per hour during sleep; however, the apneas were not characterized. We have seen one patient with mild to moderate myasthenia gravis who had daytime hypersomnolence and 10 upper airway obstructive episodes per hour during sleep with desaturation to the mid-70% range.

The Kleine-Levin syndrome is not a fully understood entity. It primarily affects adolescent males, manifesting itself with intermittent bizarre behavior, hypersexuality, and hypersomnolence. Lavie et al.[78] showed that hypopneic, central, and mixed apneic breathing occurred in these individuals during the somnolent–bizarre behavior period as well as during the nonsomnolent period. However, no mention was made of the measurements of oxygen saturation or carbon dioxide tension during the different behavioral periods.

Sleep apnea has also been associated with two rare entities, mitochondrial encephalomyopathy and olivopontocerebellar degeneration.[79,80] The olivopontocerebellar degenerative patient was treated with trazodone, which improved the paroxysmal episodes of altered state of consciousness, daytime somnolence, and sleep architecture.

Skeletal Abnormalities—Kyphoscoliosis

True kyphoscoliosis is a rare entity and most often scoliosis is the thoracic deformity that exists. The term "kyphoscoliosis" will be used here to denote either scoliosis or the combination of kyphosis and scoliosis, which cause essentially the same respiratory disorders. The pulmonary function abnormality that is seen is a restrictive pattern, i.e., reduced lung volumes. Significant ventilation-to-perfusion abnormalities are present in the awake patient, which probably accounts for the hypoxemia and increased alveolar–arterial oxygen difference.[81,82] During sleep, Mezon et al.[83] ascribed no respiratory abnormalities to severe apneas in five patients with severe kyphoscoliosis. Similar spinal deformities, abnormal pulmonary function tests, and blunted chemical drives to breathe were present in this group of patients. Two aspects separate the nocturnal pattern: males versus females with the males having apneas and the daytime clinical states. The two patients with severe daytime hypoxemia, cor pulmonale, and polycythemia demonstrated the most deranged respiration during sleep. The other three patients demonstrated fewer problem episodes during sleep and were also far less clinically symptomatic. The apneas seen were central in nature and lasted a mean duration of 64 and 19 seconds in the two patients. All patients had oxygen desaturation, with the lowest and longest episodes (apneic or nonapneic) seen during REM sleep. The low saturation values for each patient were 45, 48, 70, 73, and 87%.

In this group of patients, any degree of apneic or hypopneic breathing causes oxygen desaturation during sleep to be more severe. The restrictive lung pattern results in a decreased functional residual capacity. During sleep, particularly during REM sleep, a decrease in intercostal muscle tone could result in a further decrement in the functional residual capacity. This would diminish the limited oxygen stores and worsen ventilation-to-perfusion matching. Additionally, all patients demonstrated very blunted chemical drives to breathe, which may result in further prolongation of hypoxemic episodes during sleep instead of earlier termination and arousal. Thus, this group of patients is at a risk to develop sleep-related pulmonary hypertension, cor pulmonale, right-sided heart failure, and death.

In another study of five male patients with kyphoscoliosis, severe hypopneas and apneas of all varieties were seen in every patient.[84] Two of the patients had severe daytime somnolence, one had daytime fatigue, one had worsening cardiac failure, and another was asymptomatic during the day.

Awake oxygen saturation is a predictor of the worst nocturnal respiratory abnormalities. The three patients with the lowest awake saturation had hypopnea plus apnea index (number per hour) of 58, 63 and 68. The next worse awake saturation revealed an index of 38, and the best saturation had an index of 11 per hour. Obstructive apneas were seen in two patients. The lowest oxygen saturation levels occurred during REM sleep in all patients and ranged from 41% to 77%. It must be stressed that hypopneic episodes resulted in decreased oxygen saturation nearly as severe as that associated with the apnea. Treatment should be geared toward improving the major specific abnormality involved as described in Chapter 5.

References

1. Brunt PW, McKusick VA. Familial dysautonomia. A report of genetic and clinical studies, with a review of the literature. *Medicine* 1970; 49:343–374.

2. Lundbaek K. Recent contributions to the study of diabetic angiopathy and neuropathy. *Adv Metab Disord* 1972; 6:99–129.
3. Shy RM, Drager GA. A neurologic syndrome associated with orthostatic hypotension. *Arch Neurol* 1960; 2:511–527.
4. Frank Y, Kravath RE, Inoue K, et al. Sleep apnea and hypoventilation syndrome associated with acquired nonprogressive dysautonomia: Clinical and pathological studies in a child. *Ann Neurol* 1980; 10:18–22.
5. Bray PF, Ziter FA, Lahey ME, et al. The coincidence of neuroblastoma and acute cerebellar encephalogy. *J Pediatr* 1969; 75:983–990.
6. Moe PG, Nellhaus G. Infantile polymyoclonia-opsoclonus syndrome and neural crest tumors. *Neurology* 1970; 20:756–764.
7. Robinson MJ, Howard RN. Neuroblastoma presenting as myasthenia gravis in a child aged 3 years. *Pediatrics* 1969; 43:111–113.
8. Guilleminault C, Briskin JG, Greenfield MS, et al. The impact of autonomic nervous system dysfunction on breathing during sleep. *Sleep* 1981; 4:263–278.
9. Page MCB, Watkins PJ. Cardiorespiratory arrest in diabetic autonomic neuropathy. *Lancet* 1978; 1:14–16.
10. Garcia-Bunwel L. Cardiorespiratory arrest in diabetic autonomic neuropathy. *Lancet* 1978; 1:935–936.
11. Srinivasan G, Sanders G. Cardiorespiratory arrest in diabetes. *Lancet* 1978; 1:504–505.
12. Rees PJ, Prior JG, Cochrane GM, et al. Sleep apnoea in diabetic patients with autonomic neuropathy. *J R Soc Med* 1981; 74:192–195.
13. Lockwood AH. Shy-Drager syndrome with abnormal respirations and antidiuretic hormone release. *Arch Neurol* 1976; 33:292–295.
14. Briskin JC, Lehrman KL, Guilleminault C. Shy-Drager syndrome and sleep apnea. *In* C Guilleminault, WC Dement (eds). Sleep Apnea Syndromes. New York, Alan R. Liss, 1978, pp 317–322.
15. North J, Jewett S. Abnormal breathing patterns associated with acute brain damage. *Arch Neurol* 1974; 31:338–344.
16. Plum F, Posner JB. The Diagnosis of Stupor and Coma. Philadelphia, F.A. Davis, 1980, pp 35–36.
17. Schwartz BA, Eprinchard MJR. Cheyne-Stokes respiration and sleep: A diurnal polygraphic study. *Electroencephalogr Clin Neurophysiol* 1975; 39: 575–585.
18. Power WR, Mosko SS, Sassin JF. Sleep-stage-dependent Cheyne-Stokes respiration after cerebral infarct: A case study. *Neurology* 1982; 32:763–766.
19. Devereaux MW, Keane JR, Davis RL. Automatic respiratory failure associated with infarction of the medulla. *Arch Neurol* 1973; 29:46–52.
20. Levin BE, Maryolis G. Acute failure of autonomic respirations secondary to a unilateral brainstem infarct. *Ann Neurol* 1977; 1:583–586.
21. Askenesy JJM, Goldhammer I. Sleep apnea on a feature of bulbar stroke. *Stroke* 1988; 19:637–639.
22. Chaudhary BA, Elguindi AS, King DW. Obstructive sleep apnea after lateral medullary syndrome. *South Med J* 1982; 75:65–67.
23. Nathan PW. The descending respiratory pathway in man. *J Neurol Neurosurg Psychiatry* 1963; 26:487–499.

24. Belmusto L, Woldring S, Owens G. Localization and patterns of potentials of the respiratory pathway in the cervical spinal cord in the dog. *J Neurosurg* 1965; 22:277–283.
25. Rosomoff HL, Krieger AJ, Kuperman AS. Effects of percutaneous cervical cordotomy on pulmonary function. *J Neurosurg* 1969; 31:620–627.
26. Krieger AJ, Rosomoff HL. Sleep-induced apnea, part 1: A respiratory and autonomic dysfunction syndrome following bilateral percutaneous cervical cordotomy. *J Neurosurg* 1974; 40:168–180.
27. Krieger AJ, Standish MS, Rosomoff HL. Respiratory and autonomic dysfunction following percutaneous cervical cordotomy. *Crit Care Med* 1974; 2:91–95.
28. Krieger AJ. Sleep apnea produced by cervical cordotomy and other neurosurgical lesions in man. *In* C Guilleminault, WC Dement (eds). Sleep Apnea Syndromes. New York, Alan R. Liss, 1978, pp 273–294.
29. Krieger AJ, Rosomoff HL. Sleep-induced apnea, part 2: Respiratory failure after anterior spinal surgery. *J Neurosurg* 1974; 40:181–185.
30. Star AM, Osterman AL. Sleep apnea syndrome after spinal cord injury. *Spine* 1988; 13:116–117.
31. Plum F, Swanson AG. Abnormalities in central regulation of respiration in acute and convalescent poliomyelitis. *Arch Neurol Psychiatry* 1958; 80: 267–285.
32. Guilleminault C, Motta J. Sleep apnea syndrome as a long-term sequela of poliomyelitis. *In* C Guilleminault, WC Dement (eds). Sleep Apnea Syndromes. New York, Alan R. Liss, 1978, pp 309–315.
33. Minz M, Autret A, Laffont F, et al. A study on sleep in amyotrophic lateral sclerosis. *Biomedicine* 1979; 30:40–46.
34. Newsom Davis J, Goldman M, Loh L, et al. Diaphragm function and alveolar hypoventilation. *Q J Med* 1976; 45:87–160.
35. Skatrud J, Iber C, McHugh W. Determinants of hypoventilation during wakefulness and sleep in diaphragmatic paralysis. *Am Rev Respir Dis* 1980; 121:587–593.
36. Tussiewicz K, Moldofsky H, Bryan A, et al. Mechanics of the rib cage and diaphragm during sleep. *J Appl Physiol Respir Environ Exercise Physiol* 1977; 43:600–602.
37. Martin RJ, Sufit RL, Ringel SP, et al. Respiratory improvement by muscle training in adult-onset acid maltase deficiency. *Muscle Nerve* 1983; 6:201–203.
38. Gross D, Ladd HW, Riley EJ, et al. The effect of training on strength and endurance of the diaphragm in quadriplegia. *Am J Med* 1980; 68:27–35.
39. Buchsbaum HW, Martin WA, Turino GM, et al. Chronic alveolar hypoventilation due to muscular dystrophy. *Neurology* 1968; 18:319–327.
40. Smith PEM, Calverley PMA, Edwards RHT. Hypoxemia during sleep in Duchenne muscular dystrophy. *Am Rev Respir Dis* 1988; 137:884–888.
41. Payne CA, Greenfield JC, Jr. Electrocardiographic abnormalities associated with myotonic dystrophy. *Am Heart J* 1963; 65:436–440.
42. Caughey JE, Myrianthopoulos NC. Dystrophia Myotonica and Related Disorders. Springfield, Illinois, Thomas, 1963, p 300.
43. Miller PB. Myotonic dystrophy with electrocardiographic abnormalities: Report of case. *Am Heart J* 1962; 63:704–707.

44. DeWind LT, Jones RJ. Cardiovascular observations in dystrophia myotonica. *JAMA* 1950; 144:299–303.
45. Fisch C. Heart in dystrophia myotonica. *Am Heart J* 1951; 41:525–538.
46. Litchfield JA. A-V dissociation in dystrophia myotonica. *Br Heart J* 1953; 15:357–359.
47. Fisch C, Evans PV. Heart in dystrophia myotonica: report of autopsied case. *N Engl J Med* 1954; 251:527–529.
48. Cannon PJ. Heart and lungs in myotonic dystrophy. *Am J Med* 1962; 32:765–775.
49. Welsh JD, Lynn TN Jr, Haase GR. Cardiac findings in 73 patients with muscular dystrophy. *Arch Intern Med* 1963; 112:199–206.
50. Spurny OM, Wolf JW. Prolonged atrial flutter in myotonic dystrophy. *Am J Cardiol* 1962; 10:886–889.
51. Thomasen E. Myotonia: Thomasen's Disease (Myotonia Congenita), Paramyotonia, and Dystrophic Myotonica: A Clinical and Heredobiologic Investigation. Aarbus, Denmark, Universitets Forlaget i Aarhus, 1948, p 251.
52. Benaim S, Worster-Drought C. Dystrophia myotonica with myotonia of diaphragm causing pulmonary hypoventilation with anoxaemia and secondary polycythaemia. *Med Illus* 1954; 8:221–226.
53. Bashour F, Winchell P, Reddington J. Myotonia atrophica and cyanosis. *N Engl J Med* 1955; 252:768–770.
54. Kilburn KH, Eagan JT, Heyman A. Cardiopulmonary insufficiency associated with myotonic dystrophy. *Am J Med* 1959; 26:929–935.
55. Kohn NN, Faires JS, Rodman T. Unusual manifestations due to involvement of involuntary muscle in dystrophia myotonica. *N Engl J Med* 1964; 271:1179–1183.
56. Kaufman L. Anaesthesia in dystrophia myotonica. A review of the hazards of anesthesia. *Proc R Soc Med* 1960; 53:183–188.
57. Gillam PMS, Heaf PJD, Kaufman L, Lucas BGB. Respiration in dystrophia myotonica. *Thorax* 1964; 19:112–120.
58. Coccagna G, Mantovani M, Parchi C, et al. Alveolar hypoventilation and hypersomnia in myotonic dystrophy. *J Neurol Neurosurg Psychiatry* 1975; 38:977–984.
59. Guilleminault C, Cummiskey J, Motta J, et al. Respiratory and hemodynamic study during wakefulness and sleep in myotonic dystrophy. *Sleep* 1978; 1:19–31.
60. Hansotia P, Frens D. Hypersomnia associated with alveolar hypoventilation in myotonic dystrophy. *Neurology* 1981; 31:1336–1337.
61. Coccagna G, Martinelli P, Lugaresi E. Sleep and alveolar hypoventilation in myotonic dystrophy. *Acta Neurol Belg* 1982; 82:185–194.
62. Carroll JE, Zwillich CW, Weil JV. Ventilatory response in myotonic dystrophy. *Neurology* 1977; 27:1125–1128.
63. Begin R, Bureau MA, Lupien L, et al. Pathogenesis of respiratory insufficiency in myotonic dystrophy: The mechanical factors. *Am Rev Respir Dis* 1982; 125:312–318.
64. Armagast SJ, Ringel SP, Martin RJ. The effects of dichlorphenamide on sleep apnea in patients with myotonic dystrophy. *Clin Res* 1983; 31: 70A.

65. Lundberg N. Continuous recording and control of ventricular fluid pressure in neurosurgical practice. *Acta Psychiatr Scand* 1960; 36(149):1–153.
66. Cooper R, Hulme A. Intracranial pressure and related phenomena during sleep. *J Neurol Neurosurg Psychiatry* 1966; 29:564–570.
67. Cooper R, Hulme A. Changes of the EEG, intracranial pressure and other variables during sleep in patients with intracranial lesions. *Electroenceph Clin Neurophysiol* 1969; 27:12–22.
68. Maira G, DiRocco C, Rossi GF. Pression intraventriculaire dans l'hydrocephalie a pression 'normale' pendant la veille et le sommeil. *Neurochirurgie* 1974; 20:462–467.
69. DiRocco C, McLone D, Shimoji T, et al. Continuous intraventricular cerebrospinal fluid pressure recording in hydrocephalic children during wakefulness and sleep. *J Neurosurg* 1975; 42:683–689.
70. Munari C, Calbucci F, Versari P, et al. Pressione endocranica e variazioni del livello di vigilanza. *Riv Neurol* 1975; 45:35–44.
71. Rossi GF, Maira G, Vignati A. Intracranial pressure during sleep in man. *In* WP Koella, P Levin (eds). Second European Congress for Sleep Research, Basel, Karger, 1975, pp 169–180.
72. Rossi GF, DiRocco C, Maira G, et al. Sonno REM e pressione intracranica. *Riv Neurol* 1977; 47:570–580.
73. Munari C, Calbucci F. Pressione endocranica e sonno. *Riv Neurol* 1977; 47:591–602.
74. Munari C, Calbucci F. Correlations between intracranical pressure and EEG during coma and sleep. *Electroencephal Clin Neurophysiol* 1981; 51: 170–176.
75. Wyler AR, Wegmuller A. Epilepsy complicated by sleep apnea. *Ann Neurol* 1981; 9:403–404.
76. Bennett DR. Sleep deprivation and major motor convulsions. *Neurology* 1963; 13:953–958.
77. Spire JP, Hsu L, Holmes K, et al. Sleep patterns in myasthenia gravis. *Neurology* 1982; 32:A123.
78. Lavie P, Klein E, Gudoth N, et al. Further observations on sleep abnormalities in Kleine-Levin syndrome: Abnormal breathing pattern during sleep. *Electroencephal Clin Neurophysiol* 1981; 52:98–101.
79. Tatsumi C, Takahashi M, Yorifugi S, et al. Mitochondrial encephalomyopathy with sleep apnea. *Eur Neurol* 1988; 28:64–69.
80. Salazar-Grueso EF, Rosenberg RS, Roos RP. Sleep apnea in olivopontocerebellar degeneration: treatment with trazodone. *Ann Neurol* 1988; 23: 399–401.
81. Secker-Walker RH, Ho JE, Gill IS. Observations on regional ventilation and perfusion in kyphoscoliosis. *Am Rev Respir Dis* 1974; 110:450–457.
82. Kafer ER. Respiratory function in paralytic scoliosis. *Am Rev Respir Dis* 1974; 110:450–457.
83. Mezon BL, West P, Israels J, et al. Sleep breathing abnormalities in kyphoscoliosis. *Am Rev Respir Dis* 1980; 122:617–621.
84. Guilleminault C, Kurland G, Winkle R, et al. Severe kyphoscoliosis, breathing, and sleep. *Chest* 1981; 79:626–630.

9

Respiratory Disorders during Sleep in Pediatrics

Richard J. Martin, M.D.

Up to this point, the emphasis of this book has been on adult normal and disordered breathing. As in the adult state, infancy and childhood reveal increased frequency of abnormal breathing during sleep as more attention is focused on this disease entity. This chapter will focus on the four major pediatric respiratory sleep disturbances (Table 1): the sudden infant death syndrome, apnea of prematurity, apnea of infancy, and the sleep apnea syndrome.

Sudden Infant Death Syndrome

Although sudden infant death can be caused by arrythmias or trauma, most frequently the cause of death is unexplained, and it has thus been known as the sudden infant death syndrome (SIDS). The leading cause of death for infants between 1 month and 1 year of age in the United States is SIDS. This accounts for approximately 2 deaths per 1000 live births yearly. The time of death is usually between midnight and 6 AM.[1] The organ involvement in SIDS may be diffuse, such as mild inflammation of the upper respiratory tract and intrathoracic petechiae, but the degree of involvement is insufficient to explain death. Hypotheses explaining SIDS have focused on anatomic suffocation (due to enlarged thymus) and allergies, but these have not

Martin RJ: Cardiorespiratory Disorders During Sleep, 2nd Edition. Futura Publishing Company, Inc., Mount Kisco, NY, © 1990.

Table 1
Pediatric Sleep-Related Respiratory Disorders

Sudden infant death syndrome
No findings that by themselves explain the death
Leading cause of death between 1 month and 1 year of age
Apnea of prematurity
Affects 15% of preterm infants
Apneas are mixed, obstructive, and central
Apnea of infancy
Loosely defined syndrome
Occurs when an infant who was well exhibits episodes of apnea
Associated with multiple medical entities
Sleep apnea syndrome
Similar in symptoms and signs as the adult sleep apnea syndrome
Associated with anatomic disorders of the upper airway and neuromuscular disease

held up. More recent hypotheses have implicated abnormal respiratory and cardiac regulation. If infants die suddenly and an autopsy does not reveal the clear cause of death, then it can be hypothesized that the autonomic regulation of the cardiorespiratory system is abnormal. Generally, this is called the apnea hypothesis.

Epidemiology

A myriad of factors have been associated with SIDS before, during, and after delivery of the infant. The risk of SIDS is increased if the mother is unmarried,[2–5] poor,[3,5] and less than 20 years old.[2–4,6] During the pregnancy if the quality of prenatal care is poor,[2,4,7] if the mother has been ill,[7,8] smoked cigarettes,[6,7,9,10] or used narcotics,[11] the chances of SIDS is increased. Risk is also enhanced if the mother has had a previous fetal loss[7,12] or short intervals between pregnancies.[5,13] Interestingly, the father also plays a role in SIDS as a risk factor if he is of low social or economic level[2] or less than 20 years old.[3] In the United States, ethnicity independent of economics is important. The overall risk of SIDS is approximately 2 cases per 1000.[2] Asians have the lowest risk at 0.51 per 1000, while American Indians, Alaskan natives, and blacks have the highest rates at 5.93, 4.5, and 5.04 per 1000, respectively.[2,14,15]

Exact interpretation of this information is difficult and understanding is complicated by the lack of various controls and analyses.

Certain studies suggest that many of the above factors increase the risk of infant death due to known causes such as congenital abnormalities.[16] Other investigators have found no differences in socioeconomic factors between infants with SIDS and those who died from well-defined medical abnormalities.[17] Maternal blood types probably do not play a role in the epidemiology of SIDS. It has been thought that types B and O are at a higher risk, but strict population and ethnic controls have not been delved into.

The infant who is preterm[3,7,18–20] and at a low birth weight for gestational age[2,12] has been noted to be at increased risk of SIDS. In SIDS infants, the Apgar score is lower[7,13] and ventilatory support is required more frequently.[7] The first born has the lowest rate of SIDS compared to second or third birth orders and single-birth pregnancies are lower risks than multiple,[12,13,21] with triplets at the greatest risk. The smaller twin does not carry an increased risk,[21] but the second born does.[22] Several twin pairs, both monozygous and dizygous, have died on the same day.[12,21] This important observation suggests that an environmental process interplays with an abnormal physiologic makeup in these infants.

These infants tend to die during sleep, usually at night, and are in any sleeping position.[3,21] SIDS is the leading cause of death between 1 month and 1 year, with the peak of occurrences at 1–4 months.[6,21,23] Apparently the incidence is higher in the winter months, possibly due to upper respiratory infections.

Prior to the sudden death, infants are relatively asymptomatic, but this statement is variable from study to study. The stated symptom-free population ranges from 25% to 75%. There may be a tendency toward mild respiratory or gastrointestinal symptoms for several days before the event.[3,18,21] Occasionally the infants require hospitalization any time from birth until the SIDS occurrence.[3,8,21] Although neonatal problems are not common, an increased incidence of feeding difficulties during infancy has been noted.[7,13] Parents have described the infants as being less active and responsive, and they have an unusual cry compared to their siblings.[7,24,25]

Even though the risk of SIDS is increased in twins, as mentioned previously, and despite the fact that this entity has occurred three to four times in some families, overall, there is no evidence of genetic transmission, based on large studies. More than likely, environmental factors during pregnancy or postnatal life influence a predisposed group of infants. This observation is supported by twins who have died or had near-miss events within hours of each other.[23,26]

The parents of affected infants have either normal chemical control of breathing[27] or a decreased responsiveness.[28] In particular, parents of SIDS victims had a decreased response to inspiratory loading during carbon dioxide breathing, while controls had increased responses.[28] In infants who were near-miss (later some died[29]), ventilatory response to carbon dioxide was blunted.[30] However, the parents of these infants had normal ventilatory reponse to both hypoxia and hypercapnia.[31] There is a possibility that near-miss infants and their siblings have more periodic breathing during sleep.[32]

Infection

As mentioned previously, there is an increase in the incidence of SIDS during the winter months. At this time, upper respiratory infection is found to be the greatest reason for this and apparently potentiates SIDS. All types of viruses have been found, and none is particularly prevalent.[33,34] Mild respiratory infection is found in between 40% and 75% of the deaths.[35] A virus, respiratory syncytial virus,[36] has been associated with apnea in the young infants (see below). An interesting association with SIDS is that of amnionitis in preterm births.[37] This would suggest the possibility that intrauterine septicemia, which can cause hypoxia and ischemia, could alter the autoregulatory control of the cardiorespiratory system and potentiate mild insults to the system.

Other Possible Associated Factors

In an excellent review on SIDS, Shannon and Kelly[38] discuss a multiplicity of other factors that may or may not have some relationship to SIDS. These include liver and thyroid function, vitamins, electrolytes, anions, cations, and other body homeostatic mechanisms. Smoking and methadone addiction in the mother is strongly related to SIDS.

Pathology

Since the current definition of SIDS includes the absence of a pathologic explanation, only mild pattern changes can be pieced together. If the apnea hypothesis is correct, hypoxic changes should be noted in the two areas with highest oxygen requirements, the heart and brain stem. Although there is some evidence for hypoxic changes, cause and effect cannot be proved.

Cardiorespiratory changes are difficult to quantify as data found in one study are not consistent with that found in another or are not markedly different from controls.[38] A possible significant factor is that the pulmonary arteries in SIDS infants are not only thicker,[39] but extend farther into the lung periphery[40] than in infants who die from accidents. This raises the possibility of severe long-term hypoxia. Brain-stem gliosis, which is related to hypoxia, has been demonstrated in SIDS.[41,42] In fact, the incidence of pulmonary artery hyperplasia correlates with the astrogliosis in the brain stem.[43] The intrathoracic petechiae seen in these infants at autopsy is also indicative of hypoxia,[44] but about 30%–35% of these infants do not show these changes, indicating evidence for multiple etiologies of SIDS.

If the apnea theory is correct, then either the upper airway (obstructive apnea) or the brain stem (central and obstructive apnea) is the potential site. No specific lesion has been noted in the central nervous system to account for the possible apnea, but this is also true in adults with apneas. The upper airway in these infants has shown focal necrosis of the vocal cords,[45] but this finding is no more frequent than for acute in-hospital deaths from recognizable causes.[46] There may be more laryngeal mucous glands in the vestibular folds in SIDS,[47] which may lead to potential obstruction if inflamed.

If hypoxia as a possible result of apnea is the major abnormality in SIDS, then cardiac arrhythmias would be the terminal event. This would be particularly true if there was a conduction defect in cardiovascular control.[48] The heart rate during sleep is higher during both REM and non-REM sleep in near-SIDS infants[32] and their siblings[49] than in normal controls. The cardiovascular response to hypoxia and/or hypercapnia needs to be investigated in near-SIDS or siblings of SIDS infants.

Control of Ventilation

The control of ventilation in normals has been discussed in Chapters 2 and 3 and in sleep apnea patients in Chapter 4. This has been discussed mainly with reference to adults. A review of the important points will be presented here with an additional view of the pediatric population.

Basically, during light sleep there tends to be periodic-type breathing and occasional short apneic episodes. This type of ventilatory change is probably related to the change of state from wakefulness to sleep. As a person becomes drowsy and goes into stage 1 or 2 sleep, the arterial carbon dioxide tension set point for ventilation shifts. That is, as the normal ventilatory response during wakefulness starts to diminish at sleep onset, the alveolar ventilation decreases and there is a slight rise in the arterial carbon dioxide tension with a decrease in the arterial oxygen tension. At this point an arousal, but not necessarily an awakening, may occur, which will then increase the ventilatory drive and decrease the carbon dioxide level. The arousal is then blunted and slightly deeper sleep ensues. This cycle can be repeated, causing the periodic-type breathing that is seen in the lighter stages of sleep. Perhaps this is a more common phenomenon in older adult subjects because it takes them longer to establish sleep and to stabilize breathing. During slow-wave sleep, breathing is typically regular with rare apneas. During REM sleep, ventilatory responses to chemical stimuli are markedly decreased (see below). The decreased responsiveness to chemical and other stimuli during REM sleep probably causes the irregular, although not the periodic, pattern of breathing as well as the more frequent and longer apneas.

There is a slight but significant rise in arterial carbon dioxide (or alveolar carbon dioxide) tension during sleep in the normal population.[50–53] This increase in carbon dioxide may be due to either of two mechanisms: (1) an increase in CO_2 production or (2) a decrease in alveolar ventilation. Sleep is usually accompanied by a decrease rather than an increase in CO_2 production.[51] Thus, the mild hypercapnia of sleep is secondary to a primary alveolar hypoventilation. This is true if the alveolar ventilation is not impaired by increased mechanical impedance to breathing, even in the face of augmented respiratory drives.[54] The possibility of increased airway resistance or decreased pulmonary compliance during sleep in normal man was considered (although only in three subjects) by Robin et al.[51] There was an absence of mechanical changes in pulmonary mechanics, which supports the concept of decreased ventilatory drives and alveolar hypoventilation. A small but significant decrease in the arterial pH of 0.03–0.05 units[51–53] is associated with the hypoventilation. Hudgel et al. also showed that lung compliance and resistance do not change in normal man, but resistance in the upper airway was increased during sleep.[55]

To this point, the discussion of sleep-induced alveolar hypoventilation has been related to non-REM sleep. The measurement of alveolar ventilation during REM sleep is difficult because of the nonsteady state of ventilation. That is, tidal volume and rate vary considerably within a REM period. Thus, different conclusions, from hypoventilation to no change to hyperventilation during this sleep stage, have been reached by various investigators.

Chemical Control of Breathing

The exact relationship between the chemical control of breathing during sleep, i.e., hypercapnic and hypoxic ventilatory responses, to these irregular respiratory changes is unknown. Controversy exists about the exact control of breathing responses themselves.

In the awake state, breathing is controlled by two systems that are physically separate but function as an integrated process.[56,57] The systems are the behavioral (voluntary) control system and the metabolic (chemical) control system. The behavioral system arises in the cortical and forebrain areas. It is mainly involved in processes that use the respiratory system for nonventilatory purposes, e.g., phonation. However, this system can override the metabolic system. The metabolic system is involved in acid–base and oxygen control. The location of this control system is in the brain stem (pons and medulla) and the carotid bodies. The study of ventilatory control during sleep has mainly focused on the chemical control of breathing because it is assumed that the behavioral system is not active. This assumption may be incorrect, however.

The early reports[58–61] of ventilatory responses to hypercapnia during sleep concluded that there was a blunting of chemosensitivity during sleep. However, these studies suffer from a lack of sleep staging (probably all were non-REM studies) and failure to provide supplemental oxygen during the testing. Without the addition of oxygen to the testing system, a distinction cannot be made between a hypercapnic response and a hypercapnic–hypoxic interaction. Subsequent investigations,[62,63] using a steady-state hypercapnic response with supplemental oxygen in non-REM sleep, showed little decrease in the slope of the ventilatory response to hypercapnia. There was, rather, more of a parallel shift of the slope so that a higher carbon dioxide level was needed to elicit the same ventilatory response. Using this steady-state technique, many subjects aroused from sleep and were excluded from the study. In an extensive study, Bulow[64] found, while using a rebreathing technique, that the mean slope of change in ventilation to the change in the alveolar carbon dioxide response line decreased progressively from 1.25 L/min/mm Hg during wakefulness to 0.5 L/min/mm Hg in slow-wave sleep. He reported only one carbon dioxide response test in a subject during REM sleep which was similar to stage 1.

Phillipson et al.,[65] using a dog model, studied the effect of hypercapnia in all sleep stages. During REM sleep, the hypercapnic ventilatory response was markedly decreased in comparison to the non-REM stages. In addition, the length of the carbon dioxide rebreathing was longer and the level of alveolar carbon dioxide reached was higher during REM sleep, due to lack of arousal. The highly irregular REM breathing pattern persisted. This suggests that the progressive hypercapnia had little influence on the ventilatory control system during REM sleep, and apparently there is a change in the central respiratory control aspect of breathing during this sleep stage. Anatomically, the structure of the pontine reticular formation that is involved in REM sleep[66] is situated close to the pontine pneumotoxic center,[67] which could lead to a change in the initiating process. Another possibility that explains the irregularities of respiration is fluctuating supraspinal inhibitory and excitatory stimuli that act on the phrenic neurons of the cervical cord rather than acting centrally. It is known that other spinal motoneurons are influenced by these inhibitory–excitatory impulses that occur during REM sleep.[68]

In 12 adult human subjects (six male, six female—no difference between male and female response), the awake ventilatory response to progressive hypercapnia was 1.60 L/min/mm Hg $\pm$ 0.19 SE.[69] This response was measured at 0.69 $\pm$ 0.08 during stage 2, at 0.81 $\pm$ 0.10 during slow-wave sleep, and at 0.45 $\pm$ 0.1 during REM stages. The relationship of the hypercapnia to the irregular REM breathing patterns was not investigated. As evidenced in this study, there is marked blunting of the ventilatory response to hypercapnia during sleep. The ventilatory response to carbon dioxide measured in infants is reduced during active sleep, but the difference is not statistically significant.[70]

The ventilatory response during sleep to hypoxia has not been studied as much as the hypercapnic response. Until recently the most complete study was in dogs.[71] There was no difference in the ventilatory response from awake to all sleep stages, although the arousal response from REM sleep developed at a lower arterial oxygen saturation as compared to non-REM sleep (70.5 $\pm$ 3.4% vs. 87.5 $\pm$ 2.6%, respectively). These investigators feel that the maintenance of an intact hypoxic ventilatory response may be of importance in maintaining adequate ventilation during this stage of sleep. However, Douglas et al.[72] showed that the hypoxic drive in human subjects falls progressively and significantly from the awake state (1.07 L/min/% Δ sat ± 0.19 SE) to stage 2 (0.64 ± 0.1) to slow-wave sleep (0.62 ± 0.09) to REM sleep (0.33 ± 0.04). The different findings in the two studies appear to be species-related and obviously changes conclusions about ventilatory responses during REM and non-REM sleep in humans.

Control of Upper Airway Respiratory Muscles

The importance of the function of the musculature at the level of the larynx, pharynx, and nares is becoming more evident as all types of respiratory disorders, in particular, respiratory sleep disorders, are being more thoroughly investigated. The evolutionary development of the upper airway is complex and includes the interaction of functions such as phonation and protection of the lower airway from food and other contaminants, as well as the passage of air in and out of the lungs.[72–74] The coordination of the different functions by the upper airway muscles is complex and is controlled by interacting neural mechanisms.[75]

Early studies in animals showed that the upper airway muscles and cranial nerves act in a manner similar to the diaphragm and phrenic nerve to certain stimuli. That is, both muscle–nerve interactions increased activity to hypercapnia and responded to pulmonary stretch receptor stimulation.[76–80] Through similar activity, the upper airway muscle could stabilize the oropharyngeal structures so as to maintain airway patency during inspiration. However, there are differences that occur between the upper and lower airway (diaphragm and chest wall) muscles of respiration relative to the timing and strength of response in order to maintain upper airway patency. During inspiration, recurrent laryngeal nerve inhibiton by input from the pulmonary stretch receptors occurs earlier than phrenic nerve inhibition.[81] Furthermore, phasic electromyographic activity in the upper airway muscles begins prior to the onset of phrenic nerve activity and inspiratory airflow.[79–81] Additionally, upper airway muscle activity compared to diaphragmatic activity is preferentially stimulated by reflexes from the baroreceptors and chemoreceptors.[82–84]

The initiation of respiration occurs in the medulla, and at this level there are specific neural pools for specific respiratory muscles.[85] It appears that there is interaction between these specific areas from the medulla to the bulbar and spinal motor neurons.[86] However, until more is known about the sequence of neuromuscular activation between the upper and lower airway muscles, a precise understanding of nocturnal respiratory activity, such as sleep apnea, will not be fully investigated.

In 1978, Remmers et al.[87] accurately described the pathophysiology involved in an upper airway obstruction. In 10 patients with sleep-related upper airway obstruction, they demonstrated that the obstruction arises from oropharyngeal occlusion. This was documented by measuring the pressures generated in the posterior pharynx at the tip of the epiglottis and in the esophagus. During an upper airway obstruction, the entire alveolar-to-atmospheric pressure drop occurred in the oropharynx. Thus, the larynx and lower airways were not the primary areas of obstruction. This is also supported by nasopharyngeal intubation, which helps to alleviate the apneas to some degree. This physiologic study was in agreement with the initial clinical views of Gastaut et al.,[88] who postulated a lax tongue and mouth floor as the pathogenesis of the upper airway obstruction. There is radiographic support for the tongue and posterior pharyngeal muscle hypotonia as the anatomic process involved. This has been shown by several investigators.[89–91]

The tongue exhibits rhythmic, inspiratory activity in the upright position in man.[92] That is, the genioglossus is a muscle involved in respiration. In the supine position this muscle displays a tonic expiratory component to overcome the effects of gravity, producing occlusion. In normal sleeping individuals, the genioglossus continues to exhibit rhythmic respiratory activity during non-REM sleep. However, during REM sleep the activity declines to low levels.[93]

Considering this, Remmers and colleagues[87] were unable to find a unique relationship between the presence or absence of occlusion and genioglossal activity. However, the relationship between the peak pharyngeal pressure and peak genioglossal electromyogram activity is more important as far as the onset and cessation of an upper airway obstruction. These two variables together are sufficient in determining pharyngeal airway patency, but neither alone correlates with upper airway obstruction or ventilation. Thus, it appears that the oropharynx occludes whenever the constricting action of the transpharyngeal pressure exceeds the dilating action of the genioglossal muscle. Breath-to-breath analysis prior to the occlusion, during the occlusion, and at the resumption of ventilation can be made. Typically, the genioglossus activity precedes the pharyngeal pressure. When plotted against each other, there is a wide, flat, counterclockwise loop associated with each breath. This loop becomes narrower and more upright at the approach of the apnea because of a waning of genioglossal activity and a rise in pharyngeal pressure. As the occlusion occurs, the loops of the initial occluded efforts project more vertically than preapnea breaths, and those of subsequent respiratory attempts are progressively taller. During occlusion there are increased attempts at respiration because of changes in chemical stimulus (hypoxia and hypercapnia). This produces marked increases in the negative pleural pressure exerted, which is then reflected in the pharyngeal pressure. Therefore, the net balance of genioglossal and inspiratory muscle activity is progressively in favor of pharyngeal occlusion. There is an abrupt release of the upper airway obstruction that occurs when there is preferential activation of the genioglossus so as to develop a patent airway. There is usually an arousal or awakening associated with the termination of the apnea, which aids in the activation of the genioglossus. The exact stimulus for the arousal is unknown but may be associated with the chemical changes.

Other upper airway muscles, in addition to the genioglossus muscle, are affected in the sleep apnea syndrome. Kurtz et al.,[94] using percutaneous needle electrode inserted into the cricothyroid and chin muscles, studied seven adult patients with upper airway obstruction. In this manner, precise individual muscle recordings could be made in both the awake and sleeping states.

During wakefulness, tonic activity with phasic inspiratory reinforcements was recorded in the cricothyroid muscle. This phasic reinforcement started 200–300 msec before the onset of inspiration (lower airway) and decreased 200–300 msec before the following expiration. In sleeping patients, there were both hypopneic respiration events (decreased flow and effort) and upper airway obstruction episodes. At first there was a gradual decrease in the tonic activity associated with the hypopneas with persistence of the phasic activity. In time, the phasic activity also decreased or subsided until normal respiration resumed. During an upper airway obstruction, both the tonic and phasic activities of the cricothyroid muscle ceased. The resumption of respiration was marked by the reappearance of the phasic inspiration activity for two to three cycles and then the tonic activity returned. During disordered breathing, the chin muscles developed essentially the same patterns as the cricothyroid muscle.

However, in certain cases the phasic inspiratory activity of the chin muscles reappeared only after a prolonged period of wakefulness.

This study showed that the inhibition of the phasic inspiratory activity of the cricothyroid, despite the persistent activity of the diaphragm, reflects an impairment of the respiratory function of the laryngeal muscles. Thus it appears that many, if not all, of the upper airway muscles lose their neuro-input to stay patent in patients with upper airway obstruction. Even the facial muscles, such as the chin, are involved in this process.

Brouilette and Thach[95] studied this mechanism in rabbits to gain further knowledge of the role of the oropharyngeal muscles in maintaining extrathoracic airway patency. They found that it was easy to collapse the extrathoracic airway postmortem, but under light anesthesia, patency remained at pressures up to -80 cm H_2O. This finding suggests that a neuromuscular mechanism plays a prominent role in airway patency. Four findings arose from this study indicating that the genioglossus and geniohyoid muscles need to be active in order to pull the tongue and hyoid bone anteriorly for the prevention of occlusion. First, simple anterior movement of the hyoid bone increases the negative pressure at which the extrathoracic airway collapse occurs postmortem. This is not surprising as anesthesiologists always maintain the airway after anesthesia by pulling the patient's chin to a more anterior position. Second, after the 12th cranial nerve was severed, thereby abolishing electromyographic activity, airway closure occurred immediately with artificially occluded inspirations under anesthesia. Third, deep anesthesia depressed the muscular activity, resulting in closure of the airway with less negative pressure. Fourth, the closing pressure was linearly related to the peak integrated electromyogram of the two muscles. It was also noted that the closing pressure became more negative with progresssive asphyxia, suggesting that other muscles were recruited to help maintain that extrathoracic airway patency. Thus, for patients with upper airway obstruction, the functioning of the extrathoracic muscles relative to the intrathoracic group is of considerable importance.

In rabbits, Brouillette and Thach[96] described the relationship between the genioglossal and diaphragmatic electromyogram in normal breathing and with various stimuli. During normal respiration, the integrated genioglossal electromyogram peaked earlier in inspiration than the diaphragm. Although hypercapnia resulted in an increase in both electromyograms, the genioglossal activity reflected a greater percentage increase. Hypoxia stimulated, while hyperoxia depressed, the genioglossal activity more so than diaphragmatic activity. Varying levels of oxygenation probably relate to the peripheral chemoreceptors resulting in this muscular action.[97] It is of interest that tactile, auditory, and visual stimulation also preferentially stimulate the genioglossus.[96] Thus, in sleep apnea, the chemical and arousal stimuli appear to shift the balance of pressure forces to a portion favoring opening of the extrathoracic airway at the terminal portion of the upper airway obstruction.

The finding of decreased inspiratory motor output that occurs preapnea and then returns upon arousal at the termination of the apnea has not been fully explained. One possibility implicates the periodicity of the chemical stimuli to breathing. Many investigators feel that as the upper airway obstruction is developing, the arterial oxygen saturation rises rapidly. The saturation then falls during the apnea, and this is the signal for arousal and the breaking of the occlusion.[88,90,99,100] Onal et al. have shown that in normal awake subjects, both hypoxia and hypercapnia produce increased genioglossal and diaphragmatic muscle activity.[101,102] Another possibility is that the upper airway obstruction represents a central process with decreased input to the upper airway muscles and that the severe hypoxia that develops during sleep potentiates the problem.

Although it appears that the oscillations in saturation are of primary importance in the formation and cessation of the upper airway obstruction, the picture is not that simple. Martin et al.[103] showed that both acute and chronic hyperoxia, when compared to room air breathing, resulted in a significant decrease in the total number of apneic episodes as well as the percent apnea time (duration of apneas divided by sleep time). The length of the apneas on oxygen was slightly longer, but the total number was significantly decreased. In the eight patients studied, the response was generally positive. There was a subset who dramatically improved and another subset who remained the same or worsened. When improvement was seen, it was reflected in an improvement of the symptoms of somnolence, fatigue, and general well-being.

Two other studies support the finding that oxygenation improves the ventilatory pattern during sleep. In a man who had primary alveolar hypoventilation and central sleep apneas but no responsiveness to exogenous respiratory stimulants, low-flow nocturnal oxygen improved the sleep pattern.[104] There was a marked decrease in the number and duration of apneas and an increase in the level of ventilation, which was sustained for the 5-month follow-up period. In another study of five posttracheostomy sleep apnea patients, a dramatic decrease in the overall apnea index was seen (tracheostomy tube plugged for repeat studies).[105] Before surgery, the lowest oxygen saturation ranged between 29% and 68%, while 5 weeks posttracheostomy the lowest saturation was 86%–89%. Of interest, the ventilatory response to carbon dioxide improved in all cases following surgery. These findings, again, suggest that hypoxic brain-stem depression develops with the sleep apnea syndromes and improvement occurs when proper oxygenation is maintained.

Perhaps the respiratory muscles (upper airway and chest wall) in the pediatric population play a more involved role in the maintenance of rhythmic breathing than in adults because of the very compliant chest wall in the young. The inspiratory activity of the upper airway and chest wall muscles responds to hypercapnia and mild hypoxia.[102,106] Inspiration is facilitated by changes in airway resistance, which decreases immediately before inspiration and reaches its peak at the end of expiration[107] (shown in cats). Other interesting changes occur during expiration that actually promote narrowing of the glottic opening. These changes are the activation of thyroarytenoid, cricothyroid, and lateral cricoarytenoid muscles. Narrowing of the airway toward the end of expiration can prove to be very beneficial in infants who have very compliant chest walls. By narrowing the airway, lung volume can be maintained and oxygenation is promoted. If this mechanism of "internal positive end-expiratory pressure" is not properly functioning, a decrease in functional residual capacity, atelectasis, and hypoxemia will ensue. Thus, inspiration is facilitated by a decreased airflow resistance immediately before diaphragmatic contraction, then volume stabilization occurs during expiration by a narrowing of the upper airway muscles.

The infant is particularly vulnerable to any change that can affect ventilation. This is because the smaller the hypopharynx, the more cephalad the placement of the tongue and epiglottis,[108] resulting in a relatively unstable chest wall. This may account for the fall in functional residual capacity and oxygen tension during REM sleep in the newborn.[109] Functional residual capacity is lower in the infant than in the child or adult. Also, during apnea it falls more rapidly.[110] This rapid decrease in functional residual capacity could result from either a decrease or lack of glottic closure during expiration, an even greater chest wall compliance, or a smaller airway resistance.[107] If there is a further compromise in the respiratory system or an abnormal system to start with, then prolonged apnea possibly leading to SIDS could easily develop.

SIDS and the Apnea Hypothesis

It is difficult to make conclusive statements about an entity that has not been well delineated. What has been described, however, are episodes of apnea, periodic breathing, and abnormal ventilatory and arousal responses to hypoxia and hypercapnia in some infants who later succumb to sudden death.[111–117] These findings indicate not only a deficit in the chemical control of breathing but, more importantly, an abnormality in the arousal mechanisms.

Arousal is a complex issue that probably plays a major role in the development of sleep-related events such as SIDS. For example, both hypoxia and hypercapnia stimulate the reticular activating system and produce arousal.[119,120] However, in abnormalities of respiration and apneas that lead to significant hypoxia and hypercapnia, the reason for the failure to rapidly arouse needs to be investigated. Fink[121] demonstrated that after a period of significant hyperventilation in the awake state, subjects did not lose the normal rhythmicity of breathing, but during sleep or anesthesia, this rhythmicity following hyperventilation is absent. Sullivan et al.[122] found that in dogs laryngeal stimulation could produce apnea during sleep without any demonstration of the cough reflex. It is interesting that during wakefulness, coughing was always present, but apneas could not be induced. These two studies demonstrate that the awake state is a potent stimulus to breathing. Thus, with arousal or awakening, an appropriate overall response to respiratory stimuli does occur.

It is important that either a change in the sleep stage or total awakening occur if a respiratory problem is to be overcome. If an event such as an upper airway obstruction occurs, it would not be feasible just to exert more respiratory effort to overcome the obstruction as this would actually potentiate the problem. Upon arousal or awakening, the obstructing factors could be alleviated. The arousal response should be regarded as a separate reflex and not simply an action that is similar to the ventilatory response. In other words, patients with abnormal ventilatory drives may awaken properly if abnormal nocturnal events occur. Alternatively, it was shown that hypoxia causes a similar ventilatory response whether awake or during REM or non-REM sleep, but there is a sharp difference in the ability of hypoxia to produce arousal between those sleep stages.[71] In non-REM sleep, hypoxia rapidly led to arousal at a mean saturation of 87.5 ± 2.6% (SE), whereas it took severe hypoxia (70.5 ± 3.4%) to produce arousal during REM sleep. Perhaps this is the reason why sleep apnea patients have longer apneas with more severe desaturation during REM sleep. To lend further credence to the theory that ventilatory control and arousal are not linked, it has been shown that the hypercapnic ventilatory response is progressively diminished during sleep, but the arousal response is sustained.[65]

Asthma is another process in which arousal from sleep plays a very important role. Some asthmatic patients have severe nocturnal bronchospasm from which they only awaken by the time severe distress has developed and then quickly deteriorate to cardiopulmonary arrest. In one study,[123] two adolescent males with nocturnal arrests were studied for the arousal response during a stable period in their disease and were compared to three healthy males plus the identical twin of one of the patients who had asthma without the nocturnal arrests. The subjects wore a tight-fitting face mask to which a pneumotachograph and an occlusion device were attached. The external airway was occluded at end-expiration and released when alpha waves (indicating wakefulness) appeared on the electroencephalogram. Although there was individual variability in the response of each of the patients and control subjects, the two patients had lengthened arousal time of greater than 20 seconds in various sleep stages, while none of the normal subjects had prolonged arousal responses.

In infants and children, a positive hypoxic feedback system (i.e., hypoxia promoting further depression of ventilation) has been described in sleeping preterm infants[124] and in newborn lambs with carotid body denervation and congenital central hypoventilation.[125] Instead of the proper response of arousal and/or increased ventilation, a worsening in the physiologic response occurred. In one patient who had primary alveolar hypoventilation, breathing a hypoxic gas mixture produced acute cor pulmonale and decreased cardiac output.[125] During sleep, kittens raised in a 10% oxygen environment develop bradycardia, hypoventilation, and sudden death without arousal.[126] In general, the exact relationship of arousal, or the lack of it, to SIDS and other nocturnal cardiopulmonary disorders needs to be developed to better understand these problems.

The apnea itself can result from a total cessation of central output to the respiratory muscles, upper airway obstruction, or a combination of both preceding types. Severe hypoventilation may also be involved, producing hypercapnia and resultant hypoxemia. As stated previously, in near-SIDS (and in those who eventually died), the stimuli of hypoxia[127,128] and hypercapnia[29,129] can be abnormal. Reports have indicated that there are abnormalities in the control of the upper airway skeletal muscles, resulting in obstruction of the airway.[115,117] Similar results have been demonstrated in rabbits with denervated airways.[95] The abnormal cry that has been attributed to some SIDS infants may be due to the poor control of the upper airway musculature.[19,24,25]

As mentioned previously, mild upper respiratory infections have been associated with SIDS. Normal infants 1–3 months of age with nasopharyngitis have more apneic type breathing during non-REM sleep than when they are healthy, but fewer during REM sleep.[130] Additionally, normal infants do not always respond favorably to artificial nasal occlusion. Approximately 45% of 6-week-old infants did not breathe through their mouths with nasal occlusion of 25 seconds' duration.[131] This phenomenen was more evident during REM sleep. In near-SIDS infants, more frequent and prolonged apneas occur with nasopharyngitis than during a healthy state.[132]

Obstructive sleep apnea commonly occurs in non-SIDS infants with adenoid hypertrophy,[133] myelomeningocele,[134] Down syndrome,[135] and tracheal compression via an aberrant innominate artery.[136] This illustrates the relative ease involved in initiating periodic breathing during sleep in the young. It is interesting to note that months to years after nocturnal adenoidal obstruction was relieved, the chemoreceptor regulation was found to be blunted.[137]

Reflex apnea is a normal protective response to potentially noxious stimuli. There is a possibility that an excessive response is present in SIDS. Gastroesophageal reflux with resultant aspiration may play a role in potentiating the apneic reflex.[138] Another possibility is a vagal reflex set off by gastric contents in the esophagus only producing laryngeal spasm. Apnea is also known to follow the aortic baroreceptor reflex[139] and the Bezold-Jarisch (right atrial stretching) reflex.[140]

SIDS Pathophysiologic Hypothesis (Table 2)

Shannon and Kelly[38] summarized the available pathologic and physiologic studies to suggest the following hypothesis. Certain infants are born without the proper control mechanics of the respiratory muscles, which include the muscles of the upper airway. When a mechanical stimulus, such as a mild upper respiratory infection, or a

Table 2
SIDS Pathophysiologic Hypothesis

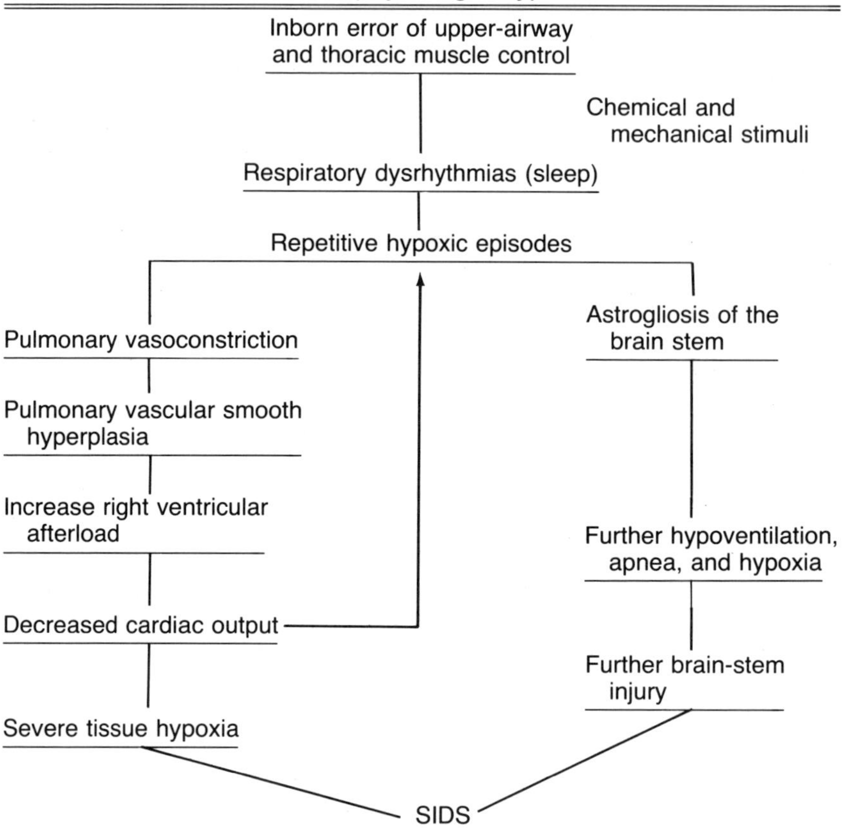

chemical alteration, such as methadone or sleep hypoxia occurs, these infants are prone to abnormal ventilatory patterns. This promotes hypoxia, which stimulates pulmonary vasoconstriction and eventually smooth muscle hypertrophy with progressive pulmonary hypertension. As a result, right ventricular failure and decreased cardiac output lead to further severe tissue hypoxia. Another life-threatening, positive feedback loop occurs when hypoxia causes astrogliosis of the brain stem. This, in turn, promotes hypoventilation and apnea with further hypoxemia. An alternative explanation is that excessive responsiveness in the pulmonary circulation to a small reduction in oxygen tension initiates a similar series of events.

Investigation and Treatment of Near-SIDS Infants

After ruling out the many causes that can prompt resuscitative measures in infants, the diagnosis of "near-SIDS" can then be entertained. It is important to recognize that among full-term infants who had only one apneic episode in the neonatal period, 5% died, while 44% died when more than one episode was documented.[141] Therefore, evaluation and treatment should be vigorously pursued.

In certain apneic states, term and preterm infants respond postively to theophylline.[142–144] However, electronic monitoring devices are needed for near-SIDS infants.[145] The parents should also be instructed in the use of cardiopulmonary resuscitation. Criticism of home monitoring units understandably revolves around its cost, psychologic trauma involved, accuracy of the equipment, and the potential for excessive use.[146,147] The home monitoring equipment is usually an impedance-type monitor. One problem that arises with this equipment occurs when the impedance change of the heartbeats exceeds the respiratory threshold. At this point, the apnea alarm does not go off. Another potential problem encountered is the occurrence of obstructive apnea where effort is made but no flow ensues; the alarm will again be delayed. A 20-second episode of total cessation of respiratory effort is necessary before the alarm sounds and, as a result, another prolonged period of apnea will occur after total effort ceases. As concerns the psychological stress on the parents, this is minimized if a well-developed 24-hour-a-day support program is available.

Apnea of Prematurity

Apnea of prematurity (AP) can occur in excess of 30% of low-birth-weight infants weighing less than 1500 g.[148] Although the etiology is unknown, it is probably related to lack of development of the respiratory and arousal centers, as tactile stimulation and respiratory stimulants improve the condition until the infant has time to grow and mature. This condition is potentially lethal because cyanosis, bradycardia, and hypotension have been documented during prolonged apneic episodes.[149–151] The apneas seen in AP are obstructive, central, and mixed. This is important diagnostically because late neurologic sequalae can develop in infants with repeated apneas that are not appropriately treated.[152,153]

Initial treatment modalities included tactile stimulation, maintenance of a low neutral zone thermal environment, and mechanical ventilation until the infant has reached a mature enough status. At the present time, theophylline is an effective and simple treatment modality.

Two studies have shown the therapeutic benefits of theophylline in AP. Shannon et al.[154] determined that oral doses of 1.5–4.0 mg/kg controlled the apneic episodes where the 2-hour serum concentrations were 6.6–11.0 meg/ml. The longer apneic episodes (those exceeding 20 seconds) were completely controlled and those lasting 10–19 seconds were markedly reduced. Any apneic-associated bradycardia was blocked. It was interesting to note in this study that the nursing staff observation, coupled with on-line alarm systems, detected only 39% of severe apneic episodes as compared to a pneumogram recording technique. This, again, illustrates the importance of proper monitoring not only for infants but children and adults. In another study,[155] low-dose theophylline therapy (2 mg/kg/d), resulting in serum concentrations of 2.8–3.9 meg/ml, was successfully employed. The apneic episodes decreased by 62% and the frequency of bradycardia decreased 73%. It was noted that no changes were observed in the ventilatory response to carbon dixoide, in the resting minute ventilation, arterial blood gases, heart rate, or serum electrolyte concentration. Therefore, the success of theophylline in treating AP works by mechanisms other than alteration of the carbon dioxide chemosensitivity.

Apnea of Infancy

Apnea of infancy (AI) is a possible premorbid clinical indication of SIDS. The standard definition for AI is a loose but fitting set of standards, "an unexplained and frightening episode of cessation of breathing for 20 seconds or longer, or a shorter respiratory pause associated with bradycardia, cyanosis, or pallor."[156] The apnea can occur when awake or asleep. Since the definition is broad-based, it delineates a clinical syndrome rather than a specific disease entity. Most frequently, the initial or only observation is noted by the parents. Frightening color changes and respiratory irregularity are important characteristics that may be noted by the parents in this disease entity.

Breathing Patterns

Since 1978, there have been several reports analyzing the respiratory patterns in AI patients. In one study of seven infants referred because of a frightening apneic episode observed by the parents, only two minor differences appeared when compared to a control population.[157] The AI patients had a lower respiratory rate postapnea than preapnea, and the respiratory pauses were more often preceded by prolonged somatic activity. In a heterogeneous population, the patterns of eight infants (five AI and three premature infants with persistent apnea) were compared to a normal population while breathing room air and 17% oxygen.[158] While breathing room air, there was no difference in these groups, but after 10 minutes of hypoxia, the infants with apnea showed a significant increase in periodic respiration. Kelly and Shannon[159] showed that AI patients had more sleep-related periodic breathing, and a greater percentage of the total time was spent in periodic breathing. Another report showed these infants to have higher respiratory rate, smaller tidal volume, and greater ventilatory response to carbon dioxide as compared to controls.[160] Guilleminault et al.[161] found that within the AI group the frequency of apneas was markedly influenced by time of the day the study was done and by the duration of uninterrupted sleep time. Therefore, the apnea frequency was low in the first 35 minutes of sleep but progressively increased thereafter.

Control of Breathing and Associated Variables

The ventilatory responses to chemical stimuli in this age group are difficult to obtain, and this may account for the wide variety of reported responses. In patients with AI, resting levels of arterial carbon dioxide[162,163] were found to be at elevated[30] levels (compared to matched group). The ventilatory response to carbon dioxide has been shown to be normal,[162] decreased,[30,163] and increased.[160] The hypoxic drive, as tested while administering 100% oxygen, is normal,[162] and with 15% oxygen, it is decreased.[163]

Arousal may also be decreased. Hunt et al.[163] found that infants with AI had less frequent arousal during hypoxia than did the control infants. In addition, the heart rate may be different; higher rates of 5–10% in both REM and non-REM sleep have been found in patients who have AI.[164] The overall variability in the rate was less in AI. Muscle tone abnormalities are also thought to be higher in AI, particularly related to shoulder hypotonia.[165] In general, apparently normal full-term infants who had greater instability of respiratory patterns during the first several weeks postpartum had lower mental and psychomotor development tested at 9 months of age than infants whose patterns were more stable.[166] Brain-stem functioning by auditory-evoked responses has been reported to be both normal[167] and abnormal[168] in AI. Overall, the neuromuscular functioning in AI infants tends to be abnormal.

Kanarek et al.[169] studied the ventilatory responses in parents of AI infants. Eight sets of parents were evaluated whose infants had proven abnormal responses to carbon dioxide. The study purposely selected for abnormal results, and their findings of normal responses in the parents strongly refutes a genetic component to chemosensitivity in this entity.

Pathophysiologic Mechanisms

Most cases of AI are thought to arise from a central basis, but obstructive apnea is also thought to play an important role. Stimulation of the laryngeal chemoreceptors can cause apnea and bradycardia. In animal studies, this reflex is more potent in the young and has the potential to be fatal.[170] Refluxed gastric contents have been suggested to be a mechanism of AI.[171–173] These infants can be relatively asymptomatic. Fixed upper airway obstruction can also occur with vocal cord paralysis, choanal stenosis, pharyngeal masses, hemangiomas, and subglottic stenosis.[174] Dynamic obstruction can occur with tracheomalacia or laryngomalacia. AI during sleep is probably related to altered ventilatory chemosensitivity.[175–177] When considering causes for cyanotic and/or apneic episodes, congenital heart disease, pulmonary vascular hyperreactivity, sepsis, meningitis, hyponatremia, hypocalcemia, hypoglycemia, and other metabolic disorders are included in the differential diagnosis.[174]

Clinical Interventions

After observation of the "frightening cyanotic or apneic" episode, the infant should be hospitalized for observation. The assumption is that the patient is at increased risk of SIDS thereafter and in a controlled environment, these infants can be observed. Alternatively, specific disease entities that cause AI can be diagnosed and treated.

In the majority of AI infants, a specific treatable entity cannot be demonstrated. In these individuals, either stimulant drugs or home monitoring of heart and/or respiratory function can be measured. There is no proof of effectiveness in either case.

The respiratory stimulants used are the methylxanthines, which include the aminophylline and theophylline preparations.[178–180] Caution must be used with these drugs in this age group because toxicity can easily develop due to delayed drug clearance.[181] Initiating theophylline doses of 2–2.5 mg/kg two to three times a day following a loading dose of 5 mg/kg is optimal.[174] In full-term infants in whom therapy was started at zero to 6 weeks, an average dose of 7.5 mg/kg/day significantly decreased the amount of periodic breathing and respiratory pauses.[181] A serum theophylline concentration of 3–11 μg/ml provides respiratory stimulation in apnea of prematurity.[154,155]

When using a theophylline preparation, caution must be observed if a possible seizure disorder was the cause of AI because this preparation will potentiate seizure activity. Lower gastroesophageal sphincter tone will be decreased, permitting reflux, which can also lead to AI. If reflux was ruled out initially as a cause of AI and theophylline is being used, then elevation of the head of the bed and assuming an upright position following feeding for 30–60 minutes will help decrease this potential problem.

The pros and cons of home monitoring of cardiorespiratory status are numerous. These have been discussed previously under SIDS. In AI, this observation should only be considered if at least one of the following is present: a family history of SIDS or AI, repetitive apneas requiring intervention to break the episode, or extreme concern by the parents or physician. Home monitoring, once initiated, should be discontinued only after the infant is at least 6 months old, has had no apneas for 2 months, has experienced an upper respiratory tract infection, and has had an immunization without resulting apneic episodes.[174]

Sleep Apnea Syndrome

The sleep apnea syndrome in children involves a complex of symptoms associated with a variety of underlying disorders (Table 3). The most common symptoms and signs are listed in Table 4. A detailed description of the pathophysiologic events that occur in the sleep apnea syndrome have been presented at the beginning of this chapter and in Chapter 4. A brief review is presented here.

The function and control of the upper airway muscles are com-

Table 3
Disorders Associated with Sleep Apnea Pediatric Syndrome

Anatomic abnormalities
Tonsillar and adenoidal hypertrophy
Craniofacial abnormalities
Septal deviation
Micro/retrognathia
Pierre-Robin syndrome
Crouzon syndrome
Treacher-Collins syndrome
Chromosomal abnormalities
Trisomy 21 (Down syndrome)
Trisomy 13
Neuromuscular disorders
Myotonic dystrophy
Chiari malformation
Syringomyelia
Cerebral palsy
Prader-Willi syndrome
Hypothyroidism

plex and are regulated by interacting neural mechanisms. Additionally, the upper airway, chest wall, and diaphragmatic musculature are interactive in a cascade of events resulting in an initially patent airway before the movement of air ensues. For a precise understanding of nocturnal respiratory activity, such as sleep apnea, further investigation into the normal sequence of medullary respiratory initiation through neuromuscular activation of the upper and lower airway muscles needs to be undertaken.

Physiological investigation into upper airway obstruction has shown that the entire alveolar-to-atmospheric pressure drop occurs in the oropharynx.[87] Thus, the larynx and lower airways are not the primary areas of obstruction. Radiographic support of the involvement of the tongue and posterior pharyngeal muscle hypotonia as the anatomic process has been shown by several investigators.[89,90]

The tongue is a respiratory muscle that exhibits rhythmic, inspiratory activity in the upright position in man.[92] In the supine position, this muscle displays a tonic expiratory component, overcoming the effects of gravity which would otherwise produce occlusion. In normal sleeping individuals, the genioglossus continues to exhibit rhythmic respiratory activity during non-REM sleep and markedly reduced levels during REM sleep.[93] Therefore, with any additional

Table 4
Sleep Apnea Syndrome Symptoms and Signs

Symptoms	
	Daytime somnolence
	Snoring
	Fitful sleep
	Frequent arousals
	Poor growth
	Change in behavior (hyperactivity, aggressive behavior) or school performance
	Delay in language development
	Morning headaches
	Enuresis
	Nocturnal diaphoresis
	Weight change (either increase or decrease)
Signs	
	Systemic hypertension
	Congestive heart failure
	Cor pulmonale
	Clubbing
	Stridor

impediment to airflow, such as hypertrophied tonsils, occlusion of the upper airway can easily occur.

Once upper airway obstruction occurs, any respiratory effort will enhance the occlusion. This is because the negative intrathoracic pressure of an inspiratory effort will tend to draw the upper airway structures over the laryngeal opening. In order to break the upper airway obstruction, there is a preferential activation of the genioglossus so as to develop a patent airway.[87] Therefore, changes in neuromuscular function during an apnea are an important signal to break the apnea. These changes are related to arousal, which is altered in patients with sleep apnea.

Patients presenting with central apneas as the predominant type of sleep-related respiratory problem comprise less than 10% in comparison to the number of patients having predominantly upper airway obstruction during sleep. Rarely, the central apneas are so severe that they occur during waking hours as well as in sleep. In this setting, cyanosis and severe hypoxia develop because the patient does not perceive the need to breathe and consequently seizures can occur.

Since central apneas are not as common as upper airway obstructions, investigation into their pathophysiology is not as extensive. In addition, central apneas, primary alveolar hypoventilation, and upper airway obstruction are frequently combined or the terms are used interchangeably in most reports, making precise separation and analysis difficult.

It appears that the chemical control of breathing (ventilatory responses to hypercapnic hyperoxia and eucapnic hypoxia) is reduced in this group of patients.[175–177] Whether the defect in ventilatory control is the primary cause of central apneas is not known. There are many other patient groups who have abnormalities in ventilatory control but who do not have central apneas during sleep. There is a possibility that this group is predisposed to the development of central apneas. Thus, during sleep, when the ventilatory responses are normally suppressed, the hypoxia that develops leads to a central blunting of the respiratory drive to breathe. This hypothesis is indirectly supported by several observations. Martin et al.[103] and McNicholas et al.[104] showed in adults that central apneas were totally eliminated or markedly improved by the use of supplemental oxygen, and Hunt[182] reported that an infant with tetralogy of Fallot was cured of central apneas and repeated "near-miss sudden infant death" episodes when oxygenation returned to normal following surgery.

Normal subjects develop periodic breathing and central apneas when taken to higher altitudes from sea level.[183,184] This type of breathing was abolished with the use of supplemental oxygen during sleep at altitude[183] and recurred about 8 minutes after the cessation of oxygen. Acetazolamide, a carbonic anhydrase inhibitor, also resulted in improvement in the ventilatory pattern and oxygenation in high-altitude sleep.[184] Acetazolamide does not heighten the slope of the ventilatory response to hypoxia but, rather, produces a parallel shift in the response curve so that ventilation is augmented at all levels of hypoxia.[186] Perhaps in this situation the subject is more responsive to a decrease in oxygen and increases respiration, thus preventing the "critical level" of hypoxia from developing and inducing periodic breathing.

In mixed apneas, there are components of both central apneas and upper airway obstruction during an apneic episode. Usually the central component precedes the obstructive one. When there are respiratory disorders during sleep, the occurrence of mixed apneas is quite common and is seen frequently throughout the night in conjunction with upper airway obstruction. The clinical presentation is similar to upper airway obstruction.

One would expect mixed apneas to be a common event in the

sleep apnea syndrome. If the drive to the neuron in the tractus solitarius is reduced, a cessation of diaphragmatic activity results, causing central apneas. If there is a decreased stimulus to an area just a few micrometers away, the upper motor neurons of the upper airway will be affected, and the result is decreased tone to the muscles that maintain extrathoracic airway patency. There is a possibility that since the anatomic regions of control are quite close, the physiologic control may be similar and, as a result, mixed apneas could easily develop. Even in an upper airway obstruction episode, there is decreased neural output to the respiratory muscles preceeding the apneas.[187]

Primary alveolar hypoventilation is defined as decreased alveolar ventilation leading to increased carbon dioxide retention that is not associated with apneas. This disorder is usually present during both wakefulness and sleep but is greatly exacerbated during sleep. Primary alveolar hypoventilation may present only during sleep.

The ventilatory responses to the chemical control of breathing are abnormal in primary alveolar hypoventilation.[188–190] This includes both a diminished response to hyperoxic hypercapnia and eucapnic hypoxia. Wolkove et al.[188] helped to explain the differences in the primary alveolar hypoventilation syndrome presenting with daytime hypercapnia or eucapnia. Both groups had past episodes of respiratory failure that could not be attributed solely to pulmonary mechanical dysfunction. When stable, one group was eucapnic during the day and the other was hypercapnic. There was no difference in pulmonary function tests and chemical respiratory control, i.e., ventilatory response and occlusion pressure responses. However, the nonchemical neural control of breathing did show differences that were assessed from the ability to duplicate tidal volumes of different sizes and to quantitate tidal volume changes. The eucapnic group was able to perform the nonchemical control testing similar to normal subjects. In contrast, the hypercapnic group was unable to maintain constant tidal volumes, and the error in estimation of tidal volume change was significantly greater than that seen in normal subjects. Thus, daytime alveolar ventilation can be controlled in nonstressed primary alveolar hypoventilation patients when the nonchemical control mechanism is intact. During sleep, it appears that this ability may be lost; however, this assumption has not been tested.

Patients with primary alveolar hypoventilation usually have normal pulmonary function tests. The development of arterial hypoxemia can be explained by the elevation in carbon dioxide levels. These patients can voluntarily hyperventilate and decrease the $PaCO_2$ toward normal, resulting in a proportional increase in PaO_2. Usually 1 minute of supervised hyperventilation while drawing a blood gas during the hyperventilation episode will be enough to document the reversal of the carbon dioxide and oxygen tensions.

In one study[191] of eight children (ages 8–14) who had sleep apnea syndrome, the difficulty in diagnosis was apparently due to lack of suspicion for this problem. Some of the children had severe symptoms for as long as 7 years before the proper diagnosis was made. The number of apneas during a night study ranged from 78 to 816, 83% of which were upper airway obstructions. As in the adult population, there was a male predominance (seven of eight). Daytime somnolence was seen in five patients, and loud snoring occurred in all patients. Enuresis was a problem in seven of eight patients. Decreased school performance was manifested in five patients, and these were the ones who also experienced morning headaches. Mood and behavioral disturbances occurred in six patients, including hallucinations in some. Hypertension was present in five, and weight change occurred in seven patients. Of interest, only two had an increase in weight while five experienced a weight reduction.

The exact cause of excessive daytime somnolence is unknown but probably is related to changes in oxygen and carbon dioxide rather than totally related to nocturnal arousals. The changes in gas tensions could possibly affect neurotransmitter synthesis in the brain, e.g., gamma-aminobutyric acid and serotonin, which could also lead to daytime somnolence.[192,193] Children are particularly embarrassed about their sleepiness and try desperately to fight this symptom. To avoid sleeping in school, the child may move about and give a false impression of being a "hyperactive" child and be thus mislabeled as such. When seated in the classroom, the child may appear awake but develops lapses of microsleep that tend to impair learning and lead to an automatic behavior syndrome.[194]

Loud snoring occurs every night and is usually the first symptom, by several years, of the sleep apnea syndrome. Initially, this sonorous noise is intermittent but eventually becomes continuous. Not uncommonly, the snoring is interrupted by silences of an apnea.

If nocturnal enuresis occurs after the child has been toilet trained, then sleep apnea should be considered. This problem does not necessarily have to occur nightly.

Morning headaches are not localized nor are they associated with other symptoms such as nausea, vomiting, fever, myalgias, etc. The typical feature of the headache is its complete cessation by late morning. The headaches may be related to the severe intrathoracic pressure swings during an upper airway obstruction. These fluctuations cause marked changes in blood flow, which can then lead to an increase in the intracranial pressure, resulting in morning headaches. The hypoxia and/or hypercapnia that develops may also cause headaches.

Systemic hypertension, pulmonary hypertension, and biventricular heart failure may all occur with this syndrome. The hypoxia and hypercapnia that develop can stimulate the release of catecholamines and other substances that produce nocturnal systemic hypertension proceeding to sustained daytime blood pressure elevation. The changes in gas tensions also produce pulmonary hypertension that ultimately induces cor pulmonale. Eventually there is left ventricular dysfunction because of the continued hypoxia.

In children older than 30 months, the sleep apnea syndrome is most often caused by enlarged tonsils and/or adenoids.[191,195] Tonsillectomy and adenoidectomy almost always produce total reversal or significant improvement in signs and symptoms; rarely, a child continues to have symptoms due to prolonged sleep apnea and may eventually need tracheostomy.[191] There is an interesting report of a child with enlarged tonsils and sickle cell anemia who was found to have severe obstructive sleep apnea.[185] This child developed strokes that were felt to be related to the apnea-associated hypoxemia with sickling of the red blood cells. Thus, in children with tonsillar hypertrophy and sickle cell anemia, sleep apnea needs to be ruled in or out and appropriate treatment undertaken.

Other treatment modalities listed in Chapter 5 for adults have not been as extensively evaluated in children but should be considered before tracheostomy, particularly if a correctable cause exists. There is a report of a 20-month old child who had the obesity–hypoventilation syndrome and abnormal beta-endorphin levels in the cerebrospinal fluid and the serum who was successfully treated at 5-day intervals with naloxone infusion.[196] The possibility of endogenous opiates or other neurotransmitters as causative factors in sleep and waking respiratory disorders needs further extensive evaluation. Corticosteroids have been reported to improve apnea in young children, and medroxyprogesterone has shown improvement in adolescents who reached Tanner IV sexual development.[197] Other general reviews on this topic can be found in Guilleminault[198] and Lembo.[199]

As in the adult population, the existence of respiratory disorders during sleep in pediatric patients can be devastating. It is imperative that a complete history and testing be done to prevent the morbidity and mortality that can occur in this age group. As further investigation continues, the abnormal mechanisms in SIDS and the apnea syndromes will be revealed, leading to better diagnostic and therapeutic intervention.

References

1. Merritt T, Valdes-Dapena M. SIDS research update. *Pediatr Ann* 1984; 13:193–207.
2. Kraus JF, Borhani NO. Post-neonatal sudden unexplained death in California: A cohort study. *Am J Epidemiol* 1972; 95:497–510.
3. Kraus JF, Borhan NO. Sudden infant death in Copenhagen 1956–1971. II. Social factors and morbidity. *Acta Paediatr Scand* 1979; 68:1–9.
4. Peterson DR, van Belle G, Chinn NM. Epidemiologic comparisons of the sudden infant death syndrome with other major components of infant mortality. *Am J Epidemiol* 1979; 110:699–707.
5. Spiers PS, Wang L. Short pregnancy interval, low birthweight and the sudden death syndrome. *Am J Epidemiol* 1976; 104:15–21.
6. Steele R, Langworth JT. The relationship of antenatal and postnatal factors to sudden unexpected death in infancy. *Can Med Assoc J* 1966; 94:1165–1171.
7. Naeye RL, Ladis B, Drage JS. Sudden infant death syndrome: A prospective study. *Am J Dis Child* 1976; 130:1207–1210.
8. Proggatt P, Lynas MA, Marshall TK. Sudden death in babies: Epidemiology. *Am J Cardiol* 1968; 22:457–468.
9. Bergman AB, Wiesnes LA. Relationship of passive cigarette-smoking on sudden infant death syndrome. *Pediatrics* 1976; 58:665–668.
10. Oakley JR, Tavare CJ, Stanton AN. Evaluation of the Sheffield system for identifying children at risk from unexpected death in infancy: Results from Birmingham and Newcastle-upon-Tyne. *Arch Dis Child* 1978; 53:649–652.
11. Rajegowda BK, Kandall SR, Falciglia H. Sudden unexpected death in infants of narcotic-dependent mothers. *Early Hum Dev* 1978; 2:219–225.
12. Arsenault PS. Maternal and antenatal factors in the risk of sudden infant death syndrome. *Am J Epidemiol* 1980; 111:278–284.
13. Carpenter RG, Gardner A, McWeeny PM, et al. Multistage scoring system for identifying infants at risk of unexpected death. *Arch Dis Child* 1977; 52:606–612.
14. Fleshman JK, Peterson DR. The sudden infant death syndrome among Alaskan natives. *Am J Epidemiol* 1977; 105:555–558.
15. Valdes-Dapena M, Birle LJ, McGovern JA, et al. Sudden unexpected death in infancy: A statistical analysis of certain socioeconomic factors. *J Pediatr* 1968; 73:387–394.
16. Kulkarni P, Hall RT, Rhodes PG, et al. Postneonatal infant mortality in infants admitted to a neonatal intensive care unit. *Pediatrics* 1978; 62: 178–183.
17. McWeeny PM, Emery JL. Unexpected postneonatal deaths (cot deaths) due to recognizable disease. *Arch Dis Child* 1975; 50:191–196.

18. Richards IDG, McIntosh HT. Confidential inquiry into 226 consecutive infant deaths. *Arch Dis Child* 1972; 47:697–706.
19. Naeye RL, Messmer J III, Specht T, et al. Sudden infant death syndrome temperament before death. *J Pediatr* 1976; 88:511–555.
20. Spiers PS. Previous fetal loss and risk of sudden infant death syndrome in subsequent offspring. *Am J Epidemiol* 1976; 103:355–361.
21. Froggart P, Lynas MA, Marshall TK. Sudden unexpected death in infants ('cot death'): report of a collaborative study in Northern Ireland. *Ulster Med J* 1971; 40:116–135.
22. Standfast SJ, Jereb S, Janerich DT. The epidemiology of sudden infant death in upstate New York. II. Birth characteristics. *Am J Public Health* 1980; 70:1061–1067.
23. Peterson DR, Chinn NM, Fisher LD. The sudden death syndrome: repetitions in families. *J Pediatr* 1980; 97:265–267.
24. Stark RE, Nathanson SN. Unusual features of cry in infant dying suddenly and unexpectedly. *In* JF Bosma, J Showace (eds). Development of Upper Respiration Anatomy and Function. Bethesda, MD, National Institutes of Health, 1975, pp 233–249.
25. Golub H, Corwin M. Infant cry: A clue to diagnosis. *Pediatrics* 1982; 69:197–201.
26. Cooke RT, Welch RG. A study in cot death. *Br Med J* 1964; 2:1549–1554.
27. Zwillich C, McCullough R, Guilleminault C, et al. Respiratory control in the parents of sudden infant death syndrome victims: Ventilatory control in SIDS parents. *Pediatr Res* 1980; 14:769–774.
28. Schiffman PL, Westlake RE, Santiago TV, et al. Ventilatory control in parents of victims of sudden-infant-death syndrome. *N Eng J Med* 1980; 302:486–491.
29. Shannon DC, Kelly D. Impaired regulation of alveolar ventilation and the sudden infant death syndrome. *Science* 1977; 197:367–368.
30. Shannon DC, Kelly DH, O'Connell K. Abnormal regulation of ventilation in infants at risk for sudden-infant-death syndrome. *N Eng J Med* 1977; 297:747–750.
31. Kanarek DJ, Kelly DH, Shannon DC. Ventilatory chemoreceptor response in parents of children at risk for sudden infant death syndrome. *Pediatr Res* 1981; 15:1402–1405.
32. Kelly DH, Walker AM, Cahen L, et al. Periodic breathing in siblings of sudden infant death syndrome victims. *Pediatrics* 1980; 66:515–520.
33. Tapp E, Jones DM, Tobin JO. Interpretation of respiratory tract histology in cot deaths. *J Clin Pathol* 1975; 28:899–904.
34. Scott DJ, Gardner PS, McQuillin J, et al. Respiratory viruses and cot death. *Br Med J* 1978; 21:2–3.
35. Beckwith JB. Observations of the pathological anatomy of the sudden infant death syndrome. *In* AB Bergman, JB Beckwith, CG Ray (eds). Sudden Infant Death Syndrome: Proceedings of the Second International Conference on Causes of Sudden Death in Infants. Seattle, University of Washington Press, 1970, pp 83–102.
36. Bruhn FW, Mokrohisky ST, McKintosh K. Apnea associated with respiratory syncytial virus infection in young infant. *J Pediatr* 1977; 90: 382–386.

37. Naeye RL. Placental abnormalities in victims of the sudden infant death syndrome. *Biol Neonate* 1977; 32:189–192.
38. Shannon DC, Kelly DH. SIDS and near SIDS. *N Eng J Med* 1982; 306: 959–965, 1022–1028.
39. Naeye RL, Whalen P, Ryser M, et al. Cardiac and other abnormalities in the sudden infant death syndrome. *Am J Pathol* 1976; 82:1–8.
40. Williams A, Vawter G, Reid L. Increased muscularity of the pulmonary circulation in victims of sudden infant death syndrome. *Pediatrics* 1979; 63:18–23.
41. Takashima S, Armstrong D, Becker L, et al. Cerebral hypoperfusion in the sudden infant death syndrome: brainstem gliosis and vasculature. *Ann Neurol* 1978; 4:257–262.
42. Takashima S, Armstrong D, Becker LE, et al. Cerebral white matter lesions in sudden infant death syndrome. *Pediatrics* 1978; 62:155–159.
43. Naeye RL. Brain-stem and adrenal abnormalities in the sudden-infant-death syndrome. *Am J Clin Pathol* 1976; 66:526–530.
44. Guntheroth WG. The significance of pulmonary petechiae in crib death. *Pediatrics* 1973; 52:601–603.
45. Pinkham HR, Beckwith JB. Vocal cord lesions in sudden infant death syndrome. *In* AB Bergman, JB Beckwith, CG Ray (eds). Sudden Infant Death Syndrome: Proceedings of the Second International Conference on Causes of Sudden Death in Infants. Seattle, University of Washington Press, 1970, pp 104–107.
46. Cullity GJ, Emery JL. Ulcerations and necrosis of vocal cords in hospital and unexpected child deaths. *J Pathol* 1975; 115:27–31.
47. Fink BR, Beckwith JB. Laryngeal mucous gland excess in victims of sudden infant death. *Am J Dis Child* 1980; 134:144–146.
48. Keeton BR, Southall E, Rutter N, et al. Cardiac conduction disorders in six infants with "near-miss" sudden infant deaths. *Br Med J* 1977; 2: 600–601.
49. Hodgman J. Polygraphic studies of normal infants and infants at risk for the sudden infant death syndrome: Heart rate and variability as a function of state. *Pediatr Res* 1978; 12:778–785.
50. Lugaresi E, Coccagna G, Cirignotta F, et al. Breathing during sleep in man in normal and pathological conditions. *Adv Exp Med Biol* 1978; 99:33–45.
51. Robin ED, Whaley RD, Crump CH, et al. Alveolar gas tensions, pulmonary ventilation and blood pH during physiologic sleep in normal subjects. *J Clin Invest* 1958; 37:981–989.
52. Birchfield RI, Sicker HO, Heyman A. Alterations in blood gases during natural sleep and narcolepsy. *Neurology* 1958; 8:107–112.
53. Birchfield RI, Sicker HO, Heyman A. Alterations in respiratory function during nocturnal sleep. *J Lab Clin Med* 1959; 54:216–222.
54. Pengelly LD, Rebuck AS, Campbell EJM. Loaded Breathing. Don Millls, Ontario, Longman, 1974.
55. Hudgel DW, Martin RJ, Johnson B. Mechanics of the respiratory system breathing pattern and lung volumes during sleep in normal man. *J Appl Physiol: Respir Environ Exercise Physiol* 1983; (in press).

56. Berger AJ, Mitchell RA, Severinghous JW. Regulation of respiration. *N Eng J Med* 1977; 297:92, 138, 194.
57. Mitchell RA, Berger AJ. Neural regulation of respiration. *Am Rev Respir Dis* 1975; 111:208–224.
58. Magnussen G. Studies on the Respiration during Sleep. London, HK Lewis, 1944.
59. Ostergaard T. The excitability of the respiratory centre during sleep and during Evipan anaesthesia. *Acta Physiol Scand* 1944; 8:1–15.
60. Birchfield RI, Sicker HO, Heyman A. Alterations in respiratory function during natural sleep. *J Lab Clin Med* 1959; 54:216–227.
61. Robin ED, Whaley RD, Crump CH, et al. Alveolar gas tensions, pulmonary ventilation and blood pH during physiologic sleep in 8 normal subjects. *J Clin Invest* 1958; 37:981–989.
62. Reed DJ, Kellogg RH. Changes in respiratory response to CO_2 during natural sleep at sea level and at altitude. *J Appl Physiol* 1958; 13:323–330.
63. Belville JW, Howland WS, Seed JC, et al. The effect of sleep on the respiratory response to carbon dioxide. *Anesthesiology* 1959; 20:628–634.
64. Bulow K. Respiration and wakefulness in man. *Acta Physiol Scand Suppl* 1963; 209:1–110.
65. Phillipson EA, Kozar LF, Rebuck AS, et al. Ventilatory and waking response to CO_2 in sleeping dogs. *Am Rev Respir Dis* 1977; 115:251–259.
66. Jouvet M. Paradoxical sleep. A study of its nature and mechanisms. *In* Progress in Brain Research, Sleep Mechanisms. Amsterdam, Elsevier, 1965, p 20.
67. Betrand F, Hugelin A. Respiratory synchronizing function of nucleus parabrachialis medelis: Pneumotoxic mechanisms. *J Neurophysiol* 1971; 34:189.
68. Pompeian O. The neurophysiological mechanisms of the postural and motor events during desynchronized sleep. *In* SS Kety, EV Evants, HL Williams (eds). Sleep and Altered States of Consciousness. Baltimore, Williams and Wilkins, 1967, p 351.
69. White DP, Douglas NJ, Pickett CK, et al. Hypoxic and hypercapnic ventilatory responses decrease during sleep in adults. *Am Rev Respir Dis* 1982; 125(2):234.
70. Fagenholz SA, O'Connell K, Shannon DC. Chemoreceptor function and sleep state in apnea. *Pediatrics* 1976; 58:31–36.
71. Phillipson EA, Sullivan CE, Read DJC, et al. Ventilatory and waking responses to hypoxia in sleeping dogs. *J Appl Physiol* 1978; 44:512–520.
72. Douglas NJ, White DP, Weil JV, et al. Hypoxic ventilatory response decrease during sleep in man. *Am Rev Respir Dis* 1982; 125:286–289.
73. Irving L. Comparative anatomy and physiology of gas transport mechanisms. *In* WO Fenn, H Rahn (eds). Handbook of Physiology: Respiration, Vol. I. Washington, DC, American Physiology Society, 1965, pp 177–212.
74. Proctor D. The upper airways. *Am Rev Respir Dis* 1977; 115:97–130.
75. Tenney SM, Bartlett D. Some comparative aspects of the control of breathing. *In* TF Hornbein (ed). Regulation of Breathing, Part I. New York, Marcel Dekker, 1981, pp 67–104.

76. Mitchinson AG, Yoffey JM. Respiratory displacement of the larynx, hyoid bone and tongue. *J Anat (London)* 1947; 81:118–120.
77. Green JH, Neil E. The respiratory function of the laryngeal muscles. *J Physiol (London)* 1955; 129:134–139.
78. Andrew B. The respiratory displacement of the larynx: a study of the accessory respiratory muscles. *J Physiol (London)* 1955; 130:474–487.
79. Ogawa T, Jefferson NC, Toman JE, et al. Action potentials of accessory respiratory muscles in dogs. *Am J Physiol* 1960; 199:569–572.
80. Eyzaguirre C, Taylor JR. Respiratory discharge of some vagal motoneurons. *J Neurophysiol* 1963; 26:61–68.
81. Cohen MI. Phrenic and recurrent laryngeal discharge patterns and the Hering-Breuer reflex. *Am J Physiol* 1975; 228:1489–1496.
82. Brouillette RT, Thach BT. Control of genioglossus inspiratory activity. *J Appl Physiol* 1981; 49:801–808.
83. Weiner D, Parker D, Mitra J, et al. Effects of blood pressure changes in hypoglossal, recurrent laryngeal and phrenic nerve activity. *Am Rev Respir Dis* 1981; 123:182.
84. Bruce EN, Cherniack NS, Mitra J, et al. Carotid sinus and medullary chemoreceptor contributions to phrenic and hypoglossal nerve responses during rebreathing. *Physiologist* 1980; 23:182.
85. Mitchell RA. Neural regulation of respiration. *In* MH Williams (ed). Clinics in Chest Medicine. Philadelphia, WB Saunders, 1980, pp 3–12.
86. Mitchell RA, Berger AJ. Neural regulation of respiration. *In* TF Hornbein (ed). Regulation of Breathing, Part I. New York, Marcel Dekker, 1981, pp 541–620.
87. Remmers JE, DeGroot WJ, Sauerland ER, et al. Pathologenesis of upper airway occlusion during sleep. *J Appl Physiol: Respir Environ Exercise Physiol* 1978; 44:931–938.
88. Gastaut H, Tassinari CA, Duron B. Polygraphic study of the episodic diural and nocturnal (hypnic and respiratory) manifestations of the Pickwick syndrome. *Brain Res* 1966; 2:167–186.
89. Smirne S, Comi G. The obstructive mechanism in Pickwickian syndrome. A serial x-ray study. *Sleep Res* 1976; 4:237.
90. Walsh RE, Michealson ED, Harkerload LE, et al. Upper airway obstruction in obese patients with sleep disturbances and somnolence. *Ann Intern Med* 1972; 76:185–192.
91. Karacan IC, Ware C, Moore C, et al. Disturbed sleep as a function of sleep apnea: Too much sleep but not enough. *Texas Med* 1977; 73:49–56.
92. Sauerland EK, Mitchell SP. Electromyographic activity of intinsic and extrinsic muscles of the human tongue. *Texas Rep Biol Med* 1975; 33: 445–455.
93. Sauerland EK, Harper RM. The human tongue during sleep: Electromyographic activity of the genioglossal muscle. *Exp Neurol* 1976; 51: 160–167.
94. Kurtz D, Krieger J, Stierle JC. EMG activity of cricothyroid and chin muscles during wakefulness and sleeping in the sleep apnea syndrome. *Electroencephalogr Clin Neurophysiol* 1978; 45:777–784.
95. Brouillette RT, Thach BT. A neuromuscular mechanism maintaining ex-

trathoracic airways patency. *J Appl Physiol: Respir Environ Exercise Physiol* 1979; 46:772–779.
96. Brouillette RT, Thach BT. Control of genioglossus muscle inspiratory activity *J Appl Physiol: Respir Environ Exercise Physiol* 1980; 49:801–808.
97. Schwieler GH. Respiratory regulation during postnatal development in cats and rabbits and some of its morphological substrate. *Acta Physiol Scand Suppl* 1968; 304:1–123.
98. Onal E, Lopata M, O'Connor T. Pathogenesis of apneas in hypersomnia sleep apnea syndrome. *Am Rev Respir Dis* 1982; 125:167–174.
99. Guilleminault C, Tilkian A, Dement WC. The sleep apnea syndromes. *Annu Rev Med* 1976; 27:465–484.
100. Motta J, Guilleminault C, Schroder JS. Tracheostomy and hemodynamic changes in sleep-induced apnea. *Ann Intern Med* 1978; 89:454–458.
101. Onal E, Lopata M, O'Connor TD. Diaphragmatic and genioglossal electromyogram responses to isocapnic hypoxia in humans. *Am Rev Respir Dis* 1981; 124:215–217.
102. Onal E, Lopata M, O'Connor TD. Diaphragmatic and genioglossal EMG responses to CO_2 rebreathing in humans. *J Appl Physiol: Respir Environ Exercise Physiol* 1981; 50:1052–1055.
103. Martin RJ, Sanders MH, Gray BA, et al. Acute and long-term ventilatory effects of hyperoxia in the adult sleep apnea syndrome. *Am Rev Respir Dis* 1982; 125:175–180.
104. McNicholas WT, Carter JL, Rutherford R, et al. Beneficial effect of oxygen in primary alveolar hypoventilation with central sleep apnea. *Am Rev Respir Dis* 1982; 125:773–775.
105. Guilleminault C, Cummiskey J. Progressive improvement of apnea index and ventilatory response to CO_2 after tracheostomy in obstructive sleep apnea syndrome. *Am Rev Respir Dis* 1982; 126:14–20.
106. Patrick GB, Rubin SB, Strohl KP, et al. Comparison of alae nasi and diaphragm activity during hypoxia, hypercapnia, and resistive loading in normal subjects. *Am Rev Respir Dis* 1981; 123(4):187 (abstract).
107. Orem J, Netick A, Dement WC. Increased upper airway resistance to breathing during sleep in the cat. *Electroencephalogr Clin Neurophysiol* 1977; 43:14–22.
108. Tonkin S. Sudden infant death syndrome; hypothesis of causation. *Pediatrics* 1975; 55:650–661.
109. Martin RJ, Okken A, Rubin D. Arterial oxygen tension during active and quiet sleep in the normal neonate. *J Pediatr* 1979; 94:271–274.
110. Henderson-Smart DJ, Read DJ. Depression of intercostal and abdominal muscle activity and vulnerability to asphyxia during active sleep in the newborn. *In* C Guilleminault, W Dement (ed). Sleep Apnea Syndromes. New York, Alan R. Liss, 1978, pp 93–118.
111. Leistner HL, Haddad GG, Epstein, et al. Heart rate and heart rate variability during sleep in aborted sudden infant death syndrome. *J Pediatr* 1980; 97:51–55.
112. Steven LH. Sudden unexplained death in infancy: Observations on a natural mechanism of adoption of the face down position. *Am J Dis Child* 1965; 110:243–247.

113. Steinschneider A. Prolonged apnea and the sudden infant death syndrome: Clinical and laboratory observations. *Pediatrics* 1972; 50:646–654.
114. Guilleminault C, Peraita R, Souquet M, et al. Apneas during sleep in infants: Possible relationship with sudden infant death syndrome. *Science* 1975; 190:677–679.
115. Steinschneider A, Rabuzzi DD. Apnea and airway obstruction during feeding and sleep. *Laryngoscope* 1976; 86:1359–1366.
116. Cornwell AC, Weitzman ED, Marmarou A. Ambulatory and in-hospital continuous recording of sleep state and cardiorespiratory parameters in 'near miss' for the sudden infant death syndrome and control infants. *Biotelemetry* 1978; 5:113–122.
117. Guilleminault C, Ariagno R, Korobkin R, et al. Mixed and obstructive sleep apnea and near miss for sudden infant death syndrome. Comparison of near miss and normal control infants by age. *Pediatrics* 1979; 64:882–891.
118. Hunt CE. Abnormal hypercapnic and hypoxic sleep arousal responses in near-miss SIDS. *Pediatr Res* 1981; 15:462–464.
119. Hugelin A, BonValet M, Dell P. Activation reticulaire et corticale d'origine chemoreceptive au cours de l'hypoxie. *Electroencephalogr Clin Neurophysiol* 1959; 11:325–340.
120. BonValet M, Hugelin A, Dell P. Sensibilite comparee du systeme reticule activateur ascendent et du centre respiratoire aux gaz du sang et a l'-adrenaline. *J Physiol (Paris)* 1955; 47:651–654.
121. Fink BR. Influence of cerebral activity in wakefulness on regulation of breathing. *J Appl Physiol* 1961; 16:15–20.
122. Sullivan CE, Murphy E, Kozar LF, et al. Waking and ventilatory responses to laryngeal stimulation in sleeping dogs. *J Appl Physiol* 1978; 45:681–689.
123. Hudgel DW, Kellum R, Martin RJ, et al. Depressed arousal response to airflow obstruction—A possible factor in near fatal nocturnal asthma. *Am Rev Respir Dis* 1982; 125(2):202.
124. Rigatto H, Brady JP, de la Torre Verduzco R. Chemoreceptor reflexes in preterm infants. I. The effect of gestational and postnatal age on the ventilatory response to inhalation of 100% and 15% oxygen. *Pediatrics* 1975; 55:604–613.
125. Shannon DC. Pathophysiologic mechanisms causing sleep apnea and hypoventilation in infants. *Sleep* 1980; 3:343–349.
126. Baker TL, McGinty DJ. Reversal of cardiopulmonary failure during active sleep in hypoxic kittens: Implications for sudden death. *Science* 1977; 198:419–421.
127. Brady JP, Ariagno RL, Watts JL, et al. Apnea, hypoxemia, and aborted sudden infant death syndrome. *Pediatrics* 1978; 62:686–691.
128. Hunt CE, McCulloch K, Brouillette RI. Diminished hypoxic ventilatory responses in near miss SIDS. *J Appl Physiol* 1981; 50:1313–1317.
129. Harding R, Johnson P, Johnston EB, et al. Cardiovascular changes in the newborn lambs during apnoea induced by stimulation of laryngeal receptors with water. *J Physiol (London)* 1976; 956:35P–36P.
130. Gould JB, Lee AFS, Cook P, et al. Apnea and sleep state in infants with nasopharyngitis. *Pediatrics* 1980; 65:713–717.

131. Swift PGF, Emery JL. Clinical observations on response to nasal occlusion in infancy. *Arch Dis Child* 1973; 48:947–951.
132. Steinschneider A. Nasopharyngitis and prolonged sleep apnea. *Pediatrics* 1975; 56:967–971.
133. Guilleminault C, Eldridge FL, Simmons FB, et al. Sleep apnea in eight children. *Pediatrics* 1976; 58:23–30.
134. Holinger PC, Holinger LD, Reichert TJ, et al. Respiratory obstruction and apnea in infants with bilateral abductor vocal cord paralysis, meningomyelocele, hydrocephalus, and Arnold-Chiari malformation. *J Pediatr* 1978; 92:368–373.
135. Loughlin G, Wynne J, Victoria B, et al. Intermittent upper airway obstruction during sleep causing accelerated pulmonary hypertension in Down's syndrome. *Chest* 1980; 78:529 (abstract).
136. Berdon WE, Baker DH, Bordiuk J, et al. Innominate artery compression of the trachea in infants with stridor and apnea: Method of roentgen diagnosis and criteria for surgical treatment. *Radiology* 1969; 92:272–278.
137. Ingram RH, Bishop JB. Ventilatory response to carbon dioxide after removal of chronic upper airway obstruction. *Am Rev Respir Dis* 1970; 102:645–647.
138. Herbst JJ, Book LS, Bray PF. Gastroesophageal reflux in the "near miss" sudden infant death syndrome. *J Pediatr* 1978; 92:73–75.
139. Talman WT, Perrone MH, Reis DJ. Evidences for L-glutamate as the neurotransmitter of baroreceptor afferent nerve fibers. *Science* 1980; 209: 813–815.
140. Dawes GS, Comroe JH Jr. Chemoreflexes from the heart and lungs. *Physiol Rev* 1954; 34:167–201.
141. Naeye RL. Neonatal apnea: underlying disorders. *Pediatrics* 1979; 63: 8–12.
142. Kelly DH, Shannon DC. Treatment of apnea and excessive periodic breathing in the full-term infant. *Pediatrics* 1981; 68:183–186.
143. Shannon DC, Gotay F, Stein IM, et al. Prevention of apnea and bradycardia in low-birthweight infants. *Pediatrics* 1975; 55:589–594.
144. Davi MJ, Sankaran K, Simons KJ, et al. Physiologic changes induced by theophylline in the treatment of apnea in preterm infants. *J Pediatr* 1978; 92:91–95.
145. Kelly DH, Shannon DC, O'Connell K. Care of infants with near-miss sudden infant death syndrome. *Pediatrics* 1978; 61:511–514.
146. Nelson NM. But who shall monitor the monitor? *Pediatrics* 1978; 61: 663–666.
147. Lucey JF. False alarms in the nursery. *Pediatrics* 1978; 61:665–666.
148. Miller HC, Behrle FC, Smull NM. Severe apnea and irregular respiratory rhythms among premature infants. *Pediatrics* 1959; 23:676.
149. Illingworth RS. Cyanotic attacks in newborn infants. *Arch Dis Child* 1957; 32:328.
150. Daily WJR, Klaus M, Meyer HBP. Apnea in premature infants: monitoring, incidence, heart rate changes and an effect of environmental temperature. *Pediatrics* 1969; 43:510.
151. Girling DJ. Changes in heart rate, blood pressure, and pulse pressure during apneic attacks in newborn babies. *Arch Dis Child* 1972; 47:405.

152. Bacola E, Behrle FC, de Schweintzl, et al. Perinatal and environmental factors in late neurogenic sequelae: I. Infants having birth weights from 1500 to 2500 grams. *Am J Dis Child* 1966; 112:359–365.
153. Bacola E, Behrle FC, de Schweintzl, et al. Perinatal and environmental factors in late neurogenic sequelae: II. Infants having birth weights from 1500 to 2500 grams. *Am J Dis Child* 1966; 112:366–371.
154. Shannon DC, Gotuy F, Stein IM, Rogers MC, et al. Prevention of apnea and bradycardia in low-birthweight infants. *Pediatrics* 1975; 55:589–594.
155. Myers TF, Milsap RL, Krauss AN, et al. Low-dose theophylline therapy in idiopathic apnea of prematurity. *J Pediatr* 1980; 96:99–103.
156. Brooks JG. Respiratory tract and mediastinum. *In* CH Kempe, HK Silver, D O'Brien (eds). Pediatric Diagnosis Treatment, 6th ed. Los Altos, CA, Lange Medical Publications, 1980, p 316.
157. Hoppenbrouwers T, Hodgman JE, Arakawa K, et al. Sleep apnea as part of a sequence of events: A comparison of three month old infants at low and increased risk for sudden infant death syndrome (SIDS). *Neuropaediatrie* 1978; 9:320–327.
158. Brady JP, Ariagno R, Watts JL, et al. Apnea, hypoxemia, and aborted sudden infant death syndrome. *Pediatrics* 1978; 62:686–691.
159. Kelly DH, Shannon DC. Periodic breathing in infants with near miss sudden infant death syndrome. *Pediatrics* 1979; 63:355–360.
160. Haddad GC, Leistner HL, Lai TL, et al. Ventilation and ventilatory pattern during sleep in aborted sudden infant death syndrome. *Pediatr Res* 1981; 15:870–883.
161. Guilleminault C, Ariagno R, Korobkin R, et al. Sleep parameters and respiratory variables in 'near miss' sudden infant death syndrome infants. *Pediatrics* 1981; 68:354–360.
162. Fagenholz SA, O'Connell K, Shannon DC. Chemoreceptor function and sleep state in apnea. *Pediatrics* 1976; 58:31–36.
163. Hunt CE, McCulloch K, Brouillette RT. Diminished hypoxic ventilatory responses in near-miss sudden infant death syndrome. *J Appl Physiol* 1981; 50:1313–1317.
164. Leistner HL, Haddad GG, Epstein RA, et al. Heart rate and heart rate variability during sleep in aborted sudden infant death syndrome. *J Pediatr* 1980; 97:51–55.
165. Korobkin R, Guilleminault C. Neurologic abnormalities in near miss for sudden infant death syndrome infants. *Pediatrics* 1979; 64:369–374.
166. Black L, Steinschneider A, Sheehe PR. Neonatal respiratory instability and infant development. *Child Dev* 1979; 50:561–564.
167. Gupta PR, Guilleminault C, Dorfman LJ. Brainstem auditory-evoked potentials in near-miss sudden infant death syndrome. *J Pediatr* 1981; 98:791–794.
168. Orlowski J, Nodar RH, Lonsdale D. Abnormal brainstem auditory evoked potentials in infants with threatened sudden infant death syndrome. *Cleveland Clin Q* 1979; 46:77–81.
169. Kanarek DJ, Kelly DH, Shannon DC. Ventilatory chemoreceptor response in parents of children at risk for sudden infant death syndrome. *Pediatr Res* 1981; 15:1402–1405.

170. Miller AJ, Dunmire C. Characterization of the post-natal development of superior laryngeal nerve fibers in the post-natal kitten. *J Neurobiol* 1976; 7:483–494.
171. Herbst JJ, Minton SD, Book LS. Gastroesophageal reflux in the 'near miss' sudden infant death syndrome. *J Pediatr* 1978; 92:73–75.
172. Leape LL. Respiratory arrest in infants secondary to gastroesophageal reflux. *Pediatrics* 1977; 60:924–928.
173. Plaxico DT, Loughlin GM. Nasopharyngeal reflux and neonatal apnea: Their relationship. *Am J Dis Child* 1981; 135:793–794.
174. Brooks JG. Apnea of infancy and sudden infant death syndrome. *Am Dis Child* 1982; 136:1012–1023.
175. Shannon DC, Marsland DW, Gould JB, et al. Central hypoventilation during quiet sleep in two infants. *Pediatrics* 1976; 57:342–346.
176. Wells HH, Kattwinkel J, Morrow JB. Control of ventilation in Ondine's curse. *J Pediatr* 1980; 96:865–897.
177. Fleming PJ, Cade D, Bryan MH, et al. Congenital central hypoventilation and sleep state. *Pediatrics* 1980; 66:425–428.
178. Kelly DH, Shannon DC, Cahen L. Effects of theophylline on apnea in young infants. *Am Rev Respir Dis* 1981; 123:85.
179. Aranda JV, Davis J, Turmen T, et al. Effect of caffeine on control of breathing in near-miss sudden infant death syndrome (SIDS). *Pediatr Res* 1981; 15:491.
180. Kelly DH, Shannon DC. Treatment of apnea and excessive periodic breathing in full-term infants. *Pediatrics* 1981; 68:183–186.
181. Rosen JP, Danish M, Pharm D, et al. Theophylline pharmacokinetics in the young infant. *Pediatrics* 1979; 64:248–251.
182. Hunt CE. Reversible central apnea in an infant with cyanotic heart disease. *Chest* 1980; 77:565–567.
183. Reite M, Jackson D, Cahoun RL, et al. Sleep physiology at high altitude. *Electroencephalogr Clin Neurophysiol* 1975; 38:463–471.
184. Sutton JR, Gray GW, Houston CS. Effects of duration at altitude and acetazolamide on ventilation and oxygenation during sleep. *Sleep* 1980; 3:455–464.
185. Robertson PL, Aldrich MS, Hansah SM, et al. Stroke associated with obstructive sleep apnea in a child with sickle cell anemia. *Ann Neurol* 1988; 23:614–616.
186. Sutton JR, Houston CS, Mansell AL, et al. Effect of acetazolamide on hypoxemia during sleep at high altitude. *N Engl J Med* 1979; 301:1329–1331.
187. Martin RJ, Pennock BE, Orr WC, et al. Respiratory mechanics and timing during sleep occlusive apnea. *J Appl Physiol: Respir Environ Exercise Physiol* 1980; 48:432–437.
188. Wolkove N, Altose MD, Kelsen SG, et al. Respiratory control abnormalities in alveolar hypoventilation. *Am Rev Respir Dis* 1980; 122:163–167.
189. Hyland RH, Jones NL, Powles ACP, et al. Primary alveolar hypoventilation treated with nocturnal electrophrenic respiration. *Am Rev Respir Dis* 1978; 117:165–172.
190. Lugliani R, Whipp BJ, Wasserman K. Doxapram hydrochloride: A res-

piratory stimulant for patients with primary alveolar hypoventilation. *Chest* 1979; 76:414–419.
191. Guilleminault C, Eldridge FL, Simmons FB, et al. Sleep apnea in eight children. *Pediatrics* 1979; 58:23–30.
192. Wood JD, Watson J, Drucker AJ. The effect of hypoxia on brain gamma amino butyric acid levels. *J Neurochem* 1968; 15:603.
193. David J, Carlsson A, MacMillan V, et al. Brain tryptophan hydroxylation dependence on arterial oxygen saturation. *Science* 1973; 182:72.
194. Guilleminault C, Billiard M, Montplaisir J, et al. Altered states of consciousness in disorders of daytime sleepiness. *J Neurol Sci* 1975; 26:377.
195. Sukerman S, Healy GB. Sleep apnea syndrome associated with upper airway obstruction. *Laryngoscope* 1979; 84:878–885.
196. Orlowski JP, Herrell DW, Moodie DS. Narcotic antagonist therapy of the obesity hypoventilation syndrome. *Crit Care Med* 1982; 10:604–607.
197. Guilleminault C, Kurobkin R, Winkle R. A review of 50 children with obstructive sleep apnea syndrome. *Lung* 1981; 159:275–287.
198. Guilleminault C. Obstructive sleep apnea syndrome and its treatment in children: Areas of agreement and controversy. *Pedia Pulmonol* 1987; 3: 429–436.
199. Lembo RM. Sleep apnea and related disorders in infants and children. *Ear, Nose Throat J* 1985; 64:8/56–27/69.

10

Sleep and Critical Care Medicine

Kevin S. Hara, M.D.,
and
John W. Shepard, Jr., M.D.

Significant respiratory and cardiovascular alterations occur during sleep, even in normal man.[1] In disease states, these alterations can produce significant stresses on oxygen delivery to the heart as well as the central nervous system.[2] The critically ill and unstable intensive care unit patient may not be able to tolerate these effects. It is therefore essential that critical care personnel have a thorough understanding of sleep and its relation to disease. In addition, critical care personnel should be familiar with the diagnosis and management of patients with primary sleep disorders such as obstructive sleep apnea. These patients are not uncommonly admitted to the intensive care unit. Even when unsuspected, the extensive respiratory and hemodynamic monitoring that occurs in intensive care units can uncover previously unrecognized sleep disorders and their effects. Lack of appreciation that these cardiopulmonary alterations are secondary to the effects of a sleep disorder can lead to their improper treatment.

Another aspect of sleep and critical care medicine is sleep deprivation. Sleep deprivation, along with its physiological and cognitive effects, is an almost universal phenomenon of intensive care units,

Martin RJ: Cardiorespiratory Disorders During Sleep, 2nd Edition. Futura Publishing Company, Inc., Mount Kisco, NY, © 1990.

both for the patients and often for the critical care personnel. While sleep deprivation has its own adverse effects, it also can mask sleep-related disorders and not allow them to be manifest until after a patient leaves the intensive care unit and is allowed to sleep. Adverse consequences may then occur during sleep in a less well-supervised setting.

This chapter will review sleep as it relates to the practice of critical care medicine. Background will first be provided by summarizing the pertinent physiologic changes that occur during sleep in normal adults. Then, the relation of sleep to the specific diseases found in the intensive care unit will be reviewed. Finally, sleep deprivation and its effects on the practice of critical care medicine will be discussed. There may be some basis for the unwritten commandment that "thou should not wean or extubate at night." We should be more careful at night because of sleep.

Sleep in Normals

Respiratory Physiology

The degree of hypoxemia and resultant hemodynamic alterations that can occur during sleep are important because of the associated risk to the cardiovascular system. In order to appreciate these effects, an understanding of the physiologic changes that occur during sleep in normal man is a prerequisite.

In normal adult humans, tidal volume (V_T) decreases by 15%–25% during sleep and is shallower during REM than non-REM sleep.[3,4] The respiratory frequency (f) increases slightly during non-REM sleep compared to wakefulness and is irregular during REM sleep. These reciprocal changes in V_T and f result in a net decrease in minute ventilation during non-REM sleep on the order of 10%. Changes in minute ventilation in REM sleep are variable, but overall fall to a similar extent. Because alveolar ventilation decreases in parallel with minute ventilation, there is an increase in the partial pressure of carbon dioxide in arterial blood ($PaCO_2$) of 2–8 mm Hg and a decrease in the partial pressure of oxygen (PaO_2) of 3–10 mm Hg.[5–8] Arterial oxygen content and oxyhemoglobin saturation (Sao_2) decrease by less than 2% during sleep because PaO_2 is positioned on the flat portion of the oxyhemoglobin dissociation in normal subjects.

These changes in arterial blood gases occur despite a 10%–15% decrease in oxygen consumption and carbon dioxide production during sleep.[6,9,10]

Apneic episodes may occur during sleep in normal adults, but they occur with a frequency of less than 5 per hour and seldom exceed 20 seconds in duration.[11,12] Studies on breath holding in normal man have been performed to explain the non-steady-state mechanisms of hypoxemia in sleep apnea and have shown that the initial lung volume, which reflects lung oxygen stores, is a major determinant of hypoxemia.[13] However, disease states that decrease arterial oxygen saturation and position on the oxyhemoglobin dissociation curve also play an important role.[14] Other factors that determine the degree of hypoxemia are the apnea duration, regional lung oxygen stores determined by ventilation/perfusion matching at apnea onset, mixed venous oxygen saturation, and cardiac output.[15]

During sleep, the upper airway dilating muscles become hypotonic, contributing to an increase in upper airway resistance.[16,17] The intercostal muscles also become hypotonic and this, along with the supine position, is associated with a decrease in functional residual capacity.[18,19] The intercostal muscles become atonic during REM sleep, resulting in further dependence of ventilation upon the diaphragm whose activity is relatively well maintained.[19,20] The dynamic compliance of the lungs does not change.[21]

The ventilatory response to hypercapnia and hypoxia are decreased during sleep, and this decreased response is more prominent in REM than non-REM sleep.[22–25] The mechanism of the decreased ventilatory responses to hypercapnia and hypoxemia during sleep are thought to be multifactorial, with increased airway resistance contributing to the reduction in ventilatory output along with decreases in central ventilatory drive.[4,17] Arousal from sleep occurs consistently with increases in $PaCO_2$ of 6–15 mm Hg.[26] In contrast, the arousal to hypoxia is weaker and often will not even occur with reductions in SaO_2 to 75%.[24,27]

Coughing does not occur during either non-REM or REM sleep in the absence of arousal. The cough response to a laryngeal stimulation is decreased during sleep and greater laryngeal stimulation is required to cause arousal and cough during REM than non-REM sleep. Therefore, an important mechanism for the clearance of aspirated pharyngeal or gastric contents is impaired during sleep. In addition, there is a decrease in mucociliary clearance during sleep.[28] In infants, laryngeal stimulation commonly results in glottis closure and obstructive apnea.

Overactivity of this reflex has been postulated to be one possible etiological mechanism for the sudden infant death syndrome.[29]

Cardiovascular Physiology

During non-REM sleep, mean systemic arterial blood pressure decreases about 5%–9% during stages 1 and 2, and approximately 8%–14% during stages 3 and 4.[30–32] During REM sleep, wide fluctuations in arterial blood pressure occur along with an average increase in pressure of 4%–6% above the non-REM sleep values. There is a small rise in the pulmonary artery pressure during sleep, but the values remain within the normal physiologic range. This averages from 18/8 mm Hg during wakefulness to 23/12 mm Hg during sleep.[33] Cardiac output has been reported to be both unchanged and decreased during sleep, falling by as much as 26% during REM sleep.[31,34,35]

In non-REM sleep the heart rate decreases by 5%–8% and becomes more regular.[31,32,35] In REM sleep, heart rate returns to awake levels and becomes highly variable.[36] These changes are produced by changes in sympathetic and parasympathetic tone.[37] Accompanying the reduction in heart rate during sleep is a reduction in ventricular ectopy.[38–40] Supraventricular arrhythmias are generally unchanged. Sinus arrhythmia and sinus bradycardia with pauses of up to 2 seconds duration are commonly observed with type 1, second-degree atrioventricular heart block occurring in up to 6% of young adult men.[38] No significant electrocardiographic changes occur in Q-T intervals, ST segments, or T-wave amplitude.[41] Sudden nocturnal death does occur in the apparently healthy.[42] Holter monitoring during sudden death in patients with cardiac disease has shown ventricular tachycardia degenerating to ventricular fibrillation to be the predominant mechanism, with bradyarrhythmias being responsible in a minority of patients.[43] It has been postulated that sudden nocturnal death can occur during sleep, with prolonged sinus arrest and ventricular tachycardia during REM sleep having been observed and proposed as possible mechanisms.[44,45]

Sleep and Diseases in the Intensive Care Unit

Critical care medicine is a multisystem specialty. The impact of sleep on this practice, however, can be broken down into the respiratory effects, cardiovascular effects, and the effects on other organ systems.

Respiratory Disorders

Obstructive Sleep Apnea

Obstructive sleep apnea (OSA) is the most important primary sleep disorder that will be present in patients admitted to the intensive care unit. Its prevalence has been estimated at 2%–4% of the general adult male population. Therefore, it will be common in patients admitted to the intensive care unit, either as the primary disorder or as a complicating disease. Because it is common, it should be looked for in all patients, especially those who are obese or have upper airway abnormalities. Patients with obstructive sleep apnea syndrome have repetitive episodes of apnea during sleep despite ventilatory efforts because of obstruction from recurrent upper airway collapse. Apneas of greater than 10 seconds' duration with an apnea index (apneas/hour of sleep) of more than 5 are criteria that have been used for the diagnosis. However, patients with clinically symptomatic OSA usually have an apnea plus hypopnea index (AHI) of greater than 30 events per hour. Patients with severe obstructive sleep apnea generally have an AHI greater than 60 per hour, with a mean apnea duration of 30 seconds and frequent arterial oxygen desaturations to less than 75%. Characteristically, these patients are overweight snorers with daytime hypersomnolence. A brief review of the respiratory and hemodynamic alterations will be discussed here. There is a more extensive review of obstructive sleep apnea in Chapter 4.

Gas exchange in patients with obstructive sleep apnea occurs under repetitive non-steady-state conditions of zero ventilation. The effects are similar to breath holding during wakefulness in normal subjects.[14] Obesity and the supine position combine to reduce end-expiratory lung volume and consequently lung oxygen stores, which must be utilized to maintain oxidative metabolism of the heart and brain during apnea. During apnea, the rate of fall and nadir of arterial oxygen saturation are determined by apnea duration, regional lung oxygen stores, mixed venous oxygen saturation, cardiac output, and baseline arterial oxygen saturation, which determines position on the oxyhemoglobin dissociation curve. The rate of fall of arterial oxygen saturation ranges from 0.23%–1.62% per second.[15]

There are cyclical increases in systemic arterial systolic and diastolic pressures during apnea.[46] The nadir of the systemic blood pressure occurs during the early to mid-portion of the apnea, after which it rises slowly, followed by an incremental increase after apnea termination (Fig. 1). The rise in systemic pressures can be severe. Schroeder et al. reported that in 22 patients with obstructive sleep apnea, six had phasic increases in systolic pressures exceeding 200 mm Hg and seven had elevations in diastolic pressures above 120 mm Hg.[46] It has also been reported that stepwise increases in systemic blood pressure can occur if there is insufficient time between apneic episodes for the return of blood pressures to baseline.[47] Sleep apnea has been associated with daytime systemic hypertension in 50%–60% of patients.[11,47] Conversely, 22%–30% of patients with essential hypertension have been found to have obstructive sleep apnea.[48–50] Urine and plasma catecholamine concentrations are increased in patients with sleep apnea and have been attributed to the repetitive stress of nocturnal oxygen desaturation.[51,52] This sustained sympathetic stimulation may be a mechanism for the development of sustained systemic hypertension. The administration of oxygen to patients with obstructive sleep apnea blunts the rise in systemic pressure.[46,53]

Patients with sleep apnea exhibit a phasic rise in pulmonary artery pressure that accompanies the hypoxia of apnea.[46,47,54,55] The magnitude of rise correlates with the degree of hypoxia and acidemia, and pulmonary artery systolic pressures exceeding 60 mm Hg have

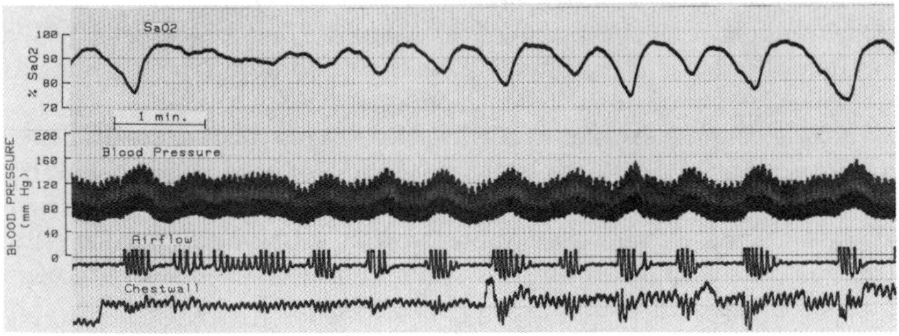

Figure 1. This tracing shows the characteristic cyclical elevations in systemic blood pressure observed in patients with obstructive sleep apnea. The last obstructive apnea with the greatest extent of oxyhemoglobin desaturation shows a characteristic gradual rise in systemic pressure throughout the latter portion of the apnea with a sudden additional increase in pressure occurring upon apnea termination.

been reported. Pulmonary edema may develop with obstructive sleep apnea.[56,57] Elevations in pulmonary artery wedge pressure occur with obstructive apnea and can reach levels contributory to the development of pulmonary edema. Buda et al. studied six patients with sleep apnea and found that the mean pulmonary artery wedge pressure increased gradually during apnea from 12 ± 2 to 20 ± 3 mm Hg.[58] Mechanisms postulated for the increase in pulmonary artery wedge pressure and myocardial dysfunction are hypoxia, right ventricular hypertension and its effect on left ventricular compliance and increased left ventricular afterload from systemic hypertension, and the markedly increased negative intrathoracic pressures. Atrial natriuretic factor has been found to be increased in obstructive sleep apnea, presumably because of repetitive atrial distension associated with negative intrathoracic pressures.[59] Atrial natriuretic factor has also been associated with high-altitude pulmonary edema and increased vascular permeability.[60]

Phasic changes in cardiac output occur with each episode of apnea. Although variable, apneas of 35–40 seconds duration are associated with a 30%–35% decrease in the cardiac output.[61] Cardiac output increases 10%–15% above baseline when ventilation resumes. This sudden increase in cardiac output at apnea termination coincides with the increases in blood pressure which occur at this point in time.

The increases in heart rate and blood pressure that occur at apnea termination result in an increase in myocardial work and oxygen consumption. However, myocardial oxygen delivery is compromised by the reduction in arterial oxygen content. This leaves myocardial oxygen delivery critically dependent on the capacity of the coronary circulation to vasodilate and provide adequate blood flow. The required levels of myocardial blood flow frequently approach coronary flow reserves, stressing myocardial oxygen balance to levels associated with maximal exercise (Fig. 2).[2,62] The bradycardia that occurs during apneas it teleologically protective as it reduces myocardial oxygen consumption and increases diastolic time, which enhances coronary arterial perfusion.

Cyclical sinus brady–tachyarrhythmia occurs in patients with sleep apnea.[63,64] Bradycardia occurs during apnea and is followed by a sudden tachycardia at apnea termination. The mechanism of bradycardia is related to enhanced vagal tone and can be blocked with atropine.[46,63,65] The degree of bradycardia is proportional to the duration of the apnea and the degree of desaturation.[65] The tachycardia

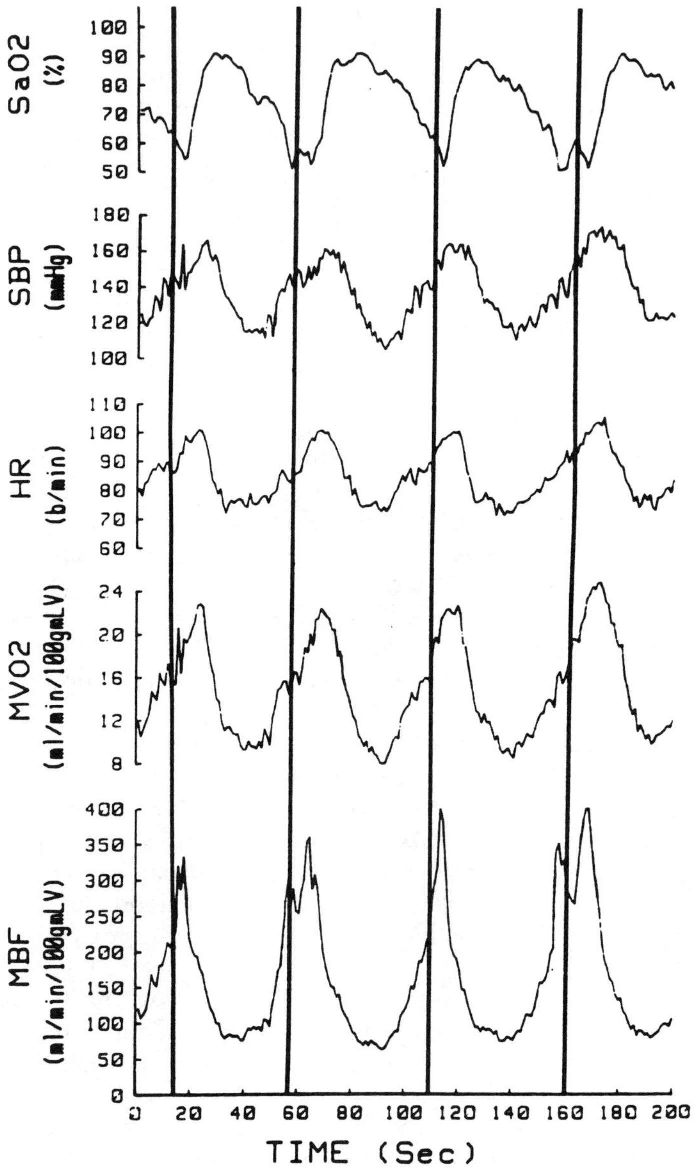

Figure 2. Sequential changes in SaO_2, systolic blood pressure (SBP), heart rate (HR), and myocardial oxygen consumption (MVO_2) estimated from the double product and myocardial blood flow (MBF) computed using the Fick equation with sequential obstructive apneas in one subject. The SaO_2 tracing has been corrected for an estimated 5-second delay in transit time from the heart to the ear. The vertical lines indicate apnea termination. (From: reference 62, with permission).

at apnea termination is due to a withdrawal of parasympathetic tone and an enhancement of sympathetic tone from the hypoxia.

Cardiac arrhythmias in patients with the obstructive sleep apnea syndrome are common. Guilleminault et al. studied 400 patients with obstructive sleep apnea with Holter monitoring and found 48% with nocturnal cardiac arrhythmias.[66] Sinus pauses exceeding 2 seconds were seen in 10%, sinus arrest of 2.5 to 13 seconds in 11%, and paroxysmal atrial fibrillation in 7%. Type 1 second-degree AV block was seen in 5% of sleep apnea patients and type 2 in 3%. Premature ventricular complexes exceeding 2 per minute were present in 20%, and ventricular tachycardia identified in 2%. Apnea-associated ventricular tachycardia occurred when the arterial oxygen saturation fell below 65%. Shepard et al. found ventricular ectopy in 74% of their patients with obstructive sleep apnea with a three-fold rise in frequency when the arterial oxygen saturation fell below a level of 60%.[67] They postulated that a critical threshold level of hypoxia was necessary for induction of myocardial irritability. It should be emphasized, however, that hypoxia probably represents only one factor in a complex relationship.

Sudden death during sleep has been described in patients with obstructive sleep apnea.[68] Presumably, some of these deaths are due to cardiac arrhythmias associated with nocturnal hypoxia, and in one patient a seizure, attributed to severe hypoxia, preceded cardiac arrest.

Patients with the obstructive sleep apnea syndrome usually present to the intensive care unit after they have developed right- or left-sided heart failure. In general, right-sided heart failure predominates in patients with concomitant lung disease, whereas left-sided heart failure develops in patients with underlying organic heart disease. Patients with obstructive sleep apnea are most commonly admitted to the intensive care unit when obstructive sleep apnea is not the primary intensive care problem, but rather a complicating or unrelated factor. When concomitant lung disease is present, obstructive sleep apnea is often overlooked and left unrecognized. If the disease is not suspected and these patients are thought to have respiratory failure from chronic obstructive pulmonary disease alone, the poor prognosis of that situation may keep these patients from receiving the appropriate treatment that they deserve. Another point to remember is that endotracheal intubation will bypass any upper airway obstruction and mask obstructive sleep apnea. Failing to recognize and treat obstructive sleep apnea as a contributing cause of respiratory failure can lead to extubation failures and prolongation of patient recovery.

Patency of the upper airway should always be considered when evaluating patients with obstructive sleep apnea. While the usual patient with OSA is simply an obese male with a short, thick neck, OSA is associated with multiple disorders in which anatomical derangements of the upper airway exist. These include macroglossia, micrognathia,[69] adenotonsillar hypertrophy,[70] lymphoma,[71] acromegaly,[72–74] myxedema,[75,76] amyloidosis,[77] and nasal obstruction.[78–82]. Edema of the upper airway following traumatic or prolonged orotracheal intubations may increase the risk of OSA. Nasotracheal intubation resulting in sinusitis, edema, and nasal occlusion postextubation will almost certainly increase this risk.

Physical examination during sleep reveals the characteristic snoring and apneic breathing pattern of obstructive sleep apnea. Paradoxical motion of the rib cage or abdomen reflecting ventilatory efforts against an occluded airway may be detected.[83] Auscultation over the upper airway in the supine position during wakefulness sometimes reveals abnormal breath sounds with wheezes or low-pitched vibratory sounds during either inspiration or expiration resembling soft snoring. The nursing and technical staff should all be instructed to observe patients' patterns of snoring and breathing during sleep, taught how to recognize apneas, and stress the importance of communicating these observations to the medical staff.

Oximetry can uncover the diagnosis by revealing the characteristic pattern of repetitive arterial oxygen desaturations during sleep. A continuous analog recording at a paper speed of 5 cm/h provides an excellent overview of the arterial oxygen saturation. The patterns of oxyhemoglobin desaturation provide major clues to the identification of sleep disordered breathing (Fig. 3). With current technology, transcutaneous oxygen and carbon dioxide monitoring has generally not been useful in adults because of increased skin thickness and the slow rate of diffusion equilibrium. Cardiac monitoring can uncover the diagnosis by displaying the cyclical sinus brady–tachyarrhythmias characteristic of obstructive sleep apnea. However, this may not be seen in patients with sinus node disease, diabetes, or those who are receiving drugs with anticholinergic activity. Cardiac monitoring may also reveal bradyarrhythmia or increased ventricular ectopy during sleep, which on closer inspection coincide with the episodes of oxygen desaturation during apnea (Fig. 4). Cyclical apnea associated blood pressure changes may be revealed by pulmonary or systemic arterial blood pressure monitoring. In addition, pulmonary artery pressures may exhibit marked respiratory variations reflecting the

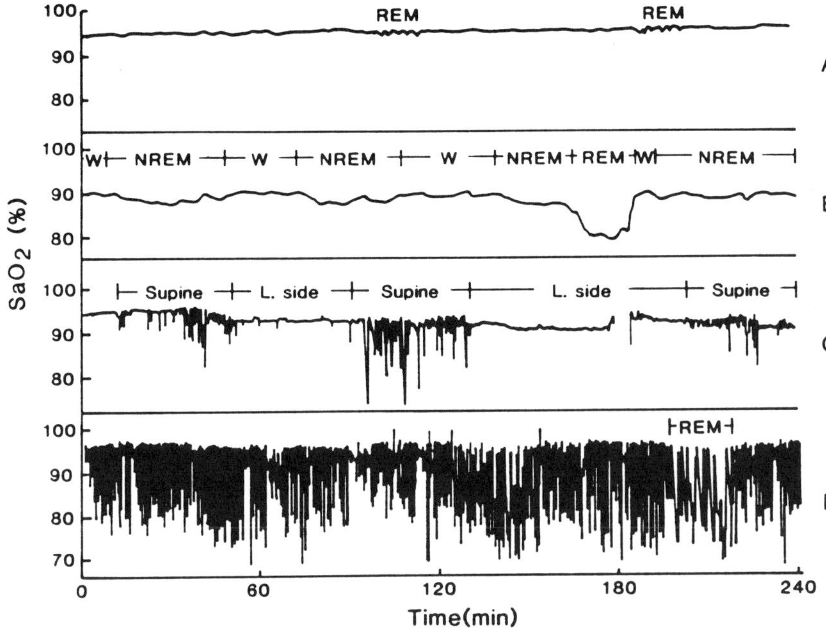

Figure 3. Ear oximetry tracings of arterial oxyhemoglobin saturation in (A) a normal subject with hypopneas during REM sleep, (B) a patient with chronic obstructive pulmonary disease demonstrating significant oxyhemoglobin desaturation during REM sleep, (C) a patient with positional obstructive sleep apnea who does not have disordered breathing events when sleeping on his left side, but has repetitive obstructive apneas and hypopneas when in the supine position, (D) a patient with nonpositional obstructive sleep apnea.

highly negative pleural pressures generated with respiratory efforts against an occluded airway.

All patients admitted to the ICU at night who have been intubated for respiratory failure or cardiopulmonary arrest are prime suspects for obstructive sleep apnea. When this occurs, elimination of the upper airway obstruction obscures the diagnosis, but results in dramatic clinical improvement.[84] Rebound deep sleep may occur and definitive diagnosis delayed until after the patient has been extubated.

The initial intensive care management of patients with severe obstructive sleep apnea focuses on the relief of the upper airway obstruction. If the diagnosis is correct, upper airway patency can be maintained with nasal continuous positive airway pressure (CPAP) or limited nasopharyngeal intubation,[85,86] thus avoiding endotracheal

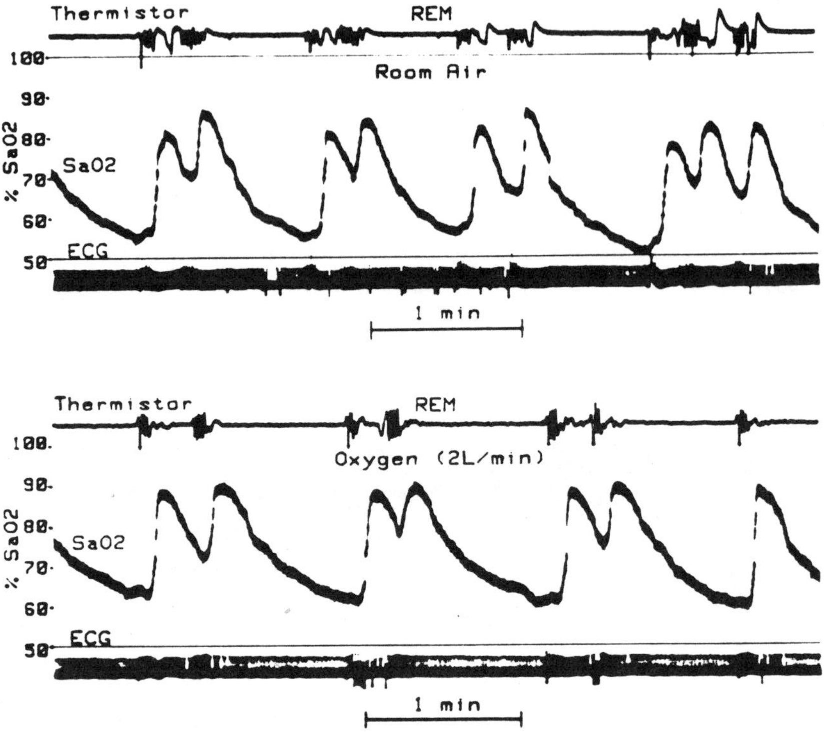

Figure 4. Tracings obtained in a patient with severe obstructive sleep apnea breathing room air, upper panel, and on supplemental oxygen, lower panel. Ventricular ectopy was present only during REM sleep when the most severe episodes of oxyhemoglobin desaturation were observed. Note that supplemental oxygen increased apnea duration, failed to eliminate the ventricular ectopy, but did ameliorate the severity of the oxyhemoglobin desaturation.

intubation. Temporarily keeping the patient awake will prevent apnea, while avoiding the supine sleep position will frequently ameliorate apnea severity. Nasal CPAP is highly effective and has become the treatment of choice for obstructive sleep apnea. The use of nasal CPAP devices can easily be implemented with the facilities available in the intensive care unit. Titration of the proper amount of CPAP ideally requires polysomnography. Pressures that are too low are ineffective. Conversely, excess pressures may be poorly tolerated and can lead to decreases in cardiac output and hypotension in hemodynamically unstable patients. In addition, excessively high levels of CPAP are occasionally associated with the development of central apneas. Pressure approximations can be achieved by beginning nasal CPAP at 5 cm H_2O and slowly increasing the pressure until snoring is eliminated and desaturations are minimized on oximetry.

Nasal CPAP is ineffective or not tolerated in a few patients. Life-threatening disease in these patients should be treated with tracheostomy. Tracheostomy cures the obstruction in obstructive sleep apnea and eliminates the associated nocturnal episodic systemic and pulmonary hypertension and dysrhythmias.[46,63,66,87] Tracheostomy in these patients, however, is not without risk.[88] Obestity and upper airway abnormalities make tracheostomy and endotracheal intubation technically difficult and surgical premedications need to be administered with extreme caution.[89–91] Therefore, elective endotracheal intubation along with stabilization of the patient should be performed before proceeding with tracheostomy. Emergency tracheostomy should rarely be necessary.

Medications such as barbiturates, narcotics, and benzodiazepines, which are respiratory depressants, should be avoided.[89,90,92] Patients have been reported to develop airway obstruction even while awake from narcotics and benzodiazepines.[89,90] The jaw thrust maneuver may be useful in temporarily supporting these patients. Oxygen should be administered with caution because of the possibility of inducing further reductions in alveolar ventilation, leading to hypercapnia acidosis. In addition, the acute administration of oxygen generally prolongs apnea duration and may not eliminate associated cardiac arrhythmias (Fig. 4).[93,94] Aminophylline has not been found to be useful in the treatment of obstructive sleep apnea.[95]

It should be emphasized that treatment of the complications of the obstructive sleep apnea syndrome should rely on treatment of the primary problem (OSA) rather than of the secondary effects. Apnea-induced bradycardia should be considered a protective mechanism with sinus pauses of 2–3 seconds being an appropriate physiological response. Longer pauses should prompt treatment of the obstruction rather than treatment with a cardiac pacemaker. Apnea-induced ventricular tachycardia should be considered life-threatening and treated definitively.

Obesity–Hypoventilation Syndrome

In 1956, Burwell et al. described a disorder of obesity and alveaolar hypoventilation that was called the Pickwickian syndrome.[96]

Since then it has been found that this syndrome usually occurs in association with obstructive sleep apnea, but it may also occur in its absence. The majority of obese patients with sleep apnea do not have alveolar hypoventilation and chronic CO_2 retention.[97] It is believed that the mechanism of alveolar hypoventilation in these patients reflects a balance between central ventilatory drive and the mechanical loads on the respiratory system.[98–102] A decrease in central ventilatory drive[99,100,101,103] and an increase in respiratory load from obesity,[104] upper airway resistence,[16,105] and concomitant lung disease[97,98,102,106] have been well documented in these patients. Another possible mechanism of alveolar hypoventilation in obesity is diaphragm dysfunction from overstretching.[107]

Daytime pulmonary hypertension occurs in a minority of patients with obstructive sleep apnea and correlates with the presence of daytime hypoxia and hypercarbia rather than with the severity of the obstructive sleep apnea.[98] Weitzenblum et al. performed right heart catheterization in 46 consecutive patients with obstructive sleep apnea.[108] Twenty percent had resting daytime pulmonary hypertension (mean PAP $\geq$ 20), but this was generally mild. These patients had a significantly lower awake Pao_2 and higher awake $Paco_2$. Apnea index, apnea duration, and lowest arterial oxygen saturation during sleep were not significantly correlated with pulmonary artery pressures. Daytime pulmonary hypertension may be seen despite a normal awake Pao_2.[46] However, clinically evident right heart failure generally does not occur in the absence of daytime hypoxia and hypercarbia.[98] Concomitant lung disease is a contributing, but not essential, factor.[108,109]

Patients with the obesity hypoventilation syndrome present to the intensive care unit when they are in decompensated right- or left-sided heart failure. Physical examination reveals obesity, cyanosis, plethora, jugular venous distension, right- or left-sided cardiac gallops, tricuspid or mitral regurgitant murmurs, rales, hepatomegaly, peripheral edema, or mental confusion. Chest radiography shows cardiomegaly and pulmonary hypertension as evidenced by an increase in central pulmonary artery size. Electrocardiography displays right-sided heart strain with P-pumonale, right ventricular hypertrophy, and right axis deviation. Hematological study shows polycythemia, while arterial blood gas analysis reveals hypoxemia and hypercapnia with or without acute respiratory acidosis. Pulmonary function studies frequently reveal restrictive or concomitant obstructive lung disease.

The hospital mortality of patients with the obesity–hypoventilation syndrome is high and has been reported to exceed 60% with common causes of death attributed to respiratory failure and pulmonary embolism.[110,111] Management of these patients in an intensive care setting should, therefore, be considered. Adequate oxygenation is of utmost priority. However, oxygen needs to be administered with caution as elimination of the hypoxic stimulus to breathe may lead to further reductions in alveolar ventilation and worsening hypercarbia with acidosis. Diuresis is necessary to treat the edema and lower mean circulatory pressures, which may contribute to elevated capillary pressures and the development of pulmonary, as well as peripheral, edema. Diuretic-associated metabolic alkalosis should be treated because of its adverse effect on ventilatory drive. Systemic hypertension and left ventricular afterload should also be controlled.

The flow-resistive and mass-elastic loads on the respiratory system need to be minimized. Upper airway resistance is lowered by avoidance of the supine position, nasal CPAP, and nasopharyngeal or endotracheal intubation. Tracheostomy is performed if the less invasive alternatives are unsuccessful. In some patients even tracheostomy may fail to completely correct the hypoventilation because of underlying deficiencies in central ventilatory drive.[90,100,112] Therapy to reduce lower airway resistance in patients with coexisting obstructive airway disease should also be undertaken. If present, gastric distension should be alleviated as it will aggravate the mass-elastic load associated with obesity. Finally, weight loss is required to decrease the respiratory load over the long term. Because success with dietary restriction alone is generally poor, surgery should be considered on an individual basis.

Central respiratory drive should be maximized. Clearly, drugs with CNS-depressant activity should be avoided. Medroxyprogesterone acetate can be used to stimulate respiratory drive and has been found helpful in managing these patients.[113,114] Acute metabolic alkalosis should be avoided and chronic metabolic alkalosis cautiously corrected if present. Acetazolamide can help in achieving this provided there is no intrinsic lung disease that would limit ventilatory output in response to an increase in central ventilatory drive.

Gross obesity makes nursing care difficult. Physical activities and ambulation are limited and special beds are often necessary to accommodate the large size of these patients. These patients are prone to develop deep venous thrombosis and pulmonary embolism because of their obesity, immobility, polycythemia, and heart failure. Adequate deep venous thrombosis prophylaxis is important for optimal management.

Periodic Breathing, Cheyne-Stokes Respiration, and Central Sleep Apnea

Periodic breathing occurs when there are fluctuations in central respiratory drive resulting in a regular crescendo–decrescendo ventilatory pattern secondary to changes in tidal ventilation with relative constancy of respiratory rate. Cheyne-Stokes respiration occurs when short episodes of apnea occur during the hypoventilatory phase of the periodic breathing pattern. Periodic breathing and Cheyne-Stokes respiration become more prominent during sleep but are also present during wakefulness. Periodic breathing occurs in normal man at sleep onset because of differences in the CO_2 set point between wakefulness and sleep. Ventilation fluctuates until non-REM stage 2 sleep is firmly established, after which ventilation becomes regular. Periodic breathing is common in the elderly population, but Cheyne-Stokes or central apneic patterns likely to develop only if there is coexisting cardiac and/or neurological disease. Periodic breathing is also accentuated by clinical stiuations that lead to the development of hypoxia, hypocapnia, and an increase in the ventilatory response to carbon dioxide.[115,116] Congestive heart failure and ascent to altitude are the classical situations in which hypocapnia and hypoxia with increased ventilatory drive contribute to periodic breathing. During REM sleep, periodic breathing may disappear as breathing comes under the behavioral control system as compared with the autonomic or chemical control system active during non-REM sleep. Circulatory slowing and a phase delay in the detection of changes in Pao_2, $Paco_2$, and pH by the central compared with the peripheral chemoreceptors may contribute to the development of periodic breathing in congestive heart failure and resolve with treatment.[117,118] Cheyne-Stokes respiration also occurs in neurologic disorders secondary to dysfunction of the respiratory control centers.

Central sleep apnea occurs when there are apneic episodes during sleep of at least 10 seconds duration due to an absence of central ventilatory drive. Central sleep apnea exists by definition when the apneic phase exceeds 10 seconds in patients with Cheyne-Stokes breathing. In contrast to these patients, in whom tidal ventilation gradually decreases and increases prior to and after the period of central apnea, there are patients in whom the central apneas have a relatively sudden onset and resumption of tidal ventilation upon apnea termination. Bradley et al. identified two groups of patients with this later type of central sleep apnea.[119] Although both groups had similar polysomnographic characteristics, one group had clinical features typical of obstructive sleep apnea with sleep disruption, excessive daytime somnolence, and normal daytime ventilatory drive and function. The other group had central sleep apnea with waking alveolar hypoventilation, hypoxemia, and decreased central ventilatory drive. There is often an overlap among central, mixed, and obstructive sleep apneas, with most patients showing a combination of these processes.

Oscillations in heart rate and cardiac rhythm have been observed to occur with the changes in oxygen saturation that result from Cheyne-Stokes respiration.[120] Heart rate and blood pressure changes also occur during central sleep apnea as they do in obstructive sleep apnea.[46,121] Oxygen administration blunts the rises in systemic pressures, but lengthens the duration of the apnea.[46]

Central sleep apnea may lead to arousals and sleep fragmentation as severe as that which occurs with obstructive sleep apnea. However, these patients usually present with a complaint of nocturnal insomnia rather than daytime hypersomnolence.[122] Treatment of central sleep apnea, Cheyne-Stokes respiration, and periodic breathing should focus on treatment of the underlying disease. For example, central sleep apnea occurring in associaton with hypothyroidism responds to thyroid replacement therapy.[123–125] The central sleep apnea that remains after treatment of obstructive sleep apnea may spontaneously resolve slowly over time.[90,100,112] Acetazolamide therapy may be useful in those patients with no identifiable brain-stem lesions and normal ventilation during wakefulness.[126] Respiratory stimulation with theophylline or medroxyprogesterone acetate may be tried but has not been found to be of much benefit. With severe oxygen desaturation and associated cardiac arrhythmias, oxygen should be administered. Oxygen therapy has also been reported to stimulate ventilation in some of these patients, presumably by relieving hypoxic brain-stem depression.[127] Oxygen may, however, prolong the duration of apneas and decrease alveolar ventilation. Nasal CPAP has been reported to be of benefit in some patients with central sleep apnea, although the mechanisms for this are not fully understood.[128,129] Generally, patients with central sleep apnea and chronic respiratory failure are difficult to treat and often require chronic positive- or negative-pressure mechanical ventilation or diaphragmatic pacing.[130–132]

Neuromuscular Disease

The relation of neuromuscular disease to sleep has been extensively reviewed in Chapter 8. The etiology of neuromuscular diseases may be diverse and includes central nervous system disorders, neuropathies, and myopathies. These patients are often admitted to the intensive care unit in respiratory failure that may result from either chronic progression of the underlying neuromuscular disease or superimposed acute decompensation secondary to aspiration, infection, or sedating medications. If the bulbar muscles are affected, obstructive sleep apnea may develop. These patients often have severe oxygen desaturation during sleep related to alveolar hypoventilation. Patients with diaphragm paralysis may decompensate during REM sleep when hypotonicity and atonicity of the chest wall musculature occurs.[133] Assisted mechanical ventilatory support is often required during the acute process. Chronic home mechanical ventilation may be needed after these patients leave the intensive care unit.[134] Nocturnal mechanical ventilation alone may be sufficient to support these patients and may improve their respiratory muscle strength, daytime ventilation, and hypersomnolence.[135–138] This can be performed with either negative- or positive-pressure ventilation. Negative-pressure ventilation, however, may result in upper airway obstruction and obstructive sleep apnea.[139] This problem is avoided with positive-pressure ventilation, and a promising new mode of administering this is through a nasal mask.[140–142]

Obstructive Lung Disease

The effects of sleep on patients with asthma and chronic obstructive pulmonary disease (COPD) have been discussed in Chapters 6 and 7. Patients requiring intensive care for these problems usually are in respiratory failure and may be on mechanical ventilation. They are thus critically ill and require optimization of all amenable factors. The effect of sleep on airway tone, ventilation, and esophageal activity should be kept in mind. Patients with chronic obstructive pulmonary disease have a high incidence of nocturnal oxygen desaturation. These patients generally will have a mean Sao_2 during sleep which is 2%–4% lower than their mean awake Sao_2. The severity of nocturnal oxyhemoglobin desaturation is greater in patients with more severe diurnal hypoxemia (Fig. 5).[52,143–149] Discreet episodes of oxyhemoglobin desaturation occur during REM sleep and will occur in about a fourth of patients to less than 85% even if the daytime Pao_2 is greater than 60 mm Hg.[52] These episodes result from transient reductions in ventilation, and oxygen therapy is effective in preventing these REM-related desaturations.[52,150] Pulmonary hyperinflation is present in patients with severe asthma and chronic obstructive pulmonary disease. When this occurs, the diaphragm is flattened and unable to function optimally. These patients, therefore, become dependent on their chest wall muscles for ventilation. During REM sleep these patients may acutely decompensate when their chest wall musculature becomes atonic.

Patients with COPD have a high incidence of ventricular ectopy. Shepard et al. reported on 42 patients with moderately severe chronic obstructive pulmonary disease ($FEV_1\%$ = 51 ± 12%).[151] Premature ventricular contractions were detected in 64% of the patients and were complex (multiform and/or repetitive) in 40%. Ventricular tachycardia, while occasionally observed, is usually asymptomatic. Pre-

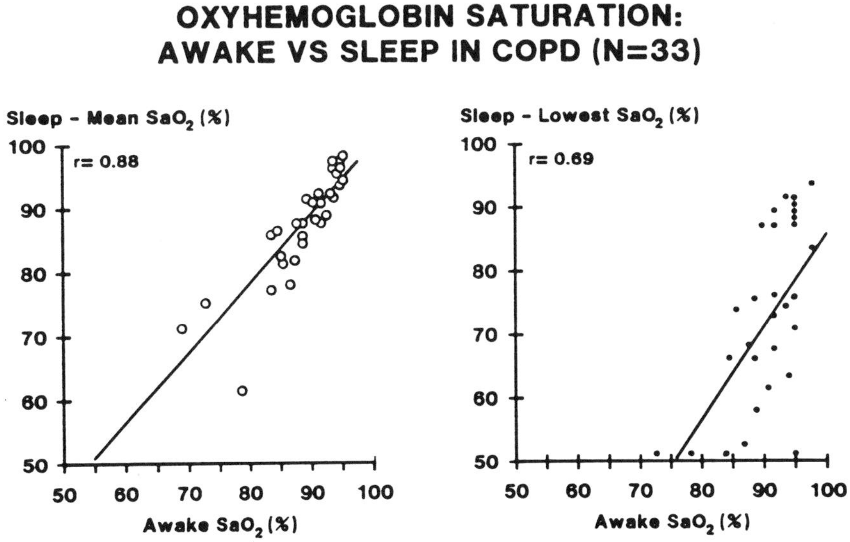

Figure 5. Relationships between mean and lowest Sao_2 during sleep compared with awake resting Sao_2 values in 33 patients with moderate to severe chronic obstructive pulmonary disease.

sumably, nocturnal desaturation can precipitate lethal ventricular arrhythmias. Fifteen patients in the series of Shepard et al. had both baseline PVCs and nocturnal desaturation to less than 80%. With the desaturation, there was a 150% increase in premature ventricular contractions in 40% of the patients (Fig. 6). The induction of arrhythmias during sleep in these patients is probably complex and due not only to hypoxia, but also to hypercapnia, acidosis, increases adrenergic activity, coexisting coronary artery disease, hypokalemia, and medications (theophylline, B-agonists, digoxin, etc.). Bradyarrhythmias are seldom observed in patients with chronic obstructive pulmonary disease, in contrast to the frequent occurrence of bradyarrhythmias in patients with obstructive sleep apnea.

Restrictive Lung Disease

Patients with interstitial lung disease generally have an increased respiratory drive, hyperventilation, and hypocapnia.[152] The hyper-

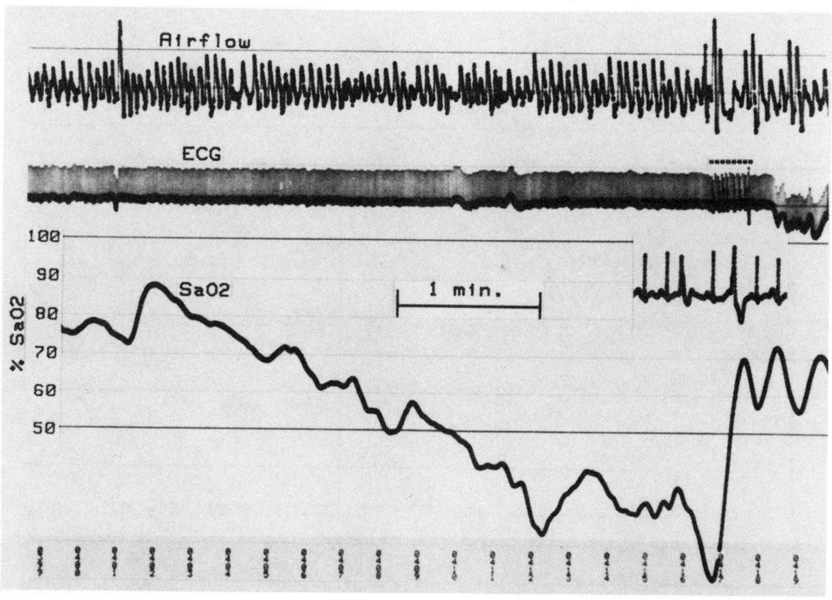

Figure 6. Episode of prolonged oxyhemoglobin desaturation during REM sleep in a patient with chronic obstructive pulmonary disease with ventricular ectopy occurring at the termination of the desaturation.

ventilation continues during non-REM sleep and apnea is uncommon.[153] When apnea does occur, oxyhemoglobin saturation falls rapidly, presumably due to small lung volumes and lung oxygen stores. During REM sleep hypoventilation and oxygen desaturation are common, with desaturation being more severe than that which occurs during maximal exercise.[154] The REM-related loss of intercostal and accessory muscle function required to maintain lung volume and ventilation in these patients is considered to be the mechanism responsible for the decompensation. Thus, as in patients with obstructive lung disease, acute respiratory decompensation may occur during sleep in a patient in the intensive care unit who is marginal during wakefulness. Sleep disruption is characteristic, especially in those with an awake oxygen saturation less than 90%, and these patients usually complain of insomnia rather than hypersomnia. Coughing contributes to the frequent nocturnal arousals and fragmented sleep that these patients demonstrate. Because of the increased respiratory drive in these patients, ventilatory stimulants are not necessary and oxygen therapy is generally not associated with hypoventilation.[155]

Patients with restrictive lung disease due to chest wall abnormalities also may have oxygen desaturation during sleep.[138,156,157] The effects of sleep on patients with severe kyphoscoliosis have already been discussed in Chapter 8. As in patients with interstitial lung diseases, these patients may have nocturnal oxygen desaturation of greatest degree during REM sleep. Chronic nocturnal mechanical ventilation may result in improvement in both symptoms and arterial blood gases during both sleep and wakefulness.[158,159]

Cardiovascular Disorders

The hypoxemia that occurs during sleep has the potential for aggravating myocardial ischemia in patients with coronary artery disease and for inducing arrhythmias in patients with myocardial irritability. These effects are further accentuated in REM sleep, sleep apnea, and lung disease because of the further alterations that occur in oxygenation, autonomic tone, and hemodynamic status. A high incidence of obstructive sleep apnea has been found in patients with coronary artery disease.[160]

Coronary Artery Disease

Nocturnal angina is a well-recognized entity. It has been shown that nocturnal angina often correlated with REM sleep.[161–163] Nowlin et al. studied four patients for a total of 12 nights and observed 39 episodes of nocturnal chest pain accompanied by significant electrocardiographic changes.[161] Thirty-two of these episodes were associated with REM sleep. Prinzmetal's variant angina has also been observed to occur during REM sleep.[163] The mechanism of nocturnal angina has been postulated to be due to the hypoxia, autonomic alterations, and increases in heart rate and blood pressure that occur during REM sleep. The same mechanisms may not be responsible for the nocturnal angina that occurs following acute myocardial infarction. Broughton and Baron reported that nocturnal angina generally occurred on days 4 and 5 after myocardial infarction during the deeper stages of non-REM sleep.[164] The mechanism of myocardial ischemia in this instance was postulated to be due to the decrease in blood pressure that occurs during these stages of sleep. Silent myocardial ischemia has been studied with continuous electrocardiographic monitoring and initially was observed to occur predominantly during sleep.[165,166] A more recent study reported that myocardial ischemia occurred most frequently within 2 hours of awakening.[167] The hourly frequency of myocardial infarction onset has been reported to increase sharply beginning at 5 AM and to reach its peak at 9 AM.[168]

Cardiac Arrhythmias

Although ventricular ectopy has been found to decrease in sleep in normal subjects,[38–40] this may not be true in patients with heart disease. Increased ventricular ectopy, including ventricular tachycardia, has been observed during REM sleep with and without associated ischemic ST-segment changes.[162,165,169] However, others have found no changes[164,170] or a decrease[171] in ventricular ectopy during sleep. It may be that subsets of patients such as those with sleep disordered breathing were those in whom ventricular ectopy increased during sleep.[67,151,170]

Congestive Heart Failure

Periodic breathing and Cheyne-Stokes respiration are common in patients with congestive heart failure and may be the presenting feature of this disorder.[172,173] These patients often have a markedly disturbed sleep with increased oxyhemoglobin desaturation, frequent arousals, nocturnal insomnia, and daytime hypersomnolence. Arousals usually coincide with the hyperventilation phase and awakenings are occasionally associated with the sensation of dyspnea.[174] When patients awaken with dyspnea following an obstructive apneic event, the sensation dissipates rapidly, whereas dyspnea associated with congestive heart failure, pulmonary edema, and cardiac asthma resolves slowly. Pulmonary edema has been reported as a presenting feature of obstructive sleep apnea.[175] The mechanism of pulmonary edema in this situation is possibly related to the mechanism of pulmonary edema that can occur with acute airway obstruction.[176–178] This has been postulated to be due to the generation of a markedly negative intrathoracic pressure and resultant transudation of fluid into the interstitium. Nocturnal ventilation improves following effective treatment of congestive heart failure[172,179]; however, the prognosis for patients with left ventricular failure and Cheyne-Stokes respiration is poor. A recent study reported a mortality rate of 40% over 6 months of follow-up.[180]

Other Disorders

Neurologic Diseases Associated with Sleep Apnea

A variety of neurologic disorders have been found to produce sleep apnea. Brain-stem infarction and neoplasms directly damage the respiratory centers and often produce dysfunction of the pharyngeal musculature. Alveolar hypoventilation and central and obstructive sleep apnea have all been observed and can result in respiratory failure requiring mechanical ventilation.[181–183] Bilateral cervical cordotomy, a procedure done for pain management, can produce central sleep apnea lasting for days to weeks after the procedure.[184] The apnea has been attributed to the disruption of ventilatory feedback pathways. Other neurologic diseases associated with sleep apnea and/or alveolar hypoventilation include syringobulbia-myelia,[185] the Arnold-Chiari malformation,[186] radiation necrosis,[187] encephalitis,[188,189] and poliomyelitis.[190–192]

Seizures

Clinical and electroencephalographic evidence of seizure activity predominantly occurs during sleep or shorly after arousal from sleep.

Sleep deprivation, which is endemic in the intensive care unit setting, is well-recognized to reduce seizure threshold.[193] In addition, nocturnal seizures may disrupt sleep, contributing to sleep deprivation. Hypoxia is probably the most prevalent clinical problem dealt with in the intensive care unit and, if sufficiently severe, leads to hypoxic encephalopathy with myoclonic activity. Fortunately, clinical experience in patients with sleep apnea has shown that transient hypoxia seldom induces seizure activity. Guilleminault et al. have described only one patient with severe obstructive sleep apnea who had a seizure and cardiac arrest presumably due to hypoxia.[68] It is surprising that the severity of the hypoxemia and elevation in intracranial pressures that have been reported in obstructive sleep apnea do not have more serious central nervous system consequences.[194]

Renal Diseases

Urine output, along with the excretion of sodium, chloride, potassium, and calcium, decreases during sleep in normal subjects.[1] This normal physiological response should be considered when evaluating decreases in urine output during sleep in patients in the intensive care unit. Obstructive sleep apnea has been found to be common in patients on chronic hemodialysis.[195] The mechanism for this is unknown but is probably not related to testosterone administration, which is common in patients with chronic renal failure.

Gastrointestinal Diseases

Gastrointestinal bleeding is a frequent problem in the intensive care unit. Although gastric acid secretion is lower during the nocturnal compared with the diurnal hours, intermittent relaxation of lower esophageal sphincter pressure allows gastroesophageal reflux to occur.[196,197] Primary peristalsis secondary to swallowing occurs at a frequency of about once a minute during wakefulness and is the primary mechanism of esophageal acid clearance, with salivary buffering contributing to the neutralization of remaining acidity.[198] During sleep, both swallowing and salivary secretion are reduced. This results in prolongation of acid clearance from the esophagus, which contributes to the development of erosive esophagitis.[199,200] The installation of acid into the distal esophagus frequently induces arousal and bursts of swallowing, which clears the acid but fragments sleep. Because the instillation of water is less likely to induce arousals, neutralization of gastric acidity throughout the night may improve sleep continuity in addition to limiting mucosal injury.

Effect of Drug Administration in the Intensive Care Unit on Sleep

A comprehensive review of the various drugs that affect sleep is beyond the scope of this chapter. A few of the drugs that are frequently used in the intensive care unit will be briefly discussed. Generally, any drug that can affect the central nervous system can also affect sleep. In general, drugs that depress the central nervous system and have a "beneficial" effect on sleep have the detrimental side effect of depressing ventilation. For this reason, sedative–hypnotics and narcotics must be used cautiously in patients with impaired respiratory status who are not on mechanical ventilatory support. These agents also affect sleep architecture. Benzodiazepines suppress slow-wave, but have little effect on REM, sleep, whereas narcotics predominantly suppress REM and, to a lesser extent, slow-wave sleep.[201,202] Tricyclic antidepressants decrease REM sleep. This effect has been considered important to the small beneficial effect of protriptyline in the treatment of obstructive sleep apnea.[203] Epidural anesthesia has also been reported to cause respiratory failure in patients with central sleep apnea.[204] However, the epidural route likely causes less respiratory suppression than intravenous narcotics and may be used with caution in patients with obstructive sleep apnea.[205]

Diuretics may have indirect effects on sleep secondary to alterations in electrolyte balance and respiratory drive. Thiazides and furosemide often contribute to the development of a metabolic alkalosis with hypokalemia. Metabolic alkalosis decreases ventilatory drive, while hypokalemia can potentiate ventricular ectopy during nocturnal hypoxemia.[151] In contrast, acetazolamide, which leads to the development of a metabolic acidosis, stimulates ventilation. This drug has been found useful in improving nocturnal sleep by decreasing periodic breathing and apneas at high altitude, as well as in the treatment of selected patients with central sleep apnea.[126,206]

The central nervous system stimulant effects of theophylline are well recognized as disrupting to sleep, especially at higher dosages. This adverse effect on sleep has been observed in patients being treated with theophylline for apnea of prematurity, obstructive sleep apnea, and nocturnal asthma.[95,207,208] Clinically, the $beta_2$ selective agonists used for airway smooth muscle relaxation are probably associated with less sleep disruption. This is most likely true when delivered via inhalation but is also possible when given orally.[209] Although they suppress REM sleep, beta blockers paradoxically increase dream recall, probably by increasing the frequency of nocturnal awakenings.[210,211] Because dopamine is an inhibitory neurotransmitter in the carotid body that acts to decrease the ventilatory response to hypoxia, caution is advised when administering dopamine to patients dependent on hypoxia as a stimulus to maintain ventilation.[212] The effects on sleep of many other drugs used in the intensive care unit, such as calcium-channel blockers and angiotensin-converting-enzyme inhibitors, have simply not been studied.

Effect of Disease and the ICU Environment on Sleep and Sleep Deprivation

Mental status changes in the critically ill are a common occurrence. Often, no organic etiology is identified, and these patients are diagnosed as having the ICU syndrome or one of its many synonyms: ICU psychosis, postoperative psychosis, cardiac psychosis, etc. The pathogenesis of this disorder is believed to involve a complex interplay of stresses from physical, psychological, and environmental factors. A major component of this process is sleep deprivaton. Prolonged sleep deprivaton in normal subjects results in irritability, disorientation, delusions, and hallucinations with overt psychosis in some individuals.[213,214] These same symptoms are observed in patients with the ICU syndrome.[215,216] Both disorders resolve rapidly with adequate sleep.[214,217] The importance of adequate sleep in the intensive care unit is exemplified by the American Association of Critical-Care Nurses' selection of research into the optimization of sleep–rest patterns and prevention of sleep deprivation in the critically ill as their top research priority.[218]

Physiological factors in the generation of sleep deprivation in the intensive care unit involve the underlying disease and the effects of therapeutic interventions. Pain is frequently a major factor that impairs sleep and is due to either the underlying disease, surgery, or invasive procedures. Patients often receive inadequate analgesia in intensive care units because of the fear of oversedation and respiratory depression. Inadequate pain control, however, is just as unacceptable. In addition, medications may directly affect sleep and the sensorium and contribute to the genesis of the ICU syndrome. Age, disease severity, surgery requiring cardiopulmonary bypass, and metabolic factors are also contributory variables.[219,220]

Important psychological factors include fear and anxiety. Their impact on sleep depends on the coping skills and premorbid psychological status of the patient. The psychological stress to the patient in the intensive care unit is immense. Fear of death and suffering is natural and can result in a vicious cycle of fear, anxiety, and insomnia. This is accentuated if mechanical ventilation is required, causing the patient to lose the ability to communicate verbally. Patients may also fear sleep because of the fear of dying during sleep.

Environmental factors in the intensive care unit that interfere with sleep involve the physical structure of the intensive care unit, along with the constant monitoring and therapeutic interventions. The intensive care unit is a busy and tense setting. Urgent interventions often have to be performed at erratic hours. Privacy is lost and patients cannot help but be affected by the status of the other patients. Ventricular tachycardia in the coronary care unit has been observed to develop in a patient following the death of a neighboring patient.[221] Noise levels in the intensive care unit have been found to exceed internationally recommended limits at all times throughout the day.[222] This is caused by staff conversations, mechanical ventilators, and the alarms of monitoring equipment.[222–224] Bright lights are another factor that disrupts sleep.[216,225] Constant intervention is performed by nurses to assess vital signs, provide body hygiene, and administer medications, as well as by respiratory therapists who assess hemodynamic parameters and adjust ventilators. These interventions interfere with sleep, as do frequent physician assessments and bedside discussions. Just the simple adjustment of intravenous infusions has been shown to cause arousal detectable on the electroencephalogram. Tests are often scheduled early in the morning for the convenience of the staff, despite necessitating patient awakening. Finally, the lack of windows can cause a time-free environment and result in the off-setting of circadian clocks.[226]

Sleep Deprivation and ICU Psychosis

These physical, psychological, and environmental factors can result in insomnia, sleep disruption, sleep deprivation, and the ICU syndrome. The incidence of postoperative psychosis has been estimated to range from less than 0.1% in general surgical patients to more than 50% in patients after open heart surgery.[217,227] The high incidence following open heart surgery probably reflects concomitant neurovascular disease associated with the procedure.[219,228] The incidence has been found to be lower in coronary care units than in surgical intensive care units, probably reflecting the calmer atmosphere in the coronary care unit where patients are able to sleep more during the day.[164,216]

Polysomnography in the intensive care unit has shown considerable variation in sleep architecture among different patients.[220,224,229,230] Total sleep time, non-REM stages 3 and 4, and REM sleep are severely diminished. In the immediate postoperative period, patients commonly do not sleep at all and sleep disruption can persist despite the administration of hypnotic medications. Poor sleep frequently persists, even after the patient leaves the intensive care unit and hospital.[225] Care givers consistently overestimate the amount of sleep obtained by patients in the intensive care unit, often to a marked degree.[230]

Treatment of sleep deprivation should focus on its prevention. The intensive care unit environment should be conducive to sleep. Noise should be minimized through staff education, avoidance of loud conversations, and the turning down of unnecessary alarms. Physical means to reduce noise levels with floor coverings and baffles can be beneficial. Even simple measures such as turning lights off and closing doors are very helpful. Sleep should be more highly considered in the scheduling of tests, procedures, and personal care. In addition, adequate analgesia and psychological support should be achieved.

Physician and Medical Staff Sleep Deprivation

Patients are not the only ones deprived of sleep in the intensive care setting. Critical care physicians and medical staff follow their patients closely for extended periods because of their unstable medical condition and the need to recognize and treat changes promptly as they occur. These personnel have erratic sleep–wake schedules, disrupted sleep, and partial sleep deprivation. Frequently, complex tasks need to be performed and difficult decisions must be made in this sleep-deprived state. The effect that this has on patient care is controversial. Previous studies have shown that the performance of sleep-deprived house officers is impaired.[231–233] More recent studies have shown changes in mood, but no effect on cognitive and psychomotor performance.[234–237] More research is needed in this area before conclusions can be made.

In conclusion, significant respiratory and cardiovascular alterations occur during sleep. These may have a significant effect in patients with disease, as well as in patients with primary sleep disorders. Disease, in turn, has a considerable impact on a patient's sleep, which can affect recovery. It is important to recognize these effects and treat them appropriately.

References

1. Orem J, Barnes CD (eds). Physiology in Sleep. New York, Academic Press, 1980.
2. Shepard JW, Schweitzer PK, Keller CA et al. Myocardial stress—exercise versus sleep in patients with COPD. *Chest* 1984; 86:366–374.
3. Douglas NJ, White DP, Pickett CK, et al. Respiration during sleep in normal man. *Thorax* 1982; 37:840–844.
4. White DP. Occlusion pressure and ventilation during sleep in normal humans. *J Appl Physiol* 1986; 61:1279–1287.
5. Birchfield RI, Sieker HO, Heyman A. Alterations in respiratory function during natural sleep. *J Lab Clin Med* 1959; 54:216–222.
6. Bulow K. Respiration and wakefulness in man. *Acta Physiol Scand* 1963; 59 (Suppl 209):1–110.
7. Reed DJ, Kellogg RH. Changes in respiratory response to CO_2 during natural sleep at sea level and at altitude. *J Appl Physiol* 1958; 13:325–330.
8. Robin ED, Whaley RD, Crump CH, et al. Alveolar gas tensions, pulmonary ventilation and blood pH during physiologic sleep in normal subjects. *J Clin Invest* 1958; 37:981–989.
9. Brebbia DR, Altschuler KZ. Oxygen consumption rate and electroencephalographic stage of sleep. *Science* 1965; 150:1621–1623.
10. Webb P, Hiestand M. Sleep metabolism and age. *J Appl Physiol* 1975; 38:257–262.
11. Guilleminault C, van den Hoed J, Mitler MM. Clinical overview of the sleep apnea syndromes. *In* C Guilleminault, W Dement (eds). Sleep Apnea Syndromes. New York, Alan R. Liss, 1978, pp 1–12.
12. Block AJ, Boysen PG, Wynne JW, et al. Sleep apnea, hypopnea and oxygen desaturation in normal subjects. *N Engl J Med* 1979; 300:513–517.
13. Findley LJ, Ries AL, Tisi GM, et al. Hypoxemia during apnea in normal subjects: Mechanisms and impact of lung volume. *J Appl Physiol* 1983; 55: 1777–1783.
14. Strohl KP, Altose MD. Oxygen saturation during breath-holding and during apneas in sleep. *Chest* 1984; 85:181–186.
15. Shepard JW. Gas exchange and hemodynamics during sleep. *Med Clin North Am* 1985; 69:1243–1264.

16. Anch AM, Remmers JE, Bunce H III. Supraglottic airway resistance in normal subjects and patients with occlusive sleep apnea. *J Appl Physiol* 1982; 53:1158–1163.
17. Skatrud JB, Dempsey JA, Badr S, et al. Effect of airway impedance on CO_2 retention and respiratory muscle activity during NREM sleep. *J Appl Physiol* 1988; 65:1676–1685.
18. Hudgel DW, Devadatta P. Decrease in functional residual capacity during sleep in normal humans. *J Appl Physiol* 1984; 57:1319–1322.
19. Tusiewicz K, Moldofsky H, Bryan AC, et al. Mechanics of the rib cage and diaphragm during sleep. *J Appl Physiol* 1977; 43:600–602.
20. Muller N, Volgyesi G, Becker L, et al. Diaphragmatic muscle tone. *J Appl Physiol* 1979; 47:279–284.
21. Hudgel DW, Martin RJ, Johnson B et al. Mechanics of the respiratory system and breathing pattern during sleep in normal humans. *J Appl Physiol* 1984; 56:133–137.
22. Berthon-Jones M, Sullivan CE. Ventilation and arousal responses to hypercapnia in normal sleeping humans. *J Appl Physiol* 1984; 57:59–67.
23. Douglas NJ, White DP, Weil JV, et al. Hypercapnic ventilatory response in sleeping adults. *Am Rev Respir Dis* 1982; 126:758–762.
24. Berthon-Jones M, Sullivan CE. Ventilatory and arousal responses to hypoxia in sleeping humans. *Am Rev Respir Dis* 1982; 125:632–639.
25. Douglas NJ, White DP, Weil JV, et al. Hypoxic ventilatory response decreases during sleep in normal men. *Am Rev Respir Dis* 1982; 125: 286–298.
26. Hedemark LL, Kronenberg RS. Ventilatory and heart rate responses to hypoxia and hypercapnia during sleep in adults. *J Appl Physiol* 1982; 53:307–312.
27. Gothe B, Goldman MD, Cherniack NS, et al. Effect of progressive hypoxia on breathing during sleep. *Am Rev Respir Dis* 1982; 126:97–102.
28. Bateman JRM, Pavia D, Clarke SW. The retention of lung secretions during the night in normal subjects. *Clin Sci Mol Med* 1978; 55:523–527.
29. Thach BT, Davies AM, Koenig JS. Pathophysiology of sudden airway obstruction in sleeping infants and its relevance for SIDS. *In* PJ Schwartz, DP Southall, M Valdes-Dapena (eds). The Sudden Infant Death Syndrome: Cardiac and Respiratory Mechanisms and Interventions. Ann NY Acad Sci 1988; 533:314–328.
30. Coccagna G, Mantovani M, Brignani F, et al. Arterial pressure changes during spontaneous sleep in man. *Electroencephalgr Clin Neurophysiol* 1971; 31:277–281.
31. Khatri IM, Freis ED. Hemodynamic changes during sleep. *J Appl Physiol* 1967; 22:867–873.
32. Snyder F, Hobson JA, Morrison DF, et al. Changes in respiration, heart rate, and systolic blood pressure in human sleep. *J Appl Physiol* 1964; 19:417–422.
33. Lugaresi E, Coccagna G, Cirignotta F, et al. Breathing during sleep in man in normal and pathological conditions. *Adv Exp Med Biol* 1978; 99:35–45.
34. Miller JC, Horvath SM. Cardiac output during human sleep. *Aviat Space Environ Med* 1976; 47:1046–1051.

35. Bristow JD, Honour AJ, Pickering TG, et al. Cardiovascular and respiratory changes during sleep in normal and hypertensive subjects. *Cardiovasc Res* 1969; 3:476–485.
36. Burdick JA, Brinton G, Goldstein L, et al. Heart-rate variability in sleep and wakefulness. *Cardiology* 1970; 55:79–83.
37. Baust W, Bohnert B. The regulation of heart rate during sleep. *Exp Brain Res* 1969; 7:169–180.
38. Brodsky M, Wu D, Denes P, et al. Arrhythmias documented by 24 hour continuous electrocardiographic monitoring in 50 male medical students without apparent heart disease. *Am J Cardiol* 1977; 39:390–395.
39. Fleg JL, Kennedy HL. Cardiac arrhythmias in a healthy elderly population. *Chest* 1982; 81:302–307.
40. Pickering TG, Johnston J, Honour AJ. Comparison of the effects of sleep, exercise and autonomic drugs on ventricular extrasystoles, using ambulatory monitoring of electrocardiogram and electroencephalogram. *Am J Med* 1978; 65:575–583.
41. Tzivoni D, Stern S. Electrocardiographic pattern during sleep in healthy subjects and in patients with ischemic heart disease. *J Electrocardiol* 1973; 6:225–229.
42. Cobb LA. Cardiac arrest during sleep. *N Engl J Med* 1984; 311:1044–1045.
43. Nikolic G, Bishop RL, Singh JB. Sudden death recorded during Holter monitoring. *Circulation* 1982; 66:218–225.
44. Guilleminault C, Pool P, Motta J, et al. Sinus arrest during REM sleep in young adults. *N Engl J Med* 1984; 311:1006–1010.
45. Lown B, Temte JV, Reich P, et al. Basis for recurring ventricular fibrillation in the absence of coronary heart disease and its management. *N Engl J Med* 1976; 294:623–629.
46. Schroeder JS, Motta J, Guilleminault C. Hemodynamic studies in sleep apnea. *In* C Guilleminault, WC Dement (eds). Sleep Apnea Syndromes. New York, Alan R. Liss, 1978, pp 177–196.
47. Tilkian AG, Guilleminault C, Schroeder JS, et al. Hemodynamics in sleep-induced apnea: Studies during wakefulness and sleep. *Ann Intern Med* 1976; 85:714–719.
48. Lavie P, Ben-Yosef R, Rubin AE. Prevalence of sleep apnea syndrome among patients with essential hypertension. *Am Heart J* 1984; 108:373–376.
49. Kales A, Bixler EO, Cadieux RJ, et al. Sleep apnoea in a hypertensive population. *Lancet* 1984; 2:1005–1008.
50. Fletcher EC, DeBehnke RD, Lovoi MS, et al. Undiagnosed sleep apnea in patients with essential hypertension. *Ann Intern Med* 1985; 103:190–195.
51. Clark RW, Boudoulas H, Schaal SF, et al. Adrenergic hyperactivity and cardiac abnormality in primary disorders of sleep. *Neurology* 1980; 30:113–119.
52. Fletcher EC, Miller J, Divine GW, et al. Nocturnal oxyhemoglobin desaturation in COPD patients with arterial oxygen tensions above 60 mm Hg. *Chest* 1987; 92:604–608.
53. Kuna S, Gillen J, Levine S. Effects of respiratory gases on the frequency and duration of obstructive apneic episodes in a patient with the sleep apnea–hypersomnolence syndrome. *Respiration* 1982; 43:108–113.

54. Coccagna G, Mantovani M, Brignani F, et al. Continuous recording of the pulmonary and systemic arterial pressure during sleep in syndromes of hypersomnia with periodic breathing. *Bull Physiol Pathol* 1972; 8:1159–1172.
55. Marrone O, Bellia V, Ferrara G, et al. Transmural pressure measurements: Importance in the assessment of pulmonary hypertension in obstructive sleep apneas. *Chest* 1989; 95:338–342.
56. Chaudhary BA, Nadimi M, Chaudhary TK, et al. Pulmonary edema due to obstructive sleep apnea. *South Med J* 1984; 77:499–501.
57. Lorch DG, Sahn SA. Post-extubation pulmonary edema following anesthesia induced by upper airway obstruction. *Chest* 1986; 90:802–805.
58. Buda AJ, Schroeder JS, Guilleminault C. Abnormalities of pulmonary artery wedge pressures in sleep-induced apnea. *Int J Cardiol* 1981; 1: 67–74.
59. Krieger J, Laks L, Wilcox I, et al. Atrial naturetic factor release during sleep in obstructive sleep apnea before and during nasal CPAP. *Am Rev Respir Dis* 1988; 137:S57 (abstract).
60. Cosby RL, Sophocles AM, Durr JA, et al. Elevated plasma atrial natriuretic factor and vasopressin in high-altitude pulmonary edema. *Ann Intern Med* 1988; 109:796–799.
61. Guilleminault C, Motta J, Mihm F, et al. Obstructive sleep apnea and cardiac index. *Chest* 1986; 89:331–334.
62. Shepard JW. Hemodynamics in obstructive sleep apnea. *In* EC Fletcher (ed). Abnormalities of Respiration During Sleep. Orlando, Florida, Grune and Stratton, 1986, pp 39–61.
63. Tilkian AG, Motta J, Guilleminault C. Cardiac arrhythmias in sleep apnea. *In* C Guilleminault, WC Dement (eds). Sleep Apnea Syndromes. New York, Alan R. Liss, 1978, pp 197–210.
64. Guilleminault C, Connolly S, Winkle R, et al. Cyclical variation of the heart rate in sleep apnoea syndrome. *Lancet* 1984; 1:126–131.
65. Zwillich C, Devlin T, White D, et al. Bradycardia during sleep apnea: Characteristics and mechanism. *J Clin Invest* 1982; 69:1286–1292.
66. Guilleminault C, Connolly SJ, Winkle RA. Cardiac arrhythmia and conduction disturbances during sleep in 400 patients with sleep apnea syndrome. *Am J Cardiol* 1983; 52:490–494.
67. Shepard JW, Garrison MW, Grither DA, et al. Relationship of ventricular ectopy to oxyhemoglobin desaturation in patients with obstructive sleep apnea. *Chest* 1985; 88:335–340.
68. Guilleminault C. Natural history, cardiac impact, and long-term follow-up of sleep apnea syndrome. *In* C Guilleminault, E Lugaresi (eds). Sleep/Wake Disorders: Natural History, Epidemiology, and Long-Term Evolution. New York, Raven Press, 1983, pp 107–125.
69. Coccagna G, di Donato G, Verucchi P, et al. Hypersomnia with periodic apneas in acquired micrognathia. *Arch Neurol* 1976; 33:769–776.
70. Orr WC, Martin RJ. Obstructive sleep apnea associated with tonsillar hypertrophy in adults. *Arch Intern Med* 1981; 141:990–992.
71. King M, Gleeson M, Rees J. Obstructive sleep apnoea and tonsillar lymphoma. *Br Med J* 1987; 294:1605–1606.

72. Perks WH, Horrocks PM, Cooper RA, et al. Sleep apnea in acromegaly. *Br Med J* 1980; 280:894–897.
73. Hart TB, Radow SK, Blackard WG, et al. Sleep Apnea in active acromegaly. *Arch Intern Med* 1985; 145:865–866.
74. Mezon BJ, West P, Maclean JP, et al. Sleep apnea in acromegaly. *Am J Med* 1980; 69:615–618.
75. Skatrud J, Iber C, Ewart R, et al. Disordered breathing during sleep in hypothyroidism. *Am Rev Respir Dis* 1981; 124:325–329.
76. Rajagopal KR, Abbrecht PH, Derderian SS, et al. Obstructive sleep apnea in hypothyroidism. *Ann Intern Med* 1984; 101:491–494.
77. Lesser BA, Leeper KV, Conway W. Obstructive sleep apnea in amyloidosis treated with nasal continuous positive airway pressure. *Arch Intern Med* 1988; 148:2285–2287.
78. Olsen KD, Kern EB, Westbrook PR. Sleep and breathing disturbance secondary to nasal obstruction. *Otolaryngol Head Neck Surg* 1981; 89: 804–810.
79. Zwillich CW, Pickett C, Hanson FN, et al. Disturbed sleep and prolonged apnea during nasal obstruction in normal men. *Am Rev Respir Dis* 1981; 124:158–160.
80. Lavie P, Fischel N, Zomer J, et al. The effects of partial and complete mechanical occlusion of the nasal passages on sleep structure and breathing in sleep. *Acta Otolaryngol* 1983; 95:161–166.
81. Suratt PM, Turner BL, Wilhoit SC. Effect of intranasal obstruction on breathing during sleep. *Chest* 1986; 90:324–329.
82. McNicholas WT, Tarlo S, Cole P, et al. Obstructive apneas during sleep in patients with seasonal allergic rhinitis. *Am Rev Respir Dis* 1982; 126: 625–628.
83. Staats BA, Bonekat HW, Harris CD, et al. Chest wall motion in sleep apnea. *Am Rev Respir Dis* 1984; 130:59–63.
84. Hall JB. The cardiopulmonary failure of sleep-disordered breathing. *JAMA* 1986; 255:930–933.
85. Afzelius L, Elmqvist D, Hougaard K, et al. Sleep apnea syndrome—an alternative to tracheostomy. *Laryngoscope* 1981; 91:285–291.
86. Nahmias JS, Karetzky MS. Treatment of the obstructive sleep apnea syndrome using a nasopharyngeal tube. *Chest* 1988; 94:1142–1147.
87. Tilkian AG, Guilleminault C, Schroeder JS, et al. Sleep-induced apnea syndrome: Prevalence of cardiac arrhythmias and their reversal after tracheostomy. *Am J Med* 1977; 63:348–358.
88. Conway WA, Victor LD, Magilligan DJ, et al. Adverse effects of tracheostomy for sleep apnea. *JAMA* 1981; 246:347–350.
89. Simmons FB, Guilleminault C, Dement WC, et al. Surgical management of airway obstructions during sleep. *Laryngoscope* 1977; 87:326–338.
90. Rafferty TD, Ruskis A, Sasaki C, et al. Perioperative considerations in the management of tracheostomy for the obstructive sleep apnoea patient. *Br J Anaesth* 1980; 52:619–621.
91. Chung F, Crago RR. Sleep apnoea syndrome and anaesthesia. *Can Anaesth Soc J* 1982; 29:439–445.
92. Hishikawa Y, Furuya E, Wakamatsu H, et al. A polygraphic study of

hypersomnia with periodic breathing and primary alveolar hypoventilation. *Bull Physiol Pathol Respir* 1970; 8:1139–1151.
93. Guilleminault C, Cummiskey J, Motta J. Chronic obstructive airflow disease and sleep studies. *Am Rev Respir Dis* 1980; 122:397–406.
94. Alford NJ, Fletcher EC, Nickeson D. Acute oxygen in patients with sleep apnea and COPD. *Chest* 1986; 89:30–38.
95. Espinoza H, Antic R, Thornton AT, et al. The effects of aminophylline on sleep and sleep-disordered breathing in patients with obstructive sleep apnea syndrome. *Am Rev Respir Dis* 1987; 136:80–84.
96. Burwell CS, Robin ED, Whaley RD, et al. Extreme obesity associated with alveolar hypoventilation—a Pickwickian syndrome. *Am J Med* 1956; 21:811–818.
97. Shepard JW. Physiologic and clinical consequences of sleep apnea. *Semin Respir Med* 1988; 9:560–568.
98. Bradley TD, Rutherford R, Grossman RF, et al. Role of daytime hypoxemia in the pathogenesis of right heart failure in the obstructive sleep apnea syndrome. *Am Rev Respir Dis* 1985; 131:835–839.
99. Garay SM, Rapoport D, Sorkin B, et al. Regulation of ventilation in the obstructive sleep apnea syndrome. *Am Rev Respir Dis* 1981; 124:451–457.
100. Rapoport DM, Garay SM, Epstein H, et al. Hypercapnia in the obstructive sleep apnea syndrome. *Chest* 1986; 89:627–635.
101. Sampson MG, Grassino A. Neuromechanical properties in obese patients during carbon dioxide breathing. *Am J Med* 1983; 75:81–90.
102. Lopata M, Onal E. Mass loading, sleep apnea, and the pathogenesis of obesity hypoventilation. *Am Rev Respir Dis* 1982; 126:640–645.
103. Zwillich CW, Sutton FD, Pierson DJ, et al. Decreased hypoxic ventilatory drive in the obesity–hypoventilation syndrome. *Am J Med* 1975; 59:343–347.
104. Luce JM. Respiratory complications of obesity. *Chest* 1980; 78:626–631.
105. Sanders MH, Moore SE. Inspiratory and expiratory partitioning of airway resistance during sleep in patients with sleep apnea. *Am Rev Respir Dis* 1983; 127:554–558.
106. Jones JB, Wilhoit SC, Findley LJ, et al. Oxyhemoglobin saturation during sleep in subjects with and without the obesity–hypoventilation syndrome. *Chest* 1985; 88:9–15.
107. Sharp JT, Druz WS, Kondragunta VR. Diaphragmatic responses to body position changes in obese patients with obstructive sleep apnea. *Am Rev Respir Dis* 1986; 133:32–37.
108. Weitzenblum E, Krieger J, Apprill M, et al. Daytime pulmonary hypertension in patients with obstructive sleep apnea syndrome. *Am Rev Respir Dis* 1988; 138:345–349.
109. Fletcher EC, Schaaf JW, Miller J, et al. Long-term cardiopulmonary sequelae in patients with sleep apnea and chronic lung disease. *Am Rev Respir Dis* 1987; 135:525–533.
110. MacGregor MI, Block AJ, Ball WC Jr. Serious complicatons and sudden death in the Pickwickian syndrome. *Hopkins Med J* 1970; 126:279–295.
111. Miller A, Granada M. In-hospital mortality in the Pickwickian syndrome. *Am J Med* 1974; 56:144–150.
112. Aubert-Tulkens G, Willems B, Veriter C, et al. Increase in ventilatory

response to CO_2 following tracheostomy in obstructive sleep apnea. *Bull Eur Physiopathol Respir* 1980; 16: 587–593.
113. Lyons HA, Huang CT. Therapeutic use of progesterone in alveolar hypoventilation associated with obesity. *Am J Med* 1968; 44:881–888.
114. Sutton FD, Zwillich CW, Creagh CE, et al. Progesterone for outpatient treatment of Pickwickian syndrome. *Ann Intern Med* 1975; 83:476–479.
115. Phillipson EA. Sleep disorders. *In* JF Murray, JA Nadel (eds). Textbook of Respiratory Medicine. Philadelphia, WB Saunders, 1988, pp 1841–1860.
116. Tobin MJ, Snyder JV. Cheyne-Stokes respiration revisited: Controversies and implications. *Crit Care Med* 1984; 12:882–887.
117. Lange RL, Hecht HH. The mechanism of Cheyne-Stokes respiration. *J Clin Invest* 1962; 41:42–52.
118. Ribeiro JP, Knutzen A, Rocco MB, et al. Periodic breathing during exercise in severe heart failure: Reversal with milrinone or cardiac transplantation. *Chest* 1987; 92:555–556.
119. Bradley TD, McNicholas WT, Rutherford R, et al. Clinical and physiologic heterogeneity of the central sleep apnea syndrome. *Am Rev Respir Dis* 1986; 134:217–221.
120. Findley LJ, Blackburn MR, Goldberger AL, et al. Apneas and oscillation of cardiac ectopy in Cheyne-Stokes breathing during sleep. *Am Rev Respir Dis* 1984; 130:937–939.
121. Martin RJ, Pickett CK, Ballard RD. Changes in heart rate associated with central sleep apnea. *Am Rev Respir Dis* 1987; 135:A37 (abstract).
122. Guilleminault C, Eldridge FL, Dement WC. Insomnia with sleep apnea: A new syndrome. *Science* 1973; 181:856–858.
123. Massumi RA, Winnacker JL. Severe depression of the respiratory center in myxedema. *Am J Med* 1964; 36:876–882.
124. Zwillich CW, Pierson DJ, Hofeldt FD, et al. Ventilatory control in myxedema and hypothyroidism. *N Engl J Med* 1975; 292:662–665.
125. Millman RP, Bevilacqua J, Peterson DD, et al. Central sleep apnea in hypothyroidism. *Am Rev Respir Dis* 1983; 127:504–507.
126. White DP, Zwillich CW, Pickett CK, et al. Central sleep apnea: Improvement with acetazolamide therapy. *Arch Intern Med* 1982; 142:1816–1819.
127. McNicholas WT, Carter JL, Rutherford R, et al. Beneficial effect of oxygen in primary alveolar hypoventilation with central sleep apnea. *Am Rev Respir Dis* 1982; 125:773–775.
128. Issa FG, Sullivan CE. Reversal of central sleep apnea using nasal CPAP. *Chest* 1986; 90:165–171.
129. Hoffstein V, Slutsky AS. Central sleep apnea reversed by continuous positive airway pressure. *Am Rev Respir Dis* 1987; 135:1210–1212.
130. Farmer WC, Glenn WWL, Gee JBL. Alveolar hypoventilation syndrome: Studies of ventilatory control in patients selected for diaphragm pacing. *Am J Med* 1978; 64:39–49.
131. Hyland RH, Jones NL, Powles ACP, et al. Primary alveolar hypoventilation treated with nocturnal electrophrenic respiration. *Am Rev Respir Dis* 1978; 117:165–172.
132. McMichan JC, Piepgras DG, Gracey DR, et al. Electrophrenic respiration. *Mayo Clin Proc* 1979; 54:662–668.

133. Skatrud J, Iber C, McHugh W, et al. Determinants of hypoventilation during wakefulness and sleep in diaphragmatic paralysis. *Am Rev Respir Dis* 1980; 121:587–593.
134. Peters SG, Viggiano RW. Home mechanical ventilation. *Mayo Clin Proc* 1988; 63:1208–1213.
135. Thorpy MJ, Schmidt-Nowara WW, Pollak CP, et al. Sleep-induced nonobstructive hypoventilation associated with diaphragmatic paralysis. *Ann Neurol* 1982; 12:308–311.
136. Marino W, Braun NMT. Reversal of the clinical sequelae of respiratory muscle fatigue by intermittent mechanical ventilation. *Am Rev Respir Dis* 1982; 125:S85 (abstract).
137. Bye PTP, Ellis ER, Donnelly PD, et al. Role of sleep in the development of respiratory failure in neuromuscular disease. *Am Rev Respir Dis* 1985; 131:A108 (abstract).
138. Goldstein RS, Molotiu N, Skrastins R, et al. Reversal of sleep-induced hypoventilation and chronic respiratory failure by nocturnal negative pressure ventilation in patients with restrictive ventilatory impairment. *Am Rev Respir Dis* 1987; 135:1049–1055.
139. Simonds AK, Branthwaite MA. Efficiency of negative pressure ventilatory equipment. *Thorax* 1985; 40:213 (abstract).
140. Ellis ER, Bye PTP, Bruderer JW, et al. Treatment of respiratory failure during sleep in patients with neuromuscular disease: Positive-pressure ventilation through a nose mask. *Am Rev Respir Dis* 1987; 135:148–152.
141. Kerby GR, Mayer LS, Pingleton SK. Nocturnal positive pressure ventilation via nasal mask. *Am Rev Respir Dis* 1987; 135:738–740.
142. Ellis ER, McCauley VB, Mellis C, et al. Treatment of alveolar hypoventilation in a six-year old girl with intermittent positive pressure ventilation through a nasal mask. *Am Rev Respir Dis* 1987; 136:188–191.
143. Trask CH, Cree EM. Oximeter studies on patients with chronic obstructive emphysema, awake and during sleep. *New Engl J Med* 1962; 266: 639–642.
144. Pierce AK, Jarrett CE, Werkle G, et al. Respiratory function during sleep in patients with chronic obstructive lung disease. *J Clin Invest* 1966; 45:631–636.
145. Koo KW, Sax DS, Snider GL. Arterial blood gases and pH during sleep in chronic obstructive pulmonary disease. *Am J Med* 1975; 58:663–670.
146. Flick MR, Block AJ. Continuous in-vivo monitoring of arterial oxygenation in chronic obstructive lung disease. *Ann Intern Med* 1977; 86:725–730.
147. Douglas NJ, Calverley PMA, Leggett RJE, et al. Transient hypoxaemia during sleep in chronic bronchitis and emphysema. *Lancet* 1979; 1:1–4.
148. Wynne JW, Block AJ, Hemenway JM, et al. Disordered breathing and oxygen desaturation during sleep in patients with chronic obstructive lung disease (COLD). *Am J Med* 1979; 66:573–579.
149. Fleetham JA, Mezon B, West P, et al. Chemical control of ventilation and sleep arterial oxygen desaturation in patients with COPD. *Am Rev Respir Dis* 1980; 122:583–589.
150. Kearley R, Wynne JW, Block AJ, et al. The effect of low flow oxygen on

sleep-disordered breathing and oxygen desaturation: A study of patients with chronic obstructive lung disease. *Chest* 1980; 78:682–685.
151. Shepard JW, Garrison MW, Grither DA, et al. Relationship of ventricular ectopy to nocturnal desaturation in patients with chronic obstructive pulmonary disease. *Am J Med* 1985:78:28–34.
152. Lourenco RV, Turino GM, Davidson LAG, et al. The regulation of ventilaton in diffuse pulmonary fibrosis. *Am J Med* 1965; 38:199–216.
153. Perez-Padilla R, West P, Lertzman M, et al. Breathing during sleep in patients with interstitial lung disease. *Am Rev Respir Dis* 1985; 132:224–229.
154. Bye PTP, Issa F, Berthon-Jones M, et al. Studies of oxygenation during sleep in patients with interstitial lung disease. *Am Rev Respir Dis* 1984; 129:27–32.
155. Kryger MH. Sleep in restrictive disorders. *Clin Chest Med* 1985; 6:675–677.
156. Mezon BL, West P, Israels J, et al. Sleep breathing abnormalities in kyphoscoliosis. *Am Rev Respir Dis* 1980; 122:617–621.
157. Guilleminault C, Kurland G, Winkle R, et al. Severe kyphoscoliosis, breathing, and sleep. *Chest* 1981; 79:626–630.
158. Hoeppner VH, Cockcroft DW, Dosman JA, et al. Nighttime ventilation improves respiratory failure in secondary kyphoscoliosis. *Am Rev Respir Dis* 1984; 129:240–243.
159. Ellis ER, Grunstein RR, Chan S, et al. Noninvasive ventilatory support during sleep improves respiratory failure in kyphoscoliosis. *Chest* 1988; 94:811–815.
160. De Olazabal JR, Miller MJ, Cook WR, et al. Disordered breathing and hypoxia during sleep in coronary artery disease. *Chest* 1982; 82:548–552.
161. Nowlin JB, Troyer WG Jr, Collins WS, et al. The association of nocturnal angina pectoris with dreaming. *Ann Intern Med* 1965; 63:1040–1046.
162. Murao S, Harumi K, Katayama S, et al. All-night polygraphic studies of nocturnal angina pectoris. *Jpn Heart J* 1972; 13:295–306.
163. King MJ, Zir LM, Kaltman AJ, et al. Variant angina associated with angiographically demonstrated coronary artery spasm and REM sleep. *Am J Med Sci* 1973; 265:419–422.
164. Broughton R, Baron R. Sleep patterns in the intensive care unit and on the ward after acute myocardial infarction. *Electroencephalogr Clin Neurophysiol* 1978; 45:348–360.
165. Araki H, Koiwaya Y, Nakagaki O, et al. Diurnal distribution of ST-segment elevation and related arrhythmias in patients with variant angina: A study by ambulatory ECG monitoring. *Circulation* 1983; 67:995–1000.
166. Chierchia S, Davies G, Berkenboom G, et al. Alpha-adrenergic receptors and coronary spasm: An elusive link. *Circulation* 1984; 69:8–14.
167. Rocco MB, Barry J, Campbell S, et al. Circadian variation of transient myocardial ischemia in patients with coronary artery disease. *Circulation* 1987; 75:395–400.
168. Muller JE, Stone PH, Turi ZG, et al. Circadian variation in the frequency of onset of acute myocardial infarction. *N Engl J Med* 1985; 313:1315–1322.

169. Rosenblatt G, Hartmann E, Zwilling GR. Cardiac irritability during sleep and dreaming. *J Psychosom Res* 1973; 17:129–134.
170. Smith R, Johnson L, Rothfeld D, et al. Sleep and cardiac arrhythmias. *Arch Intern Med* 1972; 130:751–753.
171. Lown B, Tykocinski M, Garfein A, et al. Sleep and ventricular premature beats. *Circulation* 1973; 48:691–701.
172. Dark DS, Pingleton SK, Kerby GR, et al. Breathing pattern abnormalities and arterial oxygen desaturation during sleep in the congestive heart failure syndrome. *Chest* 1987; 91:833–836.
173. Baylor P, Tayloe D, Owen D, et al. Cardiac failure presenting as sleep apnea: Elimination of apnea following medical management of cardiac failure. *Chest* 1988; 94:1298–1300.
174. Rees PJ, Clark TJH. Paroxysmal nocturnal dyspnoea and periodic respiration. *Lancet* 1979; 2:1315–1317.
175. Chaudhary BA, Ferguson DS, Speir WA Jr. Pulmonary edema as a presenting feature of sleep apnea syndrome. *Chest* 1982; 82:122–124.
176. Oswalt CE, Gates GA, Holmstrom FMG. Pulmonary edema as a complication of acute airway obstruction. *JAMA* 1977; 238:1833–1835.
177. Jackson FN, Rowland V, Corssen G. Laryngospasm-induced pulmonary edema. *Chest* 1980; 78:819–821.
178. Willms D, Shure D. Pulmonary edema due to upper airway obstruction in adults. *Chest* 1988; 94:1090–1092.
179. Crabb JE, Pingleton SK, Gollub S, et al. Sleep disordered breathing (SDB) in decompensated and compensated congestive heart failure. *Am Rev Respir Dis* 1985; 131:A104 (abstract).
180. Findley LJ, Zwillich CW, Ancoli-Israel S, et al. Cheyne-Stokes breathing during sleep in patients with left ventricular heart failure. *South Med J* 1985; 78:11–15.
181. Devereaux MW, Keane JR, Davis RL. Automatic respiratory failure associated with infarction of the medulla. *Arch Neurol* 1973; 29:46–52.
182. Levin BE, Margolis G. Acute failure of automatic respirations secondary to a unilateral brainstem infarct. *Ann Neurol* 1977; 1:583–586.
183. Chaudhary BA, Elguindi AS, King DW. Obstructive sleep apnea syndrome after lateral medullary syndrome. *South Med J* 1982; 75:65–67.
184. Krieger AJ, Rosomoff HL. Sleep-induced apnea: Part 1: A respiratory and autonomic dysfunction syndrome following bilateral percutaneous cervical cordotomy. *J Neurosurg* 1974; 39:168–180.
185. Haponik EF, Givens D, Angelo J. Syringobulbia-myelia with obstructive sleep apnea. *Neurology* 1983; 33:1046–1049.
186. Balk RA, Hiller FC, Lucas EA, et al. Sleep apnea and the Arnold-Chiari malformation. *Am Rev Respir Dis* 1985; 132:929–930.
187. Udwadia ZF, Athale S, Misra VPE, et al. Radiation necrosis causing failure of automatic ventilation during sleep with central sleep apnea. *Chest* 1987; 92:567–569.
188. White DP, Miller F, Erickson RW. Sleep apnea and nocturnal hypoventilation after Western equine encephalitis. *Am Rev Respir Dis* 1983; 127:132–133.
189. Cohn JE, Kuida H. Primary alveolar hypoventilation associated with Western equine encephalitis. *Ann Intern Med* 1962; 56:633–644.

190. Plum F, Swanson AG. Abnormalities in central regulation of respiration in acute and convalescent poliomyelitis. *Arch Neurol* 1958; 80:267–285.
191. Hill R, Robbins AW, Messing R, et al. Sleep apnea syndrome after poliomyelitis. *Am Rev Respir Dis* 1983; 127:129–131.
192. Guilleminault C, Motta J. Sleep apnea syndrome as a long-term sequela of poliomyelitis. *In* C. Guilleminault, WC Dement (eds). Sleep Apnea Syndromes. New York, Alan R. Liss, 1978, pp 309–315.
193. Degen R. A study of the diagnostic value of waking and sleep EEG's after sleep deprivation in epileptic patients on anticonvulsive therapy. *Electroencephalogr Clin Neurophysiol* 1980; 49:577–584.
194. Jennum P, Borgesen SE. Intracranial pressure and obstructive sleep apnea. *Chest* 1989; 95:279–283.
195. Millman RP, Kimmel PL, Shore ET, et al. Sleep apnea in hemodialysis patients: The lack of testosterone effect on its pathogenesis. *Nephron* 1985; 40:407–410.
196. Feldman M, Richardson CT. Total 24-hour gastric acid secretion in patients with duodenal ulcer: Comparison with normal subjects and effects of cimetidine and parietal cell vagotomy. *Gastroenterology* 1986; 90: 540–544.
197. Dent J, Dodds WJ, Friedman RH, et al. Mechanism of gastroesophageal reflux in recumbent asymptomatic human subjects. *J Clin Invest* 1980; 65:256–267.
198. Helm JF, Dodds WJ, Hogan WJ, et al. Acid neutralizing capacity of human saliva. *Gastroenterology* 1982; 83:69–74.
199. Orr WC, Robinson MG, Johnson LF. Acid clearance during sleep in the pathogenesis of reflux esophagitis. *Dig Dis Sci* 1981; 26:423–427.
200. Orr WC, Johnson LF, Robinson MG. Effect of sleep on swallowing, esophageal peristalsis, and acid clearance. *Gastroenterology* 1984; 86:814–819.
201. Roth T, Zorick F, Wittig R, et al. Pharmacological and medical considerations in hypnotic use. *Sleep* 1982; 5:S46–S52.
202. Kay DC, Eisenstein RB, Jasinski DR: Morphine effects on human REM state, waking state and NREM sleep. *Psychopharmacologia* 1969; 14:404–416.
203. Brownell LG, West P, Sweatman P, et al. Protriptyline in obstructive sleep apnea: A double-blind trial. *N Engl J Med* 1982; 307:1037–1042.
204. Lamarche Y, Martin R, Reiher J, et al. The sleep apnoea syndrome and epidural morphine. *Can Anaesth Soc J* 1986; 33:231–233.
205. Pellecchia DJ, Bretz KA, Barnette RE. Postoperative pain control by means of epidural narcotics in a patient with obstructive sleep apnea. *Anesth Analg* 1987; 66:280–282.
206. Sutton JR, Houston CS, Mansell AL, et al. Effect of acetazolamide on hypoxemia during sleep at high altitude. *N Engl J Med* 1979; 301:1329–1331.
207. Dietrich J, Krauss AN, Reidenberg M, et al. Alterations in state in apneic pre-term infants receiving theophylline. *Clin Pharmacol Ther* 1978; 24: 474–478.
208. Rhind GB, Connaughton JJ, McFie J, et al: Sustained release choline theophyllinate in nocturnal asthma. *Br Med J* 1985; 291:1605–1607.

209. Stewart IC, Rhind GB, Power JT, et al: Effect of sustained release terbutaline on symptoms and sleep quality in patients with nocturnal asthma. *Thorax* 1987; 42:797–800.
210. Betts TA, Alford C. B-blockers and sleep: A controlled trial. *Eur J Clin Pharmacol* 1985; 28:65–68 (suppl).
211. Kostis JB, Rosen RC. Central nervous system effects of B-adrenergic-blocking drugs: The role of ancillary properties. *Circulation* 1987; 75: 204–212.
212. Lahiri S, Nishino T, Mokashi A, et al. Interaction of dopamine and haloperidol with O_2 and CO_2 chemoreception in carotid body. *J Appl Physiol* 1980; 49:45–51.
213. Berger RJ, Oswald I. Effects of sleep deprivation on behaviour, subsequent sleep, and dreaming. *J Ment Sci* 1962; 108:457–465.
214. Luby ED, Frohman CE, Grisell JL, et al. Sleep deprivation: Effects on behavior, thinking, motor performance, and biological energy transfer systems. *Psychosom Med* 1960; 22:182–192.
215. Egerton N, Kay JH. Psychological disturbances associated with open heart surgery. *Br J Psychiatr* 1964; 110:433–439.
216. Helton MC, Gordon SH, Nunnery SL. The correlations between sleep deprivation and the intensive care unit syndrome. *Heart Lung* 1980; 9: 464–468.
217. Blachy PH, Starr A. Post-cardiotomy delirium. *Am J Psychiatry* 1964; 121:371–375.
218. Lewandowski LA, Kositsky AM. Research priorities for critical care nursing: A study by the American Association of Critical-Care Nurses. *Heart Lung* 1983; 12:35–44.
219. Tufo HM, Ostfeld AM, Shekelle R. Central nervous system dysfunction following open-heart surgery. *JAMA* 1970; 212:1333–1340.
220. Dohno S, Paskewitz DA, Lynch JJ, et al. Some aspects of sleep disturbance in coronary patients. *Percept Mot Skills* 1979; 48:199–205.
221. Lester BK, Block R, Gunn CG. The relation of cardiac arrhythmias to phases of sleep. *Clin Res* 1969; 11:456 (abstract).
222. Bentley S, Murphy F, Dudley H. Perceived noise in surgical wards and an intensive care area: An objective analysis. *Br Med J* 1977; 2:1503–1506.
223. Woods NF. Patterns of sleep in postcardiotomy patients. *Nurs Res* 1972; 21:347–352.
224. Richards KC, Bairnsfather L. A description of night sleep patterns in the critical care unit. *Heart Lung* 1988; 17:35–42.
225. Orr WC, Stahl ML. Sleep disturbances after open heart surgery. *Am J Cardiol* 1977; 39:196–201.
226. Hauri P. The Sleep Disorders. Upjohn, Ann Arbor, Michigan, 1982.
227. Knox SJ. Severe psychiatric disturbances in the post-operative period—a five-year survey of Belfast hospitals. *J Ment Sci* 1961; 107:1078–1096.
228. Hill JD, Aguilar MJ, Baranco A, et al. Neuropathological manifestations of cardiac surgery. *Ann Thorac Surg* 1969; 7:409–419.
229. Karacan I, Green JR Jr, Taylor WJ, et al. Sleep in post-myocardial infarction patients. *In* RS Eliot (ed). Stress and the Heart; Comtemporary Problems in Cardiology. Mt. Kisco, New York, Futura Publishing, 1974, pp 163–195.

230. Aurell J, Emlqvist D. Sleep in the surgical intensive care unit: Continuous polygraphic recording of sleep in nine patients receiving postoperative care. *Br Med J* 1985; 290:1029–1032.
231. Friedman RC, Bigger JT, Kornfeld DS. The intern and sleep loss. *N Engl J Med* 1971; 285:201–203.
232. Hart RP, Buchsbaum DG, Wade JB, et al. Effect of sleep deprivation on first-year residents' response times, memory, and mood. *J Med Educ* 1987; 62; 940–942.
233. Asken MJ, Raham DC. Resident performance and sleep deprivation: A review. *J Med Educ* 1983; 58:382–388.
234. Deaconson TF, O'Hair DP, Levy MF, et al. Sleep deprivation and resident performance. *JAMA* 1988; 260:1721–1727.
235. Bartle EJ, Sun JH, Thompson L, et al. The effects of acute sleep deprivation during residency training. Surgery 1988; 104:311–316.
236. Reznick RK, Folse JR. Effect of sleep deprivation on the performance of surgical residents. *Am J Surg* 1987; 154:520–525.
237. Deary IJ, Tait R. Effects of sleep disruption on cognitive performance and mood in medical house officers. *Br Med J* 1987; 295:1513–1516.

11

Sleep and Sleep Disorders in the Elderly

Gary C. Prechter, M.D.,
and
John W. Shepard, Jr., M.D.

In the United States 11% of the population (25 million people) are over age 65. This percentage, as well as the absolute number of elderly individuals, is expected to continue increasing.[1] With this comes the realization that their medical needs will consume a greater share of available resources.[2] Sleep disorders in the elderly are quite common and, therefore, have been an area of intense interest and research, particularly within the last decade. The focus of this chapter is directed towards the evolving concepts of sleep physiology and sleep pathology common to older individuals. Since many of the basic concepts underlying this body of knowledge are not unique to the elderly, the information presented here will be tailored to limit repetition, particularly in areas pertaining to therapy of specific disorders found in greater detail elsewhere in this text.

Age-Related Changes in Sleep

Subjective Data

Many investigators have evaluated sleep in the elderly through the use of questionnaires. Reports indicate an increased proportion of

Martin RJ: Cardiorespiratory Disorders During Sleep, 2nd Edition. Futura Publishing Company, Inc., Mount Kisco, NY, © 1990.

those over age 65 felt that their sleep was disturbed.[3–5] Perceived problems include inadequate total sleep time, increased latency to sleep onset, frequent nighttime awakening, and early morning awakening. Overall, surveys reveal that 15%–75% of the elderly are not satisfied with their sleep, with females expressing more frequent dissatisfaction than males.[6] Daytime naps are common (75%) with increasing age, more so in men than in women.[7] Nevertheless, despite a tendency toward insomnia and reduced sleep efficiency, there appears to be no evidence of reduced total sleep time during the 24-hour day. In fact, when diurnal nap time is added to nocturnal sleep time, elderly men have a longer but more variable total sleep time than younger adults.[7]

Objective Data

Polysomnographic findings in the elderly generally support the subjective data (Table 1) indicating that sleep is more fragmented and of poorer quality.[1,3,6,8–22] Sleep efficiency decreases from greater than 90% in young adults to approximately 70%–80% in the elderly.[1,13] Sleep latency increases only slightly or remains the same with age,

Table 1
Age-Related Changes in Sleep

	Changes relative to young adults
Total sleep time[a]	Unchanged
Sleep efficiency	Decreased
Sleep fragmentation (arousals and awakenings)	Increased
Latency of sleep onset	Small increase
Latency to REM sleep	Decreased
Percent non-REM stage 1	Increased
Percent non-REM stage 2	Small increase
Percent non-REM stage 3–4	Decreased[b]
Percent REM sleep	Unchanged
Auditory awakening threshold	Decreased
Sleep–wake cycle	Phase advanced
Daytime sleepiness	Increased
Daytime naps	Increased

[a]Including nap time.
[b]See text.

and the percentage of time spent in non-REM stage 1 sleep increases. This stage represents a transition stage (drowsiness) between wakefulness and solid sleep and is terminated by the appearance of non-REM stage 2. In addition, there is an increase in sleep fragmentation, manifest as frequent awakenings of brief 2- to 15-second arousals noted on EEG, as well as numerous transitions from deeper sleep stage to stage 1 sleep.[14] The percentage of stage 2 sleep shows little or no increase. Sleep spindles, which in part define stage 2, are found to be less well-formed. They are decreased in amplitude and frequency, but not duration. Although loss of spindle amplitude correlates with the degree of sulcal atrophy of the brain, there is no evidence that sleep spindle preservation is associated with maintenance of cognitive skills.[21]

One of the most consistently reported changes in sleep with aging is the reduction in slow-wave (non-REM stages 3 and 4) sleep. Reductions appear most marked in non-REM stage 4; however, recent studies based on computerized frequency analysis are not in agreement on this point.[6] The apparent discrepancy may reside in the finding that the amplitude of the slow (delta) waves declines with age so that standard criteria for amplitude of greater than 75 μV leads to a reduction in the scoring of slow-wave sleep.

The percentage of REM sleep probably does not decline in the elderly. However, the first REM period occurs earlier and subsequent REM periods tend to be more equal in duration rather than increasing in length as is seen in younger adults.[19] Auditory awakening thresholds based on arousal after a 5-second tone decline with age in stages 2, 4, and REM sleep.[23]

Elderly individuals tend to exhibit more daytime sleepiness than younger individuals, as documented by the multiple sleep latency test (MSLT),[24] but there is wide intersubject variation. Following an overnight sleep study permitting an 8.5-hour sleep allotment, the MSLT showed that one third of young adults and 90% of elderly adults had at least one test with a sleep latency less than 5 minutes.[25]

The bimodal pattern of sleep tendency as measured by the MSLT is maximal at midday and again in early morning.[24] This pattern does not mirror any known circadian rhythm and does not demonstrate a significant amplitude reduction with age in healthy elderly subjects.[24] In other aged individuals, however, there may be a disruption of the biphasic pattern, which is replaced by the polyphasic alternation of sleep and wakefulness similar to that found in children. It is not clear to what degree this change occurs by choice, but it has been ascribed to irregular habits, lack of social schedules, and aging itself.[3]

Finally, increasing age is associated with earlier times of sleep onset and wakefulness, known as phase advance, which will be discussed in greater detail below.

Etiologic Factors

The cause or causes producing age-related sleep changes in the elderly are probably multifactorial and presently incompletely defined. Loss of neuronal mass could induce EEG changes such as decreased sleep spindle and delta wave amplitude, as well as changes in the circadian oscillators responsible for lack of sleep continuity in some people.[6]

Since 85% of the elderly have at least one chronic disease,[1] it is not difficult to imagine the impact such problems and medications used to treat them have on sleep. The pain, discomfort, and anxiety arising from arthritic, cardiac, pulmonary, and urologic disorders have not been carefully studied but are frequently cited as disruptors of sleep continuity. Also suspected in this regard are the alterations in daily routine that accompany the socioeconomic changes of old age, particularly retirement. When work schedules and other regular regimens are abandoned, sleep and wake schedules also become disrupted, with daytime napping increasing the difficulties of nighttime sleep,[3] thereby producing a vicious cycle.

The role that unsuspected sleep disorders may play in the fragmentation of sleep has been recently reviewed.[16,26] In a report of noncomplaining elderly patients, 32% of women and 44% of men had five episodes or more of nocturnal apneas or hypopneas per hour.[27] Periodic leg movements (PLM) during sleep have been documented to occur in up to 57% of healthy elderly subjects, shown to increase with age, and average 4.6 episodes per hour.[19] These sleep disorders are dealt with in more detail under their respective headings in this chapter.

Defining Normality

The apparent variety of age-related changes that affect sleep and the frequency with which sleep disorders appear in the elderly make the definition of normalcy problematic.[28] However, it can be stated that daytime somnolence is not normal and, when encountered, the pursuit of a treatable sleep disorder is indicated. Apneas and PLMs are considered to have pathophysiological consequences only when their frequency exceeds threshold values, after which their actual effect on the individual must be carefully established. Even though the natural history of most sleep disorders is unknown, most experts feel that they are unremitting and worsen with age.[13] Therefore, the commonly encountered sleep disorders should not be thought of as normal accompaniments of aging but rather as abnormalities that require treatment whenever they become clinically significant.

Age-Related Changes in Ventilatory Control

Ventilatory Response to Afferent Stimuli during Wakefulness

In all humans the control of breathing during sleep shifts away from the behavioral influence of the cerebral cortex during wakefulness to the chemical control of the brain stem. The brain stem receives its information from central and peripheral receptors, which in turn respond to CO_2/H^+ concentration and O_2 tension, respectively. In the elderly there is a reduction in the hypercapnic response to 41% of younger control subjects.[29] A similar decline in hypoxic response has not been documented by all investigators when measured under isocapnic conditions,[30] but the multiplicative effect of hypercapnic and hypoxic ventilatory stimuli does diminish with age.[30]

Although these data measure the output of the central controller in terms of changes in minute ventilation, a direct conclusion concerning the decline in central neural output cannot be made without knowing that the intermediate components of the system are operating normally. Specifically, these components include the neuromuscular apparatus, chest wall, and lung. With age, the performance of the respiratory muscles decreases, as indicated by a reduction in maximal inspiratory and expiratory pressure generated under isometric conditions.[31] There is also an increase in elastic load due to a decrease in chest wall compliance with age. This is partially offset by an increase in lung compliance, but the total respiratory system compliance does decline with age.[32]

Since it is not possible to take into account accurately the impact of these age-related changes on the components of the respiratory system, a more direct method of assessing the neural response to chemical stimuli is desirable. The method of measuring the pressure generated in the first 100 msec of inspiration against an occluded airway, i.e., P_{100}, improves upon the assessment of neural drive since it is less affected by changes in lung mechanics.[33] Interestingly, this approach yields a similar reduction in hypoxic and hypercapnic response of 59% and 51%, respectively.[34] Even after normalizing for reductions in maximal inspiratory pressure, the difference between young and elderly subjects remains significant.[35] From this it would appear that the response of the central controller to these chemical stimuli declines with age (Table 2).

Central neural processing of other afferent inputs are also presumed to be altered in the elderly. Both elastic and resistive load responses are reduced with age,[36,37] but there is no change in the perception of force generation with age.[38] Furthermore, the effect that sleep imposes on the feedback from various mechanoreceptors is largely unknown. Therefore, the mechanism by which load perception is detected and the effect that sleep might have on this is unknown.

Table 2
Age-Related Changes in Ventilatory Control

Decreased hypercapnic response
Decreased combined hypoxic/hypercapnic response
Possible reduction in hypoxic response
Increased periodic breathing

Periodic Breathing during Sleep

The changes in ventilatory control in the elderly described above may affect ventilation during sleep as well. Although it is known that during non-REM sleep in normal adults there is a decrease in tidal volume and minute and alveolar ventilation, producing a rise in $PaCO_2$ of 2–8 mm Hg and a fall in $PaCO_2$ of 3–10 mm Hg, and that sensitivity to hypoxia and hypercarbia is reduced,[39–42] these changes have not been fully studied in the elderly. It is clear, however, that with advancing age there is an exaggeration of cyclical respiration, particularly during the transition phase between wakefulness and stage 1 or 2 non-REM sleep (Fig. 1). The resultant periodic breathing permits periods of apnea that last more than 10 seconds in 38% of elderly subjects.[43] These episodes occur predominantly in males during stage 1 and 2 sleep and are both central and obstructive. Periodic breathing increases with age and is particularly prominent when ventilatory oscillations are also present during wakefulness.[44] Periodic breathing appears similar to that seen in normal individuals at high altitude or breathing hypoxic gas mixtures; however, unlike these forms of environmentally induced hypoxemia, the periodic breathing of the elderly is not consistently relieved by supplemental oxygen.[45] Additionally, although a sleep-induced increase in CO_2 set point and decrease in ventilatory response to CO_2 appears to explain other forms of periodic breathing,[46] these factors have not been adequately evaluated in the elderly.

It is not known whether cardiovascular changes explain the increased periodic breathing and apnea seen in the elderly. Increased circulation time can increase periodic breathing, but a decrease in awake hypoxic and hypercapnic ventilatory response would tend to offset this change. Furthermore, it is simply not known how changes in chemoreceptor function during wakefulness alter ventilatory responses during sleep in the elderly.[47]

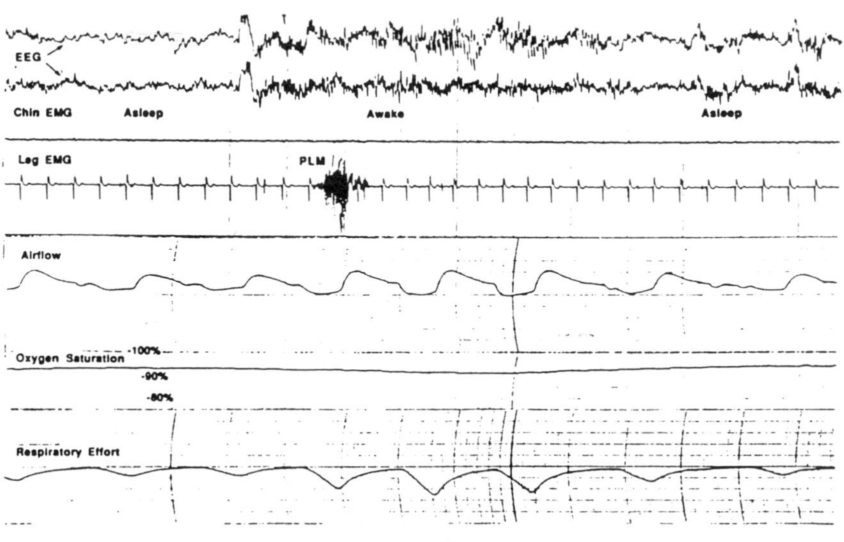

Figure 1. Periodic breathing in an elderly patient during sleep onset. Note transitions in the EEG between wakefulness (alpha waves) and non-REM stage 1 corresponding with increases and decreases in tidal ventilation. Periodic leg movements (PLMs) occur after appearance of alpha activity.

Although both apneic episodes and transient arousals are more common in the elderly, not all arousals are preceded by apneic episodes and apneas are not always followed by electroencephalographic evidence of arousal. In one study the number of arousals was no different in elderly subjects with and without apnea.[43]

Sleep Apnea

Prevalence

Within the last decade sleep apnea in the elderly has become recognized as a very common problem. Although natural history studies with adequate periods of follow-up defining the progressive prevalence of sleep apnea do not exist, there are numerous reports showing increased sleep apnea in older age groups.[14,26,27,43–45,48–69] Normal young adults have 2–10 episodes of apnea or hypopnea during a night of sleep, and these are usually in the transition phase of stage 1 or in REM sleep.[70] In noncomplaining elderly adults, 31% of women and 46% of men have five or more episodes of apnea or hypopnea per hour of sleep (apnea–hypopnea index), meeting the criteria for sleep apnea (Table 3). Most experts feel that clinically

Table 3
Prevalence and Severity of Sleep Apnea among Asymptomatic Elderly Individuals

	Total subjects		*Prevalence (%)*			*Number of subjects in categorical levels of apnea-hypopnea frequency (N/h)*			
Ref	Male	Female	Male	Female	Both	<5	5–9	10–14	≥15
43[a]	6	7			38	8	5[b]		
61	18	11			28	21	8[b]		
62	30	16			26	34	6	3	3
63[a]	68	77			28	105	26	5	9[c]
27	18	22	44	32	38	25	3	3	9
48	12	12	42	42	42	14	2	2	6
54[a]	5	5	40	20	30	7	3	0	0
56[a]	11	16	55	25	37	17	3	2	5

[a]Apnea frequency only; all others based on apnea-hypopnea frequency.
[b]Percent with apnea-hypopnea frequency greater than five per hour.
[c]Data estimated from graph.

significant daytime symptoms are generally not noticed until the apnea–hypopnea index is greater than 15. Viewed in this light, the prevalence of sleep apnea in the asymptomatic elderly is reduced to only 11% when very mild cases are omitted (Fig. 2).

Sleep apnea in the elderly seems to be associated with male sex, obesity, and the postmenopausal state.[1,57] Additionally, the prevalence of snoring, which indicates instability of the upper airway, increases with age, with 60% of men and 45% of women in their 60s being snorers.[13] Other risk factors for sleep apnea in the elderly are less well worked out. It should be true in elderly patients, as in younger individuals, that certain anatomical (macroglossia, micrognathia) or neuromuscular conditions predispose to obstructive sleep apnea. Also, cardiopulmonary disorders may lead to worsened hypoxemia in those with sleep apnea, thereby giving rise to increased cardiovascular consequences. Lastly, benzodiazepines, alcohol,[71,72] and sleep deprivation have been observed to increase sleep apnea in the elderly and, in selected individuals, the increase in apnea activity was associated with an increase in ventricular ectopy.[54]

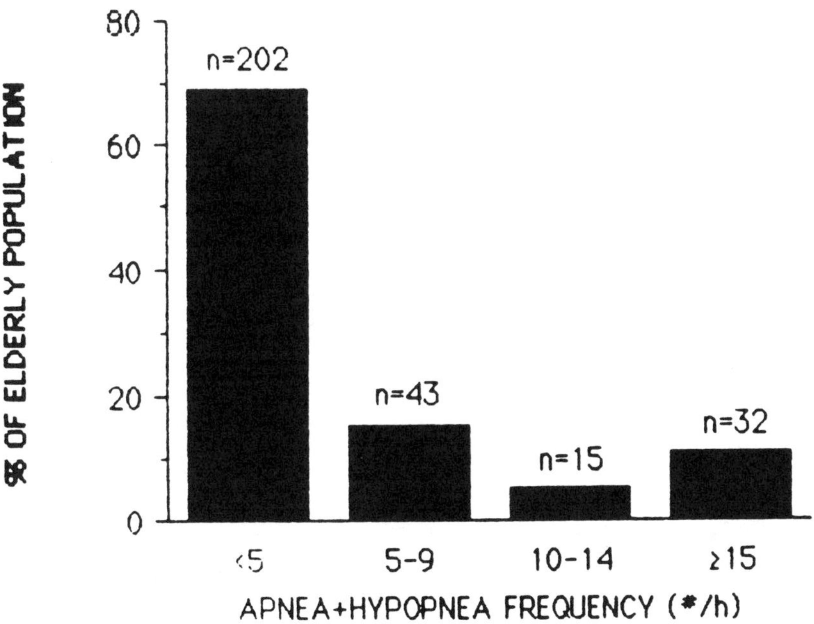

Figure 2. Frequency histogram for apnea + hypopnea incidence in elderly asymptomatic individuals. Data from references 27, 48, 54, 56, 62, 63.

Clinical Significance

Despite documentation of the frequency with which sleep apnea occurs in the elderly, it is not clear how often its presence will lead to clinically significant effects. The problem is compounded by the fact that some symptoms of sleep apnea syndrome are similar to those associated with aging. A convincing association could be made if a study demonstrating the effect of nasal CPAP on the resolution of memory loss, hypertension, arrhythmias, personality change, impotence, and other symptoms were performed. A recent report was able to show an increase in daytime sleepiness, but no difference in cardiac arrhythmias, systemic hypertension, cor pulmonale, or cognitive impairment between elderly volunteers above and below an apnea index of five per hour, despite oxyhemoglobin desaturation below 90% in all those with sleep apnea.[56] Although this was not a large study, it should serve to temper any aggressive approach to treatment of the mild apnea so prevalent in the elderly.

In contrast, studies conducted in elderly subjects with higher frequencies of sleep-disordered breathing have provided evidence for apnea related impairment. Neuropsychological testing of nondemented male subjects with a mean respiratory disturbance index (apneas plus hypopneas) of 26 per hour revealed a significant association with impaired psychometric performance.[55] In another small study of seven elderly patients with obstructive sleep apnea, indices of depression and fatigue significantly improved after 2 months of nasal CPAP treatment as compared to nontreated controls.[73] Sleep apnea has been associated with an increased mortality ratio of 2.7 in an elderly cohort of 198 subjects studied for sleep apnea and followed for up to 12 years.[58] Whether sleep apnea is actually an independent risk factor for the various clinical consequences ascribed to it awaits carefully controlled clinical trials.

Treatment Considerations

Treatment of the symptomatic elderly patient with sleep apnea proceeds generally along the lines of that described for younger adults.[74–77] Special attention should be directed towards any reversible cardiopulmonary or neuromuscular disease or structural abnormality of the upper airway. Pharmacological therapy to maximize nasal patency during sleep is advisable, along with advice to avoid the supine sleep position. Drugs that depress the central nervous system, including alcohol, sedative–hypnotics, and narcotic analgesics, should be avoided whenever possible. Although difficult to achieve, weight reduction is strongly recommended for all obese patients with sleep apnea. Tracheostomy and the use of nasal CPAP may be required with indications similar to those for younger adults. Respiratory stimulants have no proven value in the normocapic patient with obstructive sleep apnea.

Asymptomatic individuals with a low frequency of disordered breathing events (AHI $<$ 15 per hour) and only mild oxyhemoglobin desaturations into the mid-80s are probably best treated conservatively. Nasal CPAP can be considered for those asymptomatic elderly in whom oxyhemoglobin desaturation is more severe or the frequency of apneic events exceeds 15 per hour after conservative therapy.

Insomnia

Psychophysiologic Insomnia

Psychophysiologic insomnia is a common problem that results from conditioning that associates attempts to sleep with frustration, thereby encouraging arousal and persistent insomnia. Reports of patients attending sleep-disorder clinics indicate that 15%–31% of the elderly experience persistent psychophysiological insomnia.[13,78]

There is a variety of stimuli that are said to be less well tolerated in older people.[1,3,6,23,28,76,77] These include aspects of the external environment, such as noise level, and the internal environment, such as pain, urinary frequency, other medical conditions, and drugs. The influence of napping on insomnia of the elderly is controversial.[3] In younger individuals, omitting daytime naps appears to consolidate nighttime sleep. In the elderly this is not as clear. As noted previously, the elderly are sleepier by MSLT criteria[24,25] than young adults, and they nap more frequently. This may be the result of disrupted nighttime sleep or the lack of scheduled daytime activity during times when sleep tendency is greatest. The best recommendation for these patients may be to restrict daytime naps to a short period of time when sleep tendency is greatest—usually early afternoon.

Psychiatric Insomnia

Psychopathology underlying the insomnia of elderly patients seeking treatment at sleep-disorder centers is discovered in 18%–47% of cases.[3,78,79] In this population, depression is the most common psychiatric disturbance diagnosed. Depression commonly causes frequent awakenings, early morning awakening, reduction in stage 4 sleep, increased REM sleep, and short REM latency.[13,80–85]

Dementia in the elderly has been shown to be associated with increased diurnal napping, frequent nocturnal awakenings, and decreased REM and slow-wave sleep.[81,82,84,86–89] Overall, there is a breakdown and disorganization of the normal circadian rhythmicity of the sleep–wake cycle.

The usefulness of an overnight sleep study in the differentiation of elderly depressed and demented patients has received attention in recent years. Because of the different effects that these two conditions have on sleep, objective parameters have been evaluated as diagnostic discriminators. A shortened REM latency seen with depression allowed a REM latency cutoff score of 30 minutes to correctly classify 68% of depressed or demented patients.[81] Eighty percent were correctly categorized when multiple polysomnographic variables were analyzed.[84]

Drugs, Alcohol, and Medical Conditions

Withdrawal from CNS depressants such as sedative hypnotics or ethanol can produce insomnia. Although increasing serum concentrations of ethanol promote sleep, decreasing concentrations make arousal from sleep more likely. In the Stanford series of elderly patients, 21% of those with insomnia received a drug-related diagnosis.[13]

A variety of medical conditions are associated with insomnia. These include urological problems, particularly in conjunction with nocturia, nocturnal dyspnea resulting from congestive heart failure or chronic pulmonary disorders, and pain from any source, including arthritis, esophageal reflux, or peptic ulcer disease. Although not common, sleep apnea and PLMs may be the cause of insomnia by producing nighttime awakening in a patient who then has difficulty returning to sleep. Medications used to treat these and other disorders can contribute to insomnia. Theophylline and beta-agonists promote arousal; beta blockers, amantadine, and L-dopa may induce nightmares; and tricyclic antidepressants can increase the prevalence of periodic leg movements during sleep.[90]

Sedative Use and Abuse

The elderly as a group receive the largest share of sedative-hypnotic drugs intended to promote sleep.[91,92] Given the changes in drug metabolism with age,[93] it is clear that not enough is known about medication effects on sleep architecture, sleep disorders, cardiopulmonary abnormalities, or daytime function, particularly when taken over extended periods of time.[1,13] In a study of 447 elderly individuals in the Washington, DC, area, 14% were taking daily sedative–hypnotics,[13] a finding consistent with that of others.[92] In the institutionalized elderly patient, this percentage climbs to 26%–94%.[13]

Particularly disturbing effects of sleeping pills on sleep apnea in the elderly have been anecdotally documented, including a 72-year-old whose average apneic episodes lengthened from 1 minute to 3 minutes after taking 30 mg of flurazepam, with one episode lasting 5 minutes.[13] Benzodiazepines may also produce loss of balance during the daytime.[94] Recent evidence supports the contention that the use of benzodiazepines increases the risk of falling among the senior-citizen community.[95] A large case–control study of hip fractures in the elderly found twice the risk in those who had received a prescription for long-acting sedatives.[96]

The increased effect of sedative–hypnotics in the elderly is not completely explained by changes in plasma concentration. Among the commonly used sleeping pills, the difference in effect may be due in part to changes in postreceptor action.[97]

To control the use and abuse of sedative–hypnotics, it appears unreasonable to prescribe these drugs merely at a patient's request. The underlying cause for sleep difficulty must be explored and the potential for exacerbating asymptomatic sleep apnea, particularly in the setting of cardiopulmonary disease, carefully considered. Although the indications for their use are not intrinsically different in the elderly population, one's threshold for using these medications in this group should be higher and assessment of side effects more objective, including overnight sleep studies in some cases. The sedative–hypnotics with the largest safety margin are the benzodiazepines, but when utilized, they should generally be prescribed in one-half to two-thirds the usual adult dose.

Other Conditions

Periodic Leg Movements during Sleep

Periodic leg movements during sleep consist of repetitive extension of the great toe, dorsiflexion of the foot, and partial flexion at the knee and hip. The extent of the movement can range from being barely visible to violent jerking contractions. In the majority of elderly patients, the periodic increases in EMG activity detected over the anterior tibialis muscles do not lead to EEG evidence of arousal and fragmentation of nocturnal sleep (Fig. 3). In the absence of associated

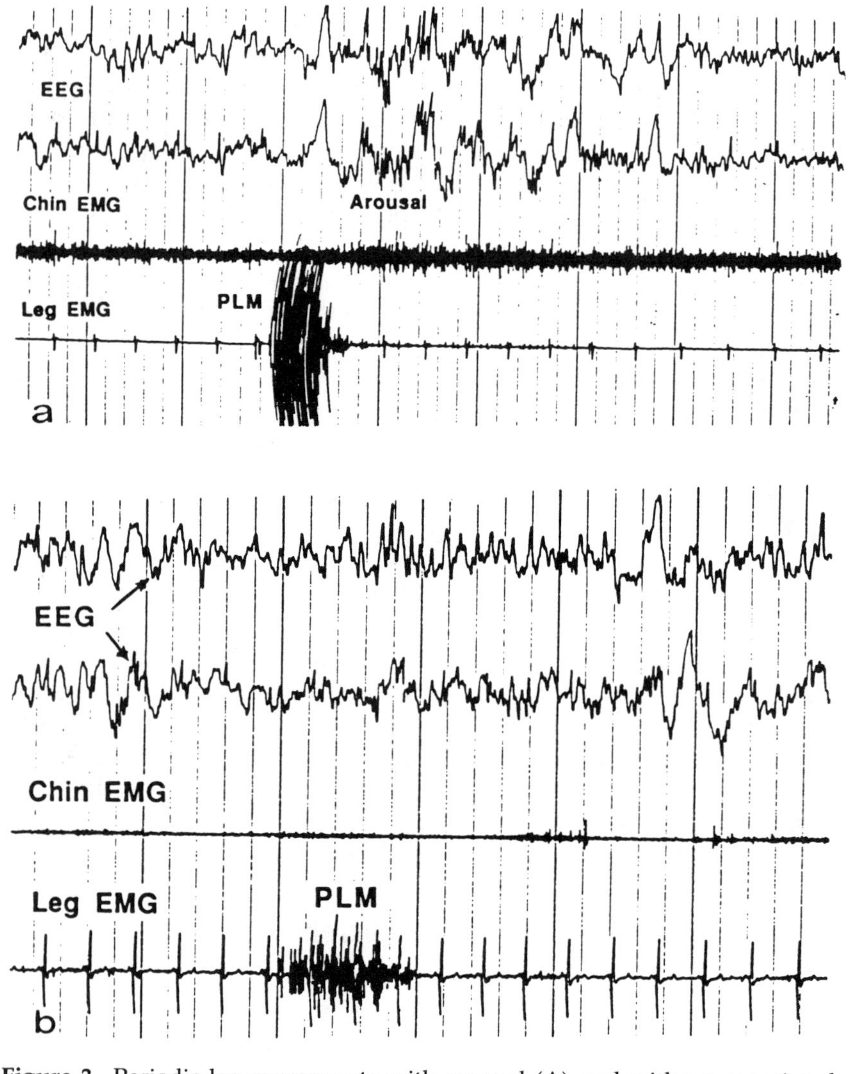

Figure 3. Periodic leg movements with arousal (A) and without associated arousal (B) in an elderly patient. Note that PLMs precede arousal in (A).

arousals, PLMs are not considered to have any clinical consequences and, therefore, do not require therapy. However, in patients with more vigorous movements and associated arousals, PLMs may result in severe sleep maintenance insomnia and daytime hypersomnolence. Clearly, treatment is indicated for symptomatic individuals with substantial PLM-associated sleep fragmentation. Benzodiazepines are generally effective, with clonazepam[98,99] and temazepam[100] having reported efficacy. Although PLMs frequently persist during therapy, movement intensity is reduced along with the frequency of arousals. Opioids are also effective, but problems with the rapid development of tolerance, addiction, and side effects limit their use. Because of the frequent presence of coexisting sleep apnea, avoidance of benzodiazepines and opioids is often advisable. In these patients L-dopa in combination with a peripheral carboxylase inhibitor is an appropriate and frequently effective form of therapy.[101–104] Studies indicate an increased prevalence with age.[3,6,13]

Restless leg syndrome (RLS) is best described as an irresistible urge to move the legs with dysesthesia, particularly noticeable at bedtime and often interfering with sleep onset. Patients with RLS invariably have PLMs, while only a small percentage of patients with PLMs have RLS. The treatment of both disorders is similar.

Advanced Sleep Phase Syndrome

A consistent finding among sleep studies of the aged is the phenomenon known as advanced sleep phase.[13,28,77] The cyclic recurrence of sleep can phase advance with age such that sleep onset tends to occur earlier in the evening and end earlier in the morning. This is usually not a problem unless an individual's socially determined sleep schedule does not coincide with a shift in the biological clock.

"Sundown" Syndrome

Nocturnal delirium manifest as confusion, agitation, and wandering is often seen in the setting of organic brain dysfunction. The treatment is first directed towards finding and correcting any organic factors. Effective, simple, nonmedical interventions can often be very helpful, including keeping the patient in familiar surroundings with a night-light to minimize visual misinterpretation and hallucinations. A drug-free period, particularly excluding sedative–hypnotics, may eliminate the problem and identify the cause. If pharmacologic therapy becomes necessary, then haloperidol is generally recommended as the drug of choice.[1]

REM Sleep Behavior Disorder

A recently described entity in which REM sleep is associated with vigorous, often violent, behavior is known as REM sleep behavior disorder. This parasomnia is marked by the loss of electromyographic atonia that normally occurs during REM sleep, allowing for the emergence of motor behavior with attempts on the part of the patient to enact his dream (Fig. 4). Jumping from bed, kicking, punching, or

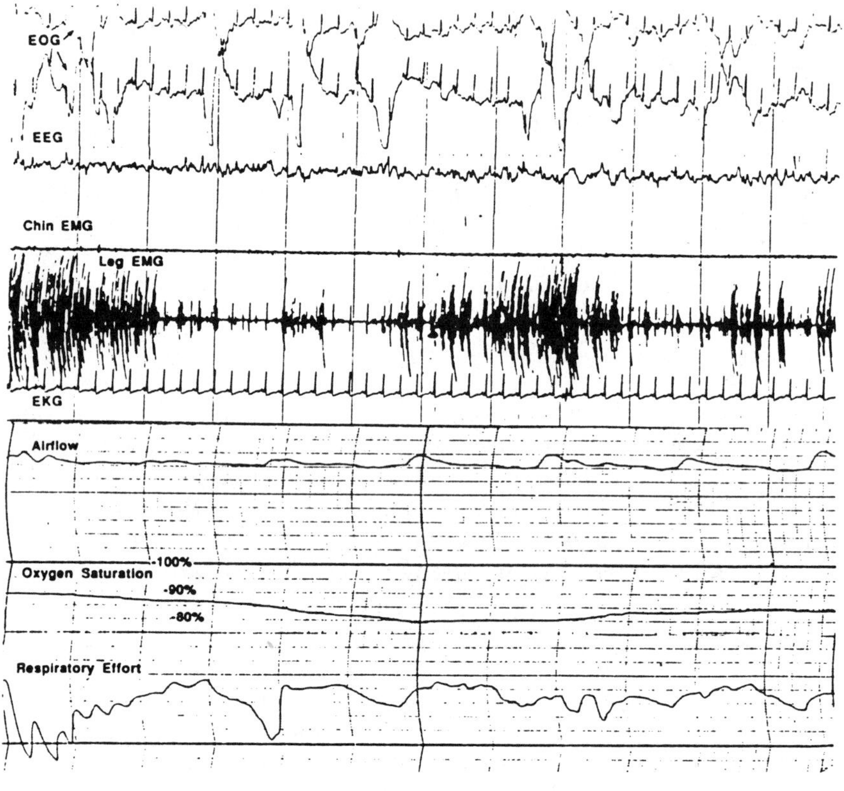

Figure 4. An elderly patient with REM behavior disorder showing unsuppressed EMG activity during REM sleep. The patient's legs were moving as though he was running, until he fell out of bed. REM sleep is clearly documented by the eye movements, atonia in the submental EMG, and irregular respiration with oxyhemoglobin desaturation.

other violent behavior can result in injury. In one study,[105] 9 of 10 patients were male and the mean age was 62. The disorder is unrelated to psychopathology but is often associated with neurologic abnormalities such as dementia or other neuropathology. While clonazepam is the drug of choice for treatment of this disorder, desipramine has also been used with temporary success.

Summary

Much of the earlier work in this field centered on subjective data gathered from questionnaires of subjects and their caretakers. More recently, overnight polysomnography, daytime nap studies, and reports of circadian factors have provided a clearer picture of sleep in the aged individual. Specific etiologic factors involved in these age-related changes of sleep and the extent to which such changes can be thought of as normal events of aging are incompletely defined. Changes in the control of breathing and its effect on sleep disorders is receiving increased attention and may provide clues to understanding the high incidence of sleep apnea in this population. The impact of social and environmental inputs, depression, dementia, medications, and medical problems on insomnia in the elderly and the use and abuse of sedatives in these individuals have been reviewed, as have periodic leg movements during sleep, advanced sleep phase syndrome, "sundown" syndrome, and the REM sleep behavior disorder. These topics are central to the understanding of sleep and aging.

References

1. Cadieux JR, Woolley DC, Kales JD. Sleep disorders in the elderly. *Psychiatr Med* 1987; 4:165–180.
2. Liftman S. Long-term care in the year 2000. *Nurs Home* 1980; 29:2–8.
3. Miles LE, Dement WC. Sleep and aging. *Sleep* 1980; 3:119–220.
4. McGhie A, Russell SM. The subjective assessment of normal sleep patterns. *J Ment Sci* 1962; 108:642–654.
5. Cohen D, Eisdorfer C, Prinz P, et al. Sleep disturbances in the institutionalized elderly. *J Am Geriatr Soc* 1983; 31:79–82.
6. Pressman MR, Fry JM. What is normal sleep in the elderly? *Clin Geriatr Med* 1988; 4:71–81.
7. Webb WB, Swinburne H. An observational study of sleep and the aged. *Percept Mot Skills* 1971; 32:895–898.

8. Kahn E, Fisher C. The sleep characteristics of the normal aged male. *J Nerv Ment Dis* 1969; 148:477–494.
9. Feinberg I. Changes in sleep cycle patterns with age. *J Psychiatr Res* 1974; 10:283–306.
10. Brezinova V. The number and duration of the episodes of the various EEG stages of sleep in young and older people. *Electroencephalogr Clin Neurophysiol* 1975; 39:273–278.
11. Smith JR, Karacon I, Yang M. Ontogeny of delta activity during human sleep. *Electroencephalogr Clin Neurophysiol* 1977; 43:229–237.
12. Weitzman ED, Czeisler CA, Zimmerman JC. Sleep duration, sleep stages, and waking time are related to circadian phase in young and older men during nonentrained conditions. *Trans Am Neurol Assoc* 1980; 105:371–374.
13. Dement WC, Miles LE, Carskadon MA. "Whitepaper" on sleep and aging. *J Am Geriatr Soc* 1982; 30:25–50.
14. Carskadon MA, Brown ED, Dement WC. Sleep fragmentation in the elderly: Relationship to daytime sleep tendency. *Neurobiol Aging* 1982; 3:321–327.
15. Hayashi Y, Endo S. All-night sleep polygraphic recordings of healthy aged persons: REM and slow-wave sleep. *Sleep* 1982; 5:277–283.
16. Webb WB. The sleep of older subjects fifteen years later. *Psychol Rep* 1982; 50:11–14.
17. Principe JC, Smith JR. Sleep spindle characteristics as a function of age. *Sleep* 1982; 5:73–84.
18. Webb WB, Schneider-Helment D. A categorical approach to changes in latency, awakening, and sleep length in older subjects. *J Nerv Ment Dis* 1984; 172:291–295.
19. Reynolds CF III, Kupfer DJ, Taska LS, et al. Sleep of healthy seniors: A revisit. *Sleep* 1985; 8:20–29.
20. Carskadon MA, Dement WC. Sleep loss in elderly volunteers. *Sleep* 1985; 8:207–221.
21. Guazzelli M, Feinberg I, Aminoff M, et al. Sleep spindles in normal elderly: Comparison with young adult patients and relation to nocturnal awakening, cognitive function, and brain atrophy. *Electroencephalogr Clin Neurophysiol* 1986; 63:526–539.
22. Ancoli-Israel S, Parker L, Sinall R, et al. Sleep fragmentation in patients from a nursing home. *J Gerontol* 1989; 44:M18–21.
23. Zepelin H, McDonald CS, Zammit GK. Effects of age on auditory awakening thresholds. *J Gerontol* 1984; 39:294–300.
24. Richardson GS, Carskadon MA, Orav EJ, et al. Circadian variation of sleep tendency in elderly and young adult subjects. *Sleep* 1982; 5:S82–S94.
25. Carskadon MA, Dement WC. Daytime sleepiness: Quantification of a behavioral state. *Neurosci Biobehav Rev* 1987; 11:307–317.
26. Smallwood RG, Vitiello MV, Giblin EC, et al. Sleep apnea: Relationship to age, sex, and Alzheimer's dementia. *Sleep* 1983; 6:16–22.
27. Carskadon MA, Dement WC. Respiration during sleep in the aged human. *J Gerontol* 1981; 36:420–423.

28. Kupfer DJ, Reynolds CF III. A critical review of sleep and its disorders from a developmental perspective. *Psychiatr Dev* 1983; 1:367–386.
29. Kronenberg RS, Drage CW. Attenuation of the ventilatory and heart rate responses to hypoxia and hypercapnia with aging in normal men. *J Clin Invest* 1973; 52:1812–1819.
30. Chapman KR, Cherniack NS. Aging effects on the interaction of hypercapnia and hypoxia as ventilatory stimuli. *J Gerontol* 1987; 42:202–209.
31. Black LF, Hyatt RE. Maximal respiratory pressures: Normal values and relationship to age and sex. *Am Rev Respir Dis* 1969; 99:696–702.
32. Turner JM, Mead J, Wohl ME. Elasticity of human lungs in relation to age. *J Appl Physiol* 1968; 25:664–671.
33. Whitelow WA, Derenne JP, Milic-Emili J. Occlusion pressure as a measure of respiratory center output in conscious man. *Respir Physiol* 1975; 23:181–199.
34. Peterson DD, Pack AI, Silage DA, et al. Effects of aging on ventilatory and occlusion pressure responses to hypoxia and hypercapnia. *Am Rev Respir Dis* 1981; 124:387–391.
35. Pack, AI, Millman RP. Changes in control of ventilation, awake and asleep, in the elderly. *J Am Geriatr Soc* 1986; 34:533–544.
36. Tack M, Altose MD, Cherniack NS. Effect of aging on respiratory sensations produced by elastic loads. *J Appl Physiol* 1981; 50:844–850.
37. Tack M, Altose MD, Cherniack NS. Effect of aging on the perception of resistive ventilatory loads. *Am Rev Respir Dis* 1982; 126:463–467.
38. Tack M, Altose MD, Cherniack NS. Effects of aging on sensation of respiratory force and displacement. *J Appl Physiol* 1983; 55:1433–1440.
39. Phillipson EA. Control of breathing during sleep. *Am Rev Respir Dis* 1978; 118:909–939.
40. Bulow K. Respiration and wakefulness in man. *Acta Physiol Scand* 1963; 59:1–110 (suppl 209).
41. Reed DL, Kellogg RH. Changes in respiratory response to CO_2 during natural sleep at sea level and at altitude. *J Appl Physiol* 1958; 13:325–330.
42. Robin ED, Whaley RD, Crump CH, et al. Alveolar gas tension, pulmonary ventilation and blood pH during physiologic sleep in normal subjects. *J Clin Invest* 1958; 37; 981–989.
43. Shore ET, Millman RP, Silage DA, et al. Ventilatory and arousal patterns during sleep in normal young and elderly subjects. *J Appl Physiol* 1985; 59:1607–1615.
44. Pack AI, Silage DA, Millman RP, et al. Spectral analysis of ventilation in elderly subjects awake and asleep. *J Appl Physiol* 1988; 64:1257–1267.
45. Millman RP, Knight H, Chung DC, et al. The effect of oxygen on sleep apnea in the elderly. *Am Rev Respir Dis* 1985; 131:A293.
46. Khoo MCK, Kronauer RE, Strohl KP, et al. Factors inducing periodic breathing in humans: A general model. *J Appl Physiol* 1982; 53:644–659.
47. Smith PL, Bleecher ER. Ventilatory control during sleep in the elderly. *Clin Geriatr Med* 1986; 2:227–240.
48. Carskadon MA, van den Hoed J, Dement WC. Sleep and daytime sleepiness in the elderly. *J Geriatr Psychiatry* 1980; 13:135–151.
49. Coleman RM, Miles LE, Guilleminault CC, et al. Sleep–wake disorders

in the elderly: A polysomnographic analysis. *J Am Geriatr Soc* 1981; 7: 289–296.
50. Ancoli-Israel S, Kripke DF, Mason W, et al. Comparison of home sleep recordings and polysomnograms in older adults with sleep disorders. *Sleep* 1981; 4:283–291.
51. Kripke DF, Ancoli-Israel S, Okudaira N. Sleep apnea and nocturnal myoclonus in the elderly. *Neurobiol Aging* 1982; 3:329–336.
52. Roehrs T, Zorick F, Sicklesteel J, et al. Age-related sleep–wake disorders at a sleep disorder center. *J Am Geriatr Soc* 1983; 31:364–370.
53. Bliwise D, Carskadon M, Carey E, et al. Longitudinal development of sleep-related respiratory disturbance in adult humans. *J Gerontol* 1984; 39:290–293.
54. Guilleminault C, Silvestri R, Mondini S, et al. Aging and sleep apnea: Action of benzodiazepine, acetazolamide, alcohol, and sleep deprivation in the healthy elderly group. *J Gerontol* 1984; 39:655–661.
55. Yesavage J, Bliwise D, Guilleminault C, et al. Preliminary communication: Intellectual deficit and sleep-related respiratory disturbance in the elderly. *Sleep* 1985; 8:30–33.
56. Knight H, Millman RP, Gur RC, et al. Clinical significance of sleep apnea in the elderly. *Am Rev Respir Dis* 1987; 136:845–850.
57. Bliwise DL, Feldman DE, Bliwise NG, et al. Risk factors for sleep disordered breathing in heterogeneous geriatric populations. *J Am Geriatr Soc* 1987; 35:132–141.
58. Bliwise DL, Bliwise NC, Partinen M, et al. Sleep apnea and mortality in an aged cohort. *Am J Public Health* 1988; 78:544–547.
59. McGinty D, Littner M, Beahm E, et al. Sleep-related breathing disorders in older men: A search for underlying mechanisms. *Neurobiol Aging* 1982; 3:337–350.
60. Ancoli-Israel S, Kripke DF, Mason W. Characteristics of obstructive and central sleep apnea in the elderly: An interim report. *Biol Psychiatry* 1987; 22:741–750.
61. Berry DTR, Phillips BA, Cook YR, et al. Sleep-disordered breathing in healthy aged persons: Possible daytime sequelae. *J Gerontol* 1987; 42: 620–626.
62. Mosko SS, Dickel MJ, Ashurst J. Night-to-night variability in sleep apnea and sleep-related periodic leg movements in the elderly. *Sleep* 1988; 11:340–348.
63. Ancoli-Israel S, Kripke DF, Mason W, et al. Sleep apnea and periodic movements in an aging sample. *J Gerontol* 1985; 40:419–425.
64. Catterall JR, Calverly PMA, Shapiro CM, et al. Breathing and oxygenation during sleep are familiar in normal men and normal women. *Am Rev Respir Dis* 1985; 132:86–88.
65. Krieger J, Turlot JC, Mangin P, et al. Breathing during sleep in normal young and elderly subjects: Hypopneas, apneas, and correlated factors. *Sleep* 1983; 6:108–120.
66. Block AJ, Wynne JW, Boysen PG. Sleep-disordered breathing and nocturnal oxygen desaturation in postmenopausal women. *Am J Med* 1980; 69:75–79.
67. Reynolds CF III, Coble PA, Black RS, et al. Sleep disturbances in a series

of elderly patients: Polysomnographic findings. *J Am Geriatr Soc* 1980; 28:164–170.
68. Ancoli-Israel S, Kripke DF, Mason W, et al. Sleep apnea and nocturnal myoclonus in a senior population. *Sleep* 1981; 4:349–358.
69. Bixler EO, Kales A, Cadieux RJ, et al. Sleep apneic activity in older healthy subjects. *J Appl Physiol* 1985; 58:1597–1601.
70. Block AJ, Boysen PG, Wynne JW, et al. Sleep apnea, hypopnea, and oxygen desaturation in normal subjects: A strong male predominance. *N Engl J Med* 1979; 300:513–517.
71. Taasan VC, Block AJ, Boysen PG, et al. Alcohol increases sleep apnea and oxygen desaturation in asymptomatic men. *Am J Med* 1981; 71: 240–245.
72. Issa FG, Sullivan CE. Alcohol, snoring and sleep apnoea. *J Neurol Neurosurg Psychiatr* 1982; 45:353–359.
73. Derderian SS, Bridenbaugh RH, Rajagopal KR. Neuropsychologic symptoms in obstructive sleep apnea improve after treatment with nasal continuous positive airway pressure. *Chest* 1988; 94:1023–1027.
74. Shepard JW Jr. Aging and sleep apnea. *In* R Strong et al. (eds). Central Nervous System Disorders of Aging: Clinical Intervention and Research. New York, Raven Press, 1988.
75. Shepard JW Jr. Cardiopulmonary disorders during sleep: Diagnosis and management. *Geriatrics* 1987; 42:51–60.
76. Quan SF, Bamford CR, Beutler LE. Sleep disturbances in the elderly. *Geriatrics* 1984; 39:42–47.
77. Howard GF III. Management of chronic sleep disorders in the elderly. *Compr Ther* 1987; 13:3–9.
78. Howard GF III, Coble PA, Black RS, et al. Sleep disturbances in a series of elderly patients: Polysomnographic findings. *J Am Geriatr Soc* 1980; 28:164–170.
79. Roehrs T, Lineback W, Zorick F, et al. Relationship of psychopathology to insomnia in the elderly. *J Am Geriatr Soc* 1982; 30:312–315.
80. Kupfer DJ, Reynolds CF III, Ulrich RF, et al. EEG sleep, depression, and aging. *Neurobiol Aging* 1982; 3:351–360.
81. Reynolds CF III, Kupfer DJ, Taska LS, et al. EEG sleep in elderly depressed, demented, and healthy subjects. *Biol Psychiatry* 1985; 20:431–442.
82. Reynolds CF III, Kupfer DJ, Hoch CC, et al. Sleep deprivation as a probe in the elderly. *Arch Gen Psychiatry* 1987; 44:982–990.
83. Rodin J, McAvay G, Timko C. A longitudinal study of depressed mood and sleep disturbances in elderly adults. *J Gerontol* 1988; 43:P45–53.
84. Reynolds CF III, Kupfer DJ, Houck PR, et al. Reliable discrimination of elderly depressed and demented patients by electroencephalographic sleep data. *Arch Gen Psychiatry* 1988; 45:258–264.
85. Buysse DJ, Reynolds CF III, Houck PR, et al. Age of illness onset and sleep EEG variables in elderly depressives. *Biol Psychiatry* 1988; 24:355–359.
86. Prinz PN, Peskind ER, Vitaliano PP, et al. Changes in the sleep and waking EEG's of nondemented and demented elderly subjects. *J Am Geriatr Soc* 1982; 30:86–93.

87. Vitiello MV, Bolson JA, Kukull WA, et al. Rapid eye movement sleep measures of Alzheimer's-type dementia patients and optimally healthy aged individuals. *Biol Psychiatry* 1984; 19:721–734.
88. Regestein QR, Morris J. Daily sleep patterns observed among institutionalized elderly residents. *J Am Geriatr Soc* 1987; 35:767–772.
89. Allen SR, Seiler WO, Stahelin HB, et al. Seventy-two hour polygraphic and behavioral recordings of wakefulness and sleep in a hospital geriatric unit: Comparison between demented and nondemented patients. *Sleep* 1987; 10:143–159.
90. Guilleminault C, Silvestin R. Aging, drugs, sleep. *Neurobiol Aging* 1982; 3:379–386.
91. Clapin-French E. Sleep patterns of aged persons in long-term care facilities. *J Adv Nurs* 1986; 11:57–66.
92. Hay D, Milne RM, Gilleard CJ. Hypnotic drugs, old people, and their habits: A general practice study. *Health Bull (Edinburgh)* 1986; 44:218–222.
93. Swift CG. Special problems relating to the use of hypnotics in the elderly. *Acta Psychiatr Scand* 1986; 73:92–98.
94. Bonnet MH, Kramer M. The interaction of age, performance, and hypnotics in the sleep of insomniacs. *J Am Geriatr Soc* 1981; 29:508–512.
95. Sorock GS, Shimkin EE. Benzodiazepine sedative and the risk of falling in a community-dwelling elderly cohort. *Arch Intern Med* 1988; 148:2441–2444.
96. Ray WA, Griffin MR, Schaffner W, et al. Psychotropic drug use and the risk of hip fracture. *N Engl J Med* 1987; 316:363–369.
97. Cook PJ. Benzodiazepine hypnotics in the elderly. *Acta Psychiatr Scand* 1986; 74:149–158.
98. Ohanna N, Peled R, Rubin AE, et al. Periodic leg movements in sleep: Effect of clonazepam treatment. *Neurology* 1985; 35:408–411.
99. Oshtory MA, Vijayan N. Clonazepam treatment of insomnia due to sleep myoclonus. *Arch Neurol* 1980; 37:119–120.
100. Mitler MH, Browman CP, Menn SJ, et al. Nocturnal myoclonus: Treatment efficacy of clonazepam and temazepam. *Sleep* 1986; 9:385–392.
101. von Scheele C. Levodopa in restless legs. *Lancet* 1986; 2:426–427.
102. Montplaisir J, Godbout R, Porier G, et al. Restless legs syndrome and periodic movements in sleep: Pathophysiology and treatment with L-dopa. *Clin Neuropharmacol* 1986; 9:456–463.
103. Guilleminault C, Mondini S, Montplaisir J, et al. Periodic leg movement, L-dopa, 5-hydroxytryptophan, and L-triptophan. *Sleep* 1987; 10:393–397.
104. Alspinar S. Restless leg syndrome treatment with dopaminergic drugs. *Clin Neuropharmacol* 1987; 10:69–79.
105. Schenk CH, Bundlie SR, Patterson AL, et al. Rapid eye movement sleep behavior disorder: A treatable parasomnia affecting older adults. *JAMA* 1987; 257:1786–1789.

Index

Martin RJ: Cardiorespiratory Disorders During Sleep, 2nd Edition. Futura Publishing Company, Inc., Mount Kisco, NY, © 1990.